NEW TRENDS IN AGING RESEARCH

NEW TRENDS IN AGING RESEARCH

Edited by:

G. Pepeu
Istituto di Farmacologia
Università di Firenze, Italy

B. Tomlinson
Dept of Pathology
Newcastle General Hospital
Newcastle upon Tyne, UK

C.M. Wischik
Medical Research Council
Laboratory of Molecular Biology
Cambridge, UK

FIDIA
RESEARCH
SERIES

Volume 15

LIVIANA PRESS
Padova

SPRINGER VERLAG
Berlin - Heidelberg
New York - Tokyo

FIDIA RESEARCH SERIES

An open-end series of publications on international biomedical research, with special emphasis on the neurosciences, published by LIVIANA Press, Padova, Italy, in cooperation with FIDIA Research Labs, Abano Terme, Italy.

The series will be devoted to advances in basic and clinical research in the neurosciences and other fields.

The aim of the series is the rapid and worldwide dissemination of up-to-date, interdisciplinary data as presented at selected international scientific meetings and study groups.

Each volume is published under the editorial responsibility of scientists chosen by organizing committees of the meetings on the basis of their active involvement in the research of the field concerned.

DISTRIBUTION

Sole distribution rights outside Italy granted to Springer - Verlag.

All orders for the Fidia Research Series should be sent to the following addresses

Italy:
LIVIANA EDITRICE S.p.A. - Via Luigi Dottesio, 1, 35138 Padova, Italia

North America:
SPRINGER - VERLAG New York, Inc. - 175 Fifth Avenue, New York, N.Y. 10010, USA

Japan:
SPRINGER - VERLAG - 37-3 Hongo 3-chome, Bunkyo-Ku, Tokyo 113, Japan

Rest of the World:
SPRINGER - VERLAG Berlin - Heidelberger Platz 3, 1000 Berlin 33, FRG

Printed in Italy

ISBN 88-7675-545-4: Liviana Editrice
ISBN 3-540-96911-X: Springer - Verlag Berlin Heidelberg New York Tokyo
ISBN 0-387-96911-X: Springer - Verlag New York Heidelberg Berlin Tokyo

---

LIVIANA Editrice S.p.A. - via Luigi Dottesio 1, 35138, Padova, Italy.

CONTENTS

III. NEUROIMMUNOLOGY

IV. BASIC RESEARCH IN SENILE DEMENTIA

V. PLASTICITY AND THERAPEUTIC POSSIBILITIES

FOREWORD

This book includes the papers presented at the International Symposium on "New Trends in Aging Research" organized in Sirmione, on the Lake Garda by the Italian Study Group on Brain Aging on April 1987 in order to celebrate and conclude its sixth year of activity.

The Group was established in 1981 by preclinical and clinical investigators involved in research on aging. The purpose, as stated in its chart, was "to foster through experimental and clinical research the knowledge on the aging mechanisms of the nervous system and to study possible diagnostic and therapeutic methods and approaches...".

In order to achieve this ambitious goal the Group has helped in disseminating relevant information through the preparation and distribution of biannual lists of references, has organized small seminars on the researches on aging in Italy and supplied a limited number of old rats.

However, these practical activities are probably not the most important contributions of the Group to the research on aging brain, a field moving very fast for the importance and number of new discoveries and their impact on the neurosciences in general. When the Group was established six years ago, most of the Italian neuroscientists were not yet fully aware that the aging of the population would make the pathology associated with the aging of the brain a major medical problem. The Group made a census of the Italian investigators involved in research on the aging brain and of their projects, became a rallying point and facilitated fruitful interactions between different laboratories. It made the Italian and international scientific communities aware of the contribution of the Italian preclinical and clinical scientists in this field. During its six years of life, the Group witnessed the birth, development and end of a Subproject of the CNR on Aging Mechanisms. The inclusion of the aging brain in the Subproject was an indirect result of the Group's existence. The Subproject will be replaced by a larger national project on aging to which members of the Group, particularly its present President Prof. G. Crepaldi, are bringing important contributions in its preparation. Furthermore, the existence of the Group with the demonstration of the original contributions of several Italian laboratories was instrumental in orienting the decision of the Ministry of Scientific Research to establish a National Research Program supporting investigations on drugs active on the aging brain.

More than one year has elapsed between the Symposium in Sirmione and the release of this book and the potential reader may wonder whether the content of the book is still up to date and worth reading. This book still offers a broad and clear overview of the trends along which research on the aging brain is moving and well documents the multidisciplinarity of this field. Aging of the brain includes morphological changes, anomalous formation and deposition of proteins, alteration of neurotransmitter systems, neuroendocrine ad immune systems. To which extent these alterations interplay needs to be clarified, but the book offers important elements of the general pictures. In this regard, particularly relevant are the chapters written by McEwen, Muller, Gottfries, Gambetti and Fuxe. All of the papers, however, contain useful information and may help the investigator to acquire the general view necessary to deal with the broad and difficult problem of understanding the aging brain and trying to answer the fundamental questions: What are the basic, initial changes of the physiological aging process in the central nervous system? What is the pathogenetic mechanism of senile dementia? What is the rational therapeutic approach to the aging brain?

Florence, October 1988

Giancarlo Pepeu, M.D.
Professor of Pharmacology
Past President of the Italian
Study Group on Brain Aging

Section I

NEUROCHEMISTRY

New Trends in Aging Research
G. Pepeu, B. Tomlinson, C.M. Wischik (eds)
Fidia Research Series, vol. 15
Liviana Press, Padova © 1988

EVIDENCE FOR SELECTIVE CHANGES IN PEPTIDE AND MONOAMINE SYNAPSES AND THEIR INTERACTIONS IN THE AGING RAT BRAIN. POSSIBLE LOSS OF HOMEOSTATIC RESPONSES AND OF TROPHIC SIGNALS

Kjell Fuxe, Luigi F. Agnati[1], Isabella Zini[1], Emilio Merlo Pich[1], Antonio Cintra, Isao Kitayama, Anders Härfstrand, Gabriel v. Euler, Wiley Vale[2], Gino Toffano[1] and Menek Goldstein[3]

Department of Histology, Karolinska Institutet, Stockholm, Sweden;
[1]Department of Human Physiology, University of Modena, Italy;
[2]The Salk Institute, La Jolla, California, USA; and
[3]Department of Psychiatry, New York University Medical Center, New York, USA

INTRODUCTION

Our previous immunocytochemical and autoradiographical studies in combination with morphometrical and microdensitometrical procedures demonstrated selective changes in the pre- and postsynaptic properties of central monoaminergic and peptidergic neuron in the aged rat brain (Agnati et al., 1984a; 1985a; 1985b; 1986a; 1986b; 1986c; 1987; Zoli et al., 1987; Fuxe et al., 1986a; 1986b). Transmitter stores, transmitter recognition sites and transduction mechanisms as measured by analysis of cyclic AMP and calcium induced phosphorylation were found to be impaired in several brain areas in the 24-month-old male rat compared with the 3-month-old male rat. One major finding has been that the peptidergic messengers in the monoamine neurons may often be preferentially reduced in the aged rat brain compared with the classical transmitter and its synthesizing enzymes (for review, see Fuxe et al., 1986b; Agnati et al., 1986c). Furthermore, within the mediobasal hypothalamus highly discrete changes have been observed in the peptide neurons, which may contribute to the aging induced changes in neuroendocrine function (Agnati et al., 1985a; Fuxe et al., 1986a). The most marked change was a marked loss in the number of tyrosine hydroxylase (TH) immunoreactive nerve cell bodies in the periarcuate area and the ventrolateral part of the arcuate nucleus.

In the present paper this work has been continued by analyzing changes in levels and turnovers of D2 and α2-adrenergic receptors in discrete brain areas of the aged male rat using as a tool to study receptor turnover the peptide coupling agent N-ethoxy-carbonyl-2-ethoxy-1,2-dihydroquinoline (EEDQ) (Hamblin and Creese, 1983; Meller et al., 1985; Fuxe et al., 1986d), which produces marked and irreversible inactivation of monoamine receptors *in vivo* in the rat brain. By the use of EEDQ we have also analyzed if the possible regulation by monoamine receptors of mu and delta opiate receptors and ^{3}H-imipramine binding sites is altered in the aged rat brain. Early work by Agnati et al. (1984c) indicated that the CCK-8 modulation of D2 receptors in striatal membranes was altered in the 24-month-old male rat brain compared with the 3-month-old male rat. In this study evaluation of growth hormone releasing factor (GRF) immunoreactive (IR) nerve terminals of the median eminence have been continued in the aged male rat brain by use of immunocytochemistry in combination with morphometrical and microdensitometrical procedures (Agnati et al., 1984b) in order to further elucidate the previous findings on loss of TH IR in GRF IR cell bodies in the arcuate and periarcuate region (see Fuxe et al., 1986a).

MATERIAL AND METHODS

Three- and 24-month-old male Sprague-Dawley rats have been studied. The rats were given food pellets and water *ad libitum* and kept under standardized humidity, temperature and lighting conditions (lights on at 8 a.m. and lights off at 8 p.m.).

Studies on Monoamine Receptors and Turnovers

The D2 receptor antagonist ^{3}H-Spiperone was used to label D2 receptors and the α2-adrenoreceptor agonist ^{3}H-paraminoclonidine to study α2-adrenergic receptors. The incubation conditions were based on the protocols by Creese et al. (1977) and of Rouot and Snyder (1979). ^{3}H-Spiperone was used in a concentration of 2nM and ^{3}H-paraminoclonidine in a concentration of 10 nM. At these concentrations far above the Kd values the respective binding sites are almost saturated. Therefore, a change in the binding observed probably mainly reflects a change in the density of receptors in the area measured. Furthermore, the incubation time was such as to allow equilibrium conditions to develop.

The irreversible monoamine receptor blocking agent EEDQ was used to inactivate monoamine receptors. The dose of EEDQ was 6 mg/kg given i.p. EEDQ (Aldrich, Milwaukee, USA) was dissolved in ethanol and subsequently diluted in propylene glycol and water to give a final ratio of 1:1:2 (v/v/v). Control rats were given the solvent. A change in D2 and α2-adrenergic receptor turnover was studied by comparing the rate of recovery of ^{3}H-Spiperone binding and ^{3}H-paraminoclonidine binding in various brain areas in 3-month-old and 24-month-old male rat. For this purpose the EEDQ treated rats were sacrificed 1, 2 and 4 days after the treatment (see Fig. 1). The number of rats in each experimental group was 4.

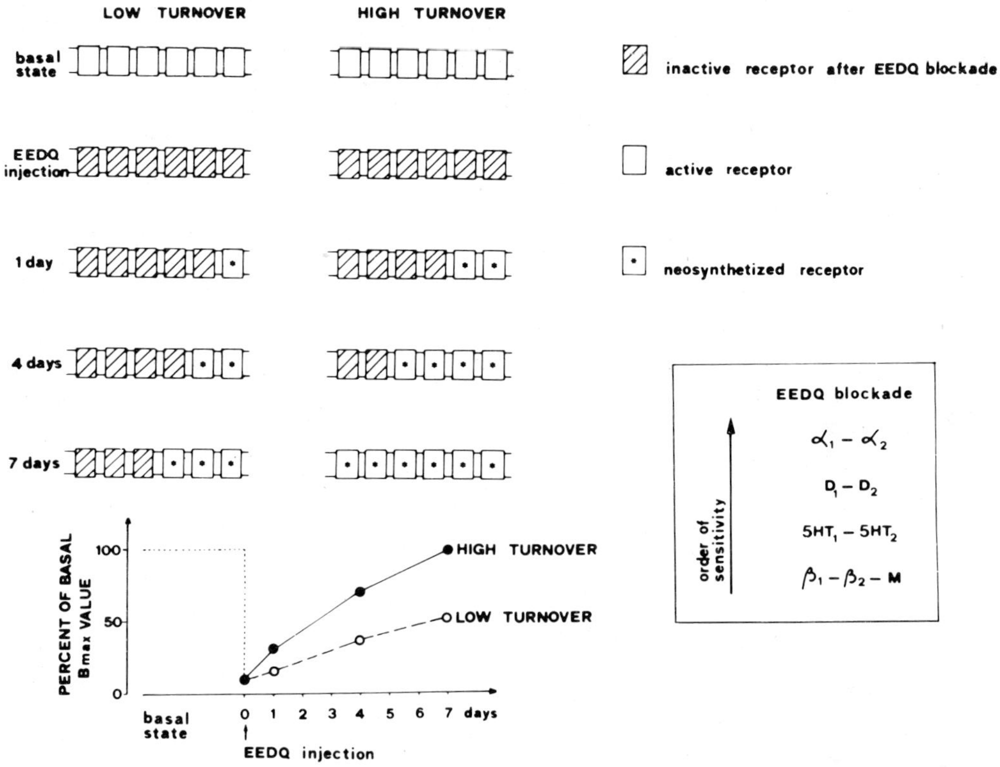

Figure 1. Schematic illustration of the method to study monoamine receptor turnover by means of the EEDQ technique.

Mu and Delta Type of Opiate Receptors, ^{3}H-imipramine Binding Sites and their Interaction with Monoamine Receptors

As a radioligand for mu opiate receptors ^{3}H-etorphin was used (60 ci/mmol; New England Nuclear, Boston, USA) in a concentration of 2 nM. As a radioligand for delta opiate receptors ^{3}H-D-ser-L-leu-L-thr-enkephalin ^{3}H-DSTLE (30.5 ci/mmol; New England Nuclear, Boston, USA) was used at a concentration of 11.5 nM. For details on the binding procedures, see Agnati et al. (1984a). Equilibrium conditions were allowed to develop, since incubation time was carried out at room temperature for 60 min for both radioligands (see also Agnati et al., 1984a). The incubation buffer was Tris HCl 170 mM, pH 7.4 for ^{3}H-etorphin and Tris HCl 170 mM, pH 7.4 containing EDTA 1 mM and bacitracin 40 mg/l for ^{3}H-DSTLE. Non specific binding was defined as the binding in the presence of naloxone (1 μM) for ^{3}H-etorphin and of Levalorphan (1 μM) for ^{3}H-DSTLE binding.

^{3}H-imipramine (78.1 Ci/mmol, NEN) binding was performed as described in Fuxe et al. (1983), using a radioligand concentration of 20 nM. Unspecific binding was defined as the binding in the presence of 10 μM of desipramine.

To study if monoamine receptors can modulate mu and delta type of opiate receptors in various brain areas as well as ^{3}H-imipramine binding sites, located on the 5-HT nerve terminals (see Langer and Briley, 1981; Fuxe et al., 1983), EEDQ treatment was performed as described above. This monoamine receptor blocking agent has no direct effect on the peptide receptors nor on the ^{3}H-imipramine binding sites. However, if an interaction exists between the monoamine and subtypes of opiate receptors and the 5-HT-autoreceptors and the ^{3}H-imipramine binding sites, irreversible blockade of monoamine receptors should influence the ^{3}H-etorphin, ^{3}H-DSTLE and ^{3}H-imipramine binding. The EEDQ treated animals were analyzed 1, 2 and 4 days after the injection of EEDQ. The number of rats in each experimental group was 6.

In all experiments the rats were anaesthetised with Brietal (75 mg/kg i.p.) and perfused with ice-cold saline followed by 300 ml of ice-cold 0.1% paraformaldehyde in 0.1 M-phosphate buffer (pH 7.4). The brains were dissected out and immediately frozen and sectioned in a cryostat at various rostrocaudal levels but mainly at levels bregma $\pm$ 0.7 mm according to the Paxinos and Watson atlas. Coronal sections were made and the thickness was 14 μm. Tritium sensitive film (Ultra film; LKB, Stockholm, Sweden) was used and the exposure time ranged from 4-6 weeks at −20°C. The films were developed in Eastman Kodak D19 film developer (4 min at 22°C). Quantitative receptor autoradiography was performed by means of computer assisted microdensitometry (IBAS image analyser, Zeiss Kontron, Munich, West-Germany) and appropriate standards (Benfenati et al., 1986).

Immunocytochemical Experiments

Three- and 24-month-old male specific pathogen free Sprague-Dawley rats were used (four rats per group). The rabbit antiserum against rat GRF has been previously well characterized (see Cintra et al., 1987). The primary antiserum was diluted 1:1000. As control serum was used the antiserum absorbed with GRF (50 μg/ml diluted antiserum). The incubation was performed over night at 4°C. The rats were anaesthetized with methohexital sodium (75 mg/kg) and killed by transcardiac perfusion with 0.9% NaCl followed by a 30 min perfusion with 500 ml of ice-cold 0.1 M sodium phosphate buffer (pH 7.4) containing 4% (w/v) paraformaldehyde. The biotin-avidin method was used to demonstrate the GRF immunoreactivity in coronal vibratome sections (30 μm thick) of the medial basal hypothalamus. The biotinylated goat antirabbit antibody was used followed by incubation with avidin biotinylated peroxidase (Vectastain). As chromogene was used diaminobenzidine.

The GRF immunoreactive nerve terminal areas of the medial palisade zone and the lateral palisade zone of the median eminence were determined following discrimination in the IBAS analyzer to obtain the specific field area of the nerve terminal networks. Furthermore, to obtain an index of the relative antigen contents in the GRF IR nerve terminals of the median eminence the mean grey value was determined by means of a microdensitometrical procedure (see Agnati et al., 1978; Agnati et al., 1987). The total GRF IR is then obtained by multiplying the field area with the mean grey value (see also Kitayama et al., 1987).

RESULTS

RECEPTOR AUTORADIOGRAPHICAL EXPERIMENTS

Studies on D2-dopamine Receptors

The results are summarized in Figures 2 and 3. A twenty to forty per cent reduction is observed in ^{3}H-Spiperone binding in the nucleus caudatus putamen, nucleus accumbens and tuberculum olfactorium while the ^{3}H-Spiperone binding in the claustrum is not significantly reduced in the 24-month-old male rat. A comparison of receptor turnovers of D2 receptors in the young and old male rat was obtained by studying the recovery of the ^{3}H-Spiperone binding after EEDQ induced inactivation of monoamine receptors as evaluated from the ratio of the binding of ^{3}H-Spiperone observed 4 days after EEDQ treatment and ^{3}H-Spiperone binding in the basal state. It was found that the recovery of ^{3}H-Spiperone binding was reduced within the medial and central part of the nucleus caudatus putamen, in the nucleus accumbens and in the claustrum in the 24-month-old male rat. No difference between the young and old rat was found in the tuberculum olfactorium with regard to recovery of ^{3}H-Spiperone binding after EEDQ induced inactivation.

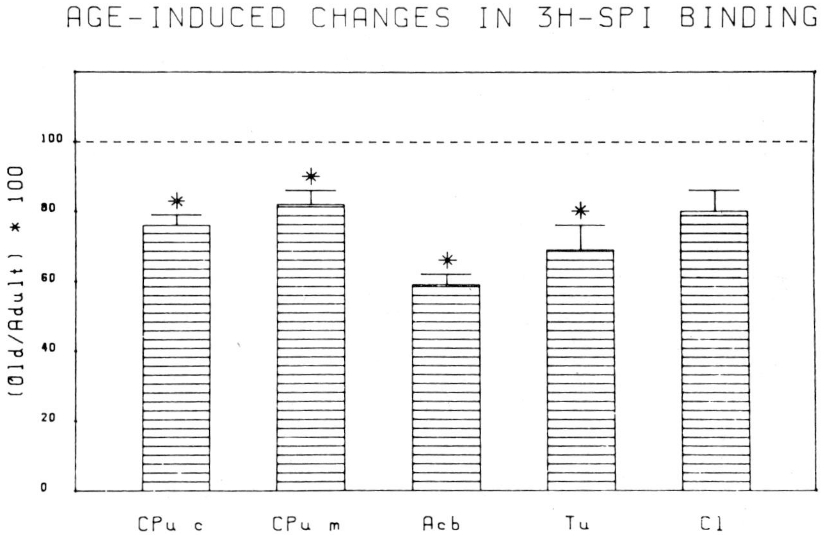

Figure 2. ^{3}H-spiperone binding in various forebrain regions of the 24-month-old male rat as expressed in % of the binding in the 3-month-old male rat (adult). Means ± s.e.m. are shown out of 6 rats. Student's t test. *$p<0.05$. Abbreviations used: CPu c = nucleus caudatus putamen, central part; CPu m = nucleus caudatus putamen, medial part; Acb = nucleus accumbens; Tu = tuberculum olfactorium; Cl = claustrum.

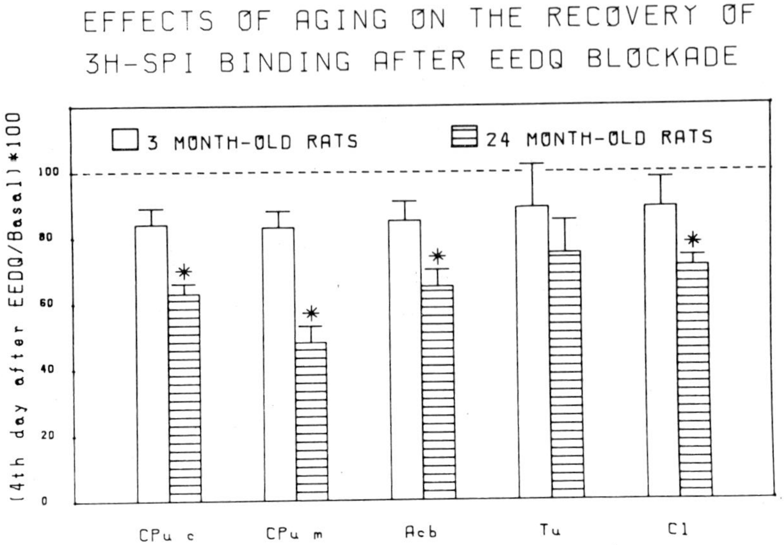

Figure 3. Effects of aging on the turnover of D-2 receptors in various regions of the forebrain (see text to Fig. 2). Evaluation of D-2 receptor turnover has been obtained by expressing the binding of ^{3}H-spiperone on the fourth day after EEDQ treatment (6 mg/kg i.p.) in % of the basal state (no EEDQ treatment). Means ± s.e.m. are shown out of 6 rats. Student's t test. $^*p<0.05$.

Studies on α2-adrenergic Receptors

The results are summarized in Figures 4 and 5. A 20-40% reduction in ^{3}H-paraminoclonidine (PAC) binding was observed in a large number of areas of the 24-month-old male rat as compared with the 3-month-old male rat (Fig. 4). The areas showing a reduced ^{3}H-PAC binding were as follows: the cingulate cortex (Cg), the external and internal layers of frontoparietal cortex (Ctxe and Ctxi), the nucleus caudatus putamen (Pu), nucleus accumbens (Acb), tuberculum olfactorium (Tu), the substantia gelatinosa of the nucleus tractus spinalis nervi trigemini (SV) and the nucleus supraopticus (SO) which had the most marked change in ^{3}H-PAC binding. The nucleus entopiriformis (En) and the nucleus tractus solitarius (nTS), however, showed no changes in ^{3}H-PAC binding, when the young and old rats were compared.

As in the case with ^{3}H-Spiperone binding a reduced recovery of ^{3}H-PAC binding was observed in several brain regions after the EEDQ induced inactivation of monoamine receptors in the 24-month-old male rat compared with the 3-month-old male rat (Fig. 5). As evaluated from the ratio of ^{3}H-PAC binding on the 4th day after EEDQ treatment and ^{3}H-PAC binding under basic conditions (no EEDQ treatment), recovery of ^{3}H-PAC binding in the old rat was significantly reduced in the nucleus caudatus putamen, nucleus accumbens and tuberculum olfactorium but not in the cortical regions studied. Recovery was also reduced in the entopiriform nucleus, the nucleus tractus solitarius and the substantia gelatinosa of the nucleus tractus spinalis nervi trigemini (SV). However, recovery of ^{3}H-PAC binding in the nucleus supraopticus was similar in the young and the old rat.

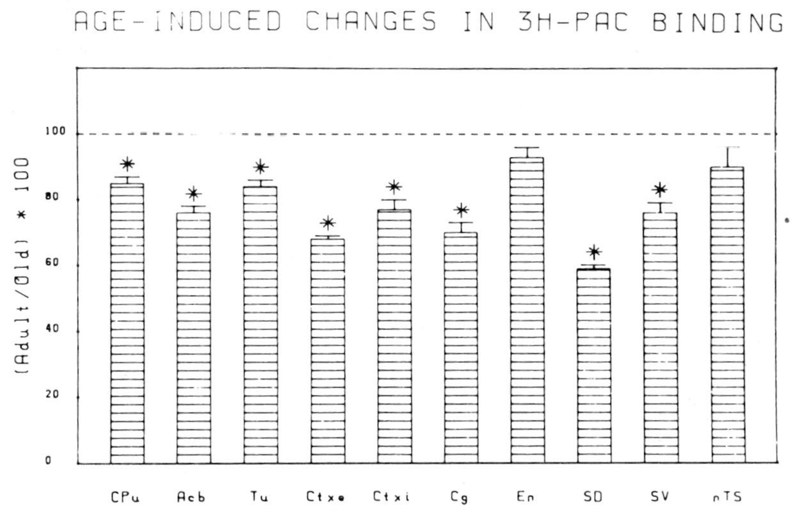

Figure 4. Effects of aging on ^{3}H-paraminoclonidine binding in various regions of the 24-month-old male rat. The ^{3}H-PAC binding is expressed in % of the binding found in the corresponding region in the 3-month-old male rat (adult). Means ± s.e.m. are shown out of 6 rats. Student's t test. *$p<0.05$. For some abbreviations, see text to Figure 2. Ctxe = frontoparietal cortex, external layer; Ctxi = frontoparietal cortex, internal layer; Cg = cingulate cortex; En = entopiriform nucleus; SO = nucleus supraopticus; SV = substantia gelatinosa of the nucleus tractus spinalis nervi trigemini; NTS = nucleus tractus solitarius.

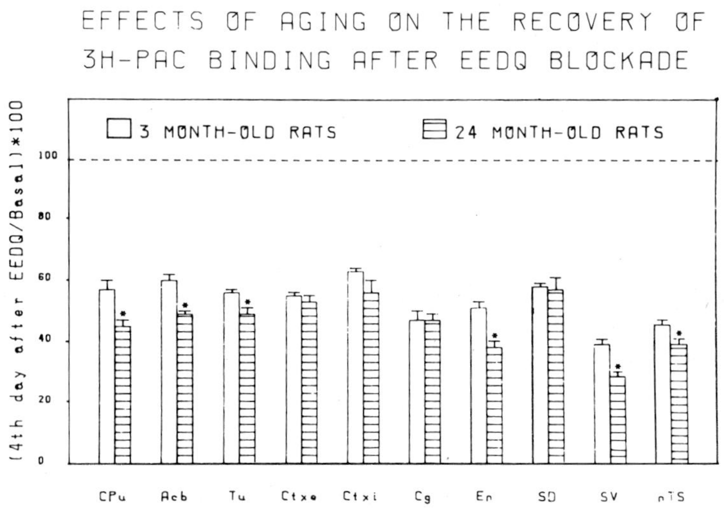

Figure 5. Effects of aging on the turnover of α_2-adrenergic receptors in various brain areas of the 24-month-old male rat. The α_2-adrenergic receptor turnover was evaluated by measurement of the ^{3}H-PAC binding on the fourth day after EEDQ treatment (6 mg/kg i.p.) expressed in % of the respective basal state (no EEDQ treatment). Means ± s.e.m. are shown. Student's t test. *$p<0.05$. For abbreviations see text to Figure 4.

Studies on ^{3}H-etorphin and ^{3}H-DSTLE Binding

The results are summarized in Table 1 and Figures 6 and 7. It is shown that both ^{3}H-etorphin and ^{3}H-DSTLE binding within the various parts of the striatum and in the cortical regions are reduced by 10-25% (see also Agnati et al., 1984a). Only ^{3}H-DSTLE

Table 1. *Autoradiographical studies on ^{3}H-etorphin and ^{3}H-DSTLE binding in various brain areas of adult (3 months) and old (24 months) rats*

Region	^{3}H-etorphin			^{3}H-DSTLE		
	Adult	Old	(O/A) *100	Adult	Old	(O/A) *100
CPu	707.9±15.7	648±10.9**	91.6±1.5	609.6±14.4	490.0±30.7**	80.3±5.0
Acb	758.3±16.5	593±19.1**	78.2±2.5	555.6±9.5	435.3±11.0**	78.3±1.9
Tu	630.9±27.0	481±14.2**	76.4±2.2	479.0±9.0	398.4±9.8 **	84.8±2.1
Cl	713.8±21.5	632±25.5**	88.6±3.6	708.4±20.0	684.7±26.3	96.6±3.7
FrPa	486.9±12.5	423±6.0 **	86.9±1.2	395.7±10.9	396.1±18.9	93.2±4.8
Cg	538.1±12.5	488±9.5 **	90.7±1.8	–	–	–

The mean values (± s.e.m.) are expressed in fmol/mg protein. The comparisons between the mean values observed in each region in adult and old rats were carried out by means of Student's t test (* = $p<0.05$; ** = $p<0.01$). List of abbreviations: CPu = caudate putamen, Acb = n. accumbens, Tu = tuberculum olfactorium, Cl = claustrum, FvPa = frontoparietal cortex, Cg = cingulate cortex.

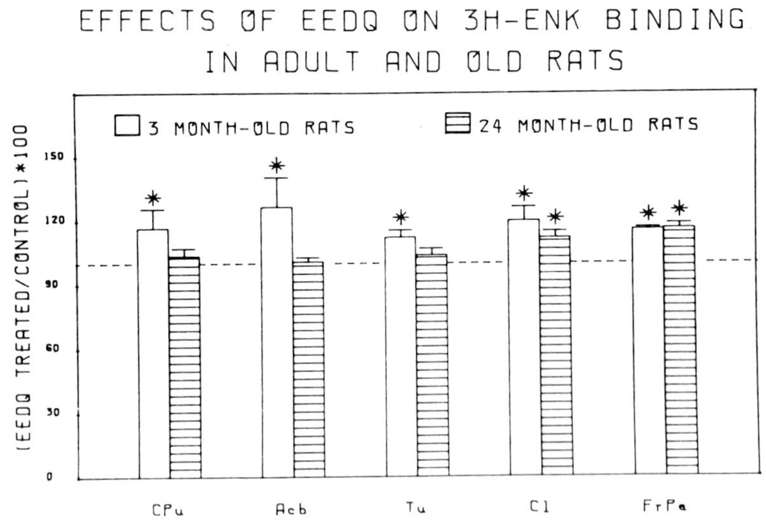

Figure 6. Effects of aging on the EEDQ induced increase in ^{3}H-DSTLE binding in various forebrain regions. EEDQ was given in doses of 6 mg/kg i.p. 48 h before killing. The ^{3}H-DSTLE binding obtained after EEDQ treatment is expressed in % of the respective control group mean value. Means ± s.e.m. out of 6 rats. Student's t test. *$p<0.05$. For abbreviations see text to Figure 4.

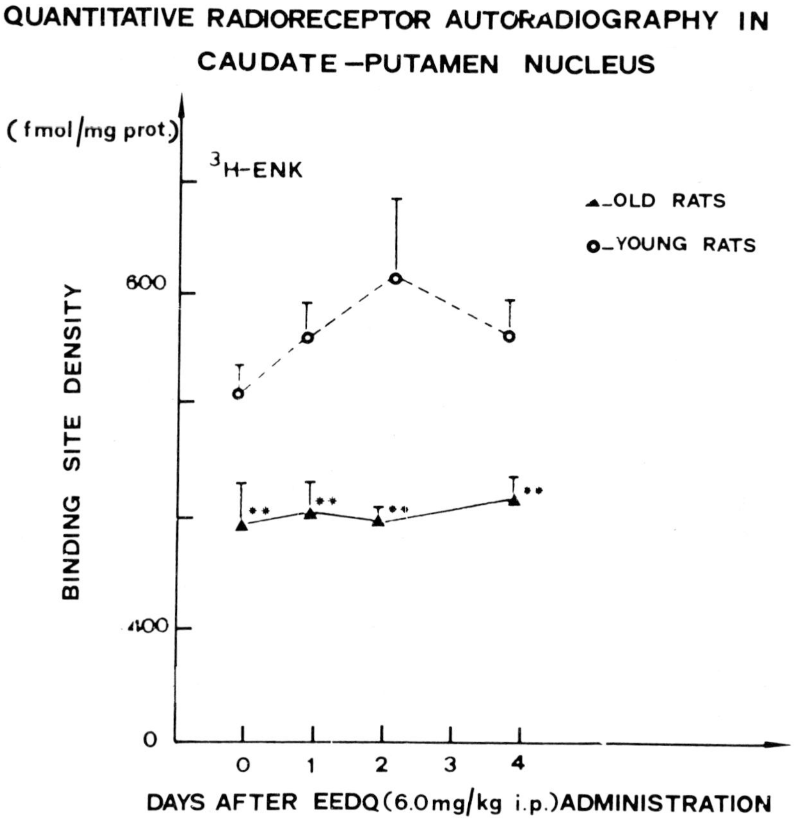

Figure 7. Effects of EEDQ treatment on the ^{3}H-DSTLE binding in the nucleus caudatus putamen in the young and old male rat (3- and 24-month-old male rat respectively). Various time intervals after EEDQ treatment have been analyzed. Means $\pm$ s.e.m. are shown. n=4. Student's t test. **$p<0.01$. The statistical comparisons have been performed at the respective time intervals after EEDQ treatment between the binding obtained in the old and the young rat.

binding in the claustrum and in the frontoparietal cortex was unaffected in the 24-month-old male rat compared with the 3-month-old male rat. EEDQ treatment was found to produce an increase in ^{3}H-DSTLE binding by 10-25% in all the forebrain areas analyzed of the young rat (Fig. 6). However, in the old rat EEDQ treatment only increased ^{3}H-DSTLE binding within the claustrum and the frontal parietal cortex and not within the CPu, Acb and Tu. The results shown in Figure 6 were obtained at the 48-hour time interval after EEDQ treatment. At the 24-hour time interval the EEDQ induced increase in ^{3}H-DSTLE binding in the Cpu was not evident in the adult rats, but they were still observed on the 4th day after EEDQ treatment (Fig. 7). At no time interval after EEDQ treatment was a modulation in ^{3}H-DSTLE binding observed in the nucleus caudatus putamen (Fig. 7), nucleus accumbens and tuberculum olfactorium of the old rat.

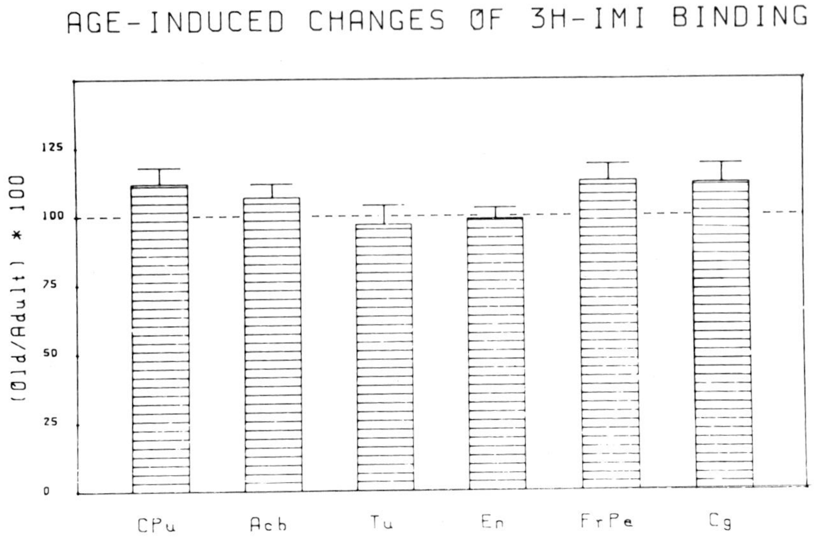

Figure 8. ^{3}H-imipramine binding in various forebrain regions in the 24-month-old male rat. The binding is expressed in % of the corresponding value obtained in the 3-month-old male rat (adult). Means ± s.e.m. are shown. No statistical differences were found as evaluated by means of Student's t test. For abbreviations, see text to previous figures.

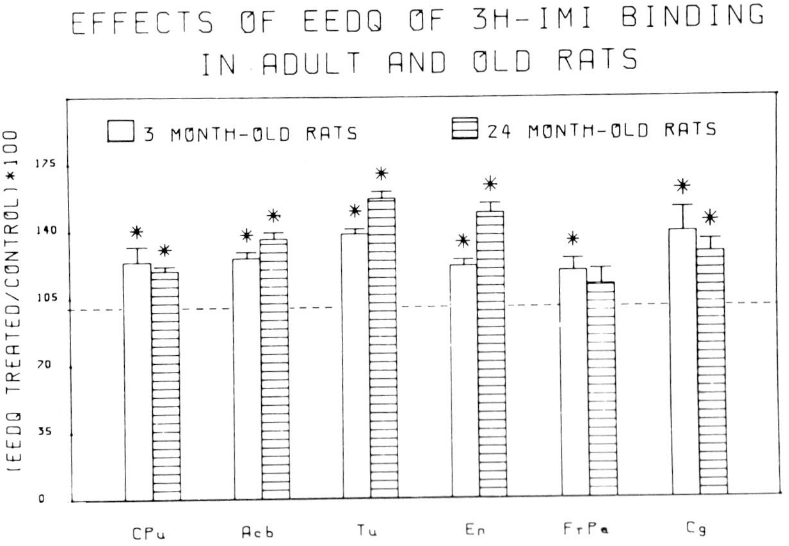

Figure 9. Effects of EEDQ treatment on ^{3}H-imipramine binding in various forebrain regions of the 3- and 24-month-old male rat. EEDQ was administered in a dose of 6 mg/kg i.p. 48 h before killing. The results are expressed in % of the respective control group mean value (no EEDQ treatment). Means ± s.e.m. are shown out of 6 rats. Student's t test. *$p<0.05$. For abbreviations, see text to previous figures.

Studies on ^{3}H-imipramine Binding

The results are summarized in Figures 8 and 9. As seen the ^{3}H-imipramine binding is not reduced in any area of the forebrain studied in the aged male rat. Furthermore, EEDQ treatment as evaluated at the 48-hour time interval is found to produce significant 15-25% increases in ^{3}H-imipramine binding in the CPu, Acb and Tu, the frontoparietal (FrPa), cingulate cortex (Cg) and in the entopiriform nucleus (En). The EEDQ induced increases of ^{3}H-imipramine binding were also demonstrated in the aged male rat (24-month-old rat).

IMMUNOCYTOCHEMICAL EXPERIMENTS

The results from the studies on the GRF immunoreactive nerve terminals of the median eminence are illustrated in Figure 10 and summarized in Table 2. In the medial palisade zone (MPZ) a marked reduction is observed in the mean grey value and in the immunoreactive area of GRF-like IR, leading to a significant reduction also of the total IR. In the lateral palisade zone (LPZ) a marked reduction in the aged rat is only observed in the mean grey value but not in the immunoreactive area of the GRF IR. However, due to the marked change in the mean grey value a substantial change in total immunoreactivity is still observed in the LPZ of the 24-month-old male rat.

DISCUSSION

The 24-month-old male rat must be regarded as a very old animal, since in the Sprague-Dawley strain analyzed it is difficult for the rats to live for a substantially longer period. The neurochemical alterations observed in the present and previous papers (Agnati et al., 1984a; 1985a; 1985b; 1986a; 1986b; 1986c; Fuxe et al., 1986a; 1986b) on this strain of rats must therefore be regarded as reflecting changes in the brain at the end of the aging process. In agreement with previous work (see *inter alia* Agnati et al., 1984a) widespread reductions of D2 receptor binding, of α2-adrenoreceptor binding and of mu and delta opiate receptor binding were observed in the 24-month-old male rat compared with the 3-month-old male rat. The changes were *inter alia* found both in the cortical regions and in the dorsal and ventral striatum. In agreement with previous work (Leff et al., 1984; Farabegoli et al., 1987) indications of a reduced D2 receptor turnover were obtained within the nucleus caudatus putamen. In addition, evidence for a reduced D2 receptor turnover was obtained in the nucleus accumbens and in the claustrum. In the present experiments we have also obtained indications based on the EEDQ experiments for a reduced α2-adrenergic receptor turnover within the dorsal and ventral striatum and in certain brain stem nuclei but not within the cortical areas (both limbic and neocortex). These results give evidence for a reduced plasticity of the D2 and α2-adrenergic receptors in several brain areas in the 24-month-old male rat. However, with regard to the α2-adrenergic receptors this loss of plasticity does not include the cerebral cortex.

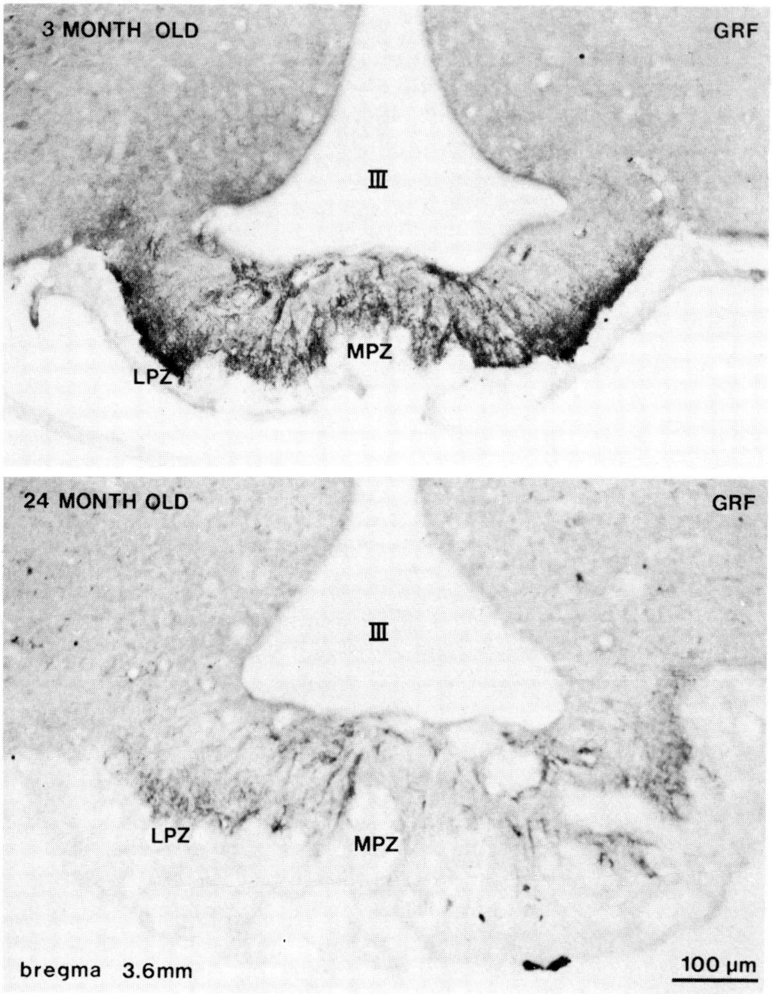

Figure 10. GRF IR in the mediobasal hypothalamus of the 3-month-old and 24-month-old male rat. Transverse section; Bregma level 3.6 mm. Antiserum dilution 1:1000. The biotin-avidin immunoperoxidase procedure was used (Vectastain). A marked reduction of GRF IR present in nerve terminals is found both in the medial and lateral palisade zone (MPZ and LPZ).

It has been demonstrated that this loss of D2, α2-adrenergic and opiate receptors is associated also with a loss of regional catecholamine stores, and of regional enkephalin and beta-endorphin like IR (see Agnati et al., 1984a; 1986c). It therefore seems likely in view of the presence of losses of both transmitter stores and their corresponding transmitter receptors that a deficit exists in the 24-month-old male rat with regard to D2 operated dopamine transmission, α2-adrenergic operated transmission and mu and delta opiate receptor operated transmission. This interpretation is also in agreement with

Table 2. *Effects of aging on GRF IR in the medial and lateral palisade zone of the median eminence as evaluated by computer assisted morphometrical and microdensitometrical analyses*

	GRF-IR			
	MPZ		LPZ	
	Young	Old	Young	Old
Mean gray value (GV)	58±7.1*	39.4±4.4	66±7.4*	38.9±4.2
IR-area (μm²)	2430±184*	1422±76	1028±8	1176±143
Total unweighted IR ($\bar{x}$·IR-area)	454.062±56.380*	117.414±39.381	320.200±76.840*	94.189±7.458

other observations such as, e.g. reduced capability of morphine to induce hypothermia in the old rat (McDougal et al., 1981; Roth, 1983).

Previous findings have indicated the existence of interactions between opiate receptors and dopamine receptors in the nucleus accumbens and striatum (Kalivas and Bronson, 1985; Stinus et al., 1985; Esposito et al., 1987; Schoffelmeer et al., 1986). 6-OH-DA induced lesions of the mesolimbic dopamine neurons as well as blockade of dopamine receptors by neuroleptics produce a behavioural supersensitivity to microinjections of enkephalin analogues in the nucleus accumbens. Furthermore, injections of 6-OH-DA into the nucleus accumbens result in an increase of delta opiate binding sites but not in mu opiate binding sites. Our studies give further support for an interaction between delta opioid and dopamine receptors in dorsal and ventral striatum. Thus, irreversible blockade of probable dopamine receptors by EEDQ induced a delayed increase 48 hours later in delta but not in mu opiate receptor binding sites in the nucleus accumbens and in the nucleus caudatus putamen. These results also indicate that second messengers may be involved in this receptor-receptor interaction in view of the delayed increase in delta opiate receptor binding. The change was most marked in the nucleus accumbens and maximal at the 48 hour time interval. At the 4-day time interval, when a substantial recovery of D2 receptor binding sites has taken place, the increases are substantially less but still significant. In the old brain this receptor-receptor interaction is lost within the nucleus caudatus putamen, the nucleus accumbens and the tuberculum olfactorium. Thus, receptor plasticity in the aged brain is also lost with regard to their ability to interact with other receptors. However, in the cortical areas interactions between monoamine receptors and delta opiate receptors appear to persist. The special vulnerability of the receptor interactions in the basal ganglia may be caused by the deficit in DA D2 receptors present in the 24-month-old male rat as indicated in the present and previous studies (Agnati et al., 1984c). Under all conditions the present results indicate that the cortical plasticity, but not the striatal plasticity, may be maintained in terms of interactions between monoamine and delta opiate receptors.

The present observations that ^{3}H-imipramine binding is increased by EEDQ treatment may be explained on the basis that EEDQ blocks 5-HT autoreceptors on the

5-HT nerve terminal membrane, where also the ^{3}H-imipramine binding sites are located and linked to the ionic transporter (see Langer and Briley, 1981). This leads to the assumption that an interaction exists between the 5-HT autoreceptor and the ^{3}H-imipramine binding sites. The present results indicate that the 5-HT autoreceptor exerts an inhibitory modulation of ^{3}H-imipramine binding, an interaction which may make it possible for the 5-HT autoreceptor, inhibiting of 5-HT release, to regulate the 5-HT uptake capacity of the membrane. The present results show that this interaction is intact in the 24-month-old male rat showing that some receptor-receptor interactions are more vulnerable to the aging process than others.

These results, taken together with previous observations showing that cyclic AMP and calcium induced protein phosphorylation is reduced in the aged brain (the striatum and the cerebral cortex) (Agnati et al., 1986a), suggest that the aging process in its end stage results in deficits at all levels of the synapse, that is deficits in the synthesis and release of transmitters and cotransmitters and especially peptide cotransmitters, deficits in the receptor sites, their turnovers and their interactions with other receptors, and deficits in the transduction mechanism as seen in the studies on protein phosphorylation. Thus, homeostatic responses will be impaired leading to e.g. deterioration in the ability of the brain to respond to stress (see Agnati et al., 1986b). A reduced synaptic plasticity can also lead to a decreased function of heterostatic mechanisms in synaptic transmission, since the above synaptic mechanisms may be basic to the regulation of the setpoint of the overall negative feedback activity, controlling the efficacy of the various transmission lines (Agnati et al., 1985b; Fuxe et al., 1984; 1986c). This loss in synaptic plasticity could be the basis for the loss of memory traces and their formation in the aged brain.

Finally, in the present paper we have extended our previous obsevations that GRF IR neurons of the arcuate nucleus innervating the median eminence may be severely affected by the aging process (Fuxe et al., 1986a). Thus, GRF IR was severely reduced within the lateral and medial palisade of the median eminence suggesting an impairment of growth hormone (GH) secretion and thus in the trophic effects of (GH) in peripheral tissues. The hypothesis may be introduced that the impairment of GRF synthesis and release and even the degeneration of GRF IR neurons leads to a reduced trophic support to peripheral tissues and to an acceleration of the aging process.

SUMMARY

By means of quantitative receptor autoradiography in combination with inactivation of monoamine receptors by N-ethoxycarbonyl-2-ethoxy-1,2-dihydroquinoline (EEDQ) it was shown that the D2 receptor levels are reduced by 20-40% in the nucleus caudatus putamen, nucleus accumbens and tuberculum olfactorium in the 24-month-old male rat, whereas the D2 receptor levels in the claustrum were not significantly reduced. The reduction of D2 receptor levels was associated with a significant reduction of D2 receptor turnover. Studies on ^{3}H-paraminoclonidine (PAC) binding also demonstrated reductions of α2-adrenergic agonist binding sites in many brain areas of aged male rat, also associated with reductions of α2 adrenoceptor turnovers. By means of the radioligand ^{3}H-etorphin, which in low concentrations preferentially labels mu opiate receptors, and ^{3}H-D-ser-L-leu-L-thr-enkephalin (DSTLE), which preferentially labels delta opiate receptors, further evidence was obtained that these two types of opiate binding sites are reduced by 15-25% in various forebrain regions in the 24-month-old male rat. An irreversible blockade of monoamine receptors, probably of dopamine receptors, by EEDQ, resulted in 10-20% increases in the ^{3}H-DSTLE binding but not in ^{3}H-etorphin binding in the nucleus caudatus putamen, nucleus accumbens and tuberculum olfactorium of the 3-month-old male rat but not in the 24-month-old male rat. The EEDQ induced increase in delta opiate binding was in several areas only observed two days after EEDQ treatment. These results suggest an interaction between D-2 and delta opiate receptors, operating mainly via second messenger mechanisms, and which are absent in the aged brain.

The ^{3}H-imipramine binding sites, however, appeared to be unaltered in several forebrain regions of the aged rat. Furthermore, the EEDQ induced increase in ^{3}H-imipramine binding observed 1-4 days after EEDQ treatment in many forebrain regions was found to be present also in the aged brain. These results may be explained by an interaction between the ^{3}H-imipramine binding sites, located on the 5-HT nerve terminals, and adjacent 5-HT autoreceptors which may exert an inhibitory influence on the ^{3}H-imipramine binding sites linked to the ion transporter for 5-HT uptake.

By means of semiquantitative immunocytochemistry in combination with automatic image analysis further evidence was obtained for a disappearence of GRF immunoreactive nerve terminal networks of the external layer of the medial eminence of the 24-month-old rat. These results are in agreement with our previous work and indicate a reduced synthesis of GRF in the aged brain, possibly associated with a degeneration of GRF immunoreactive neurons of the arcuate nucleus. Thus, reduced serum growth hormone levels may exist in the aged rat, leading to reduced trophic effects on various peripheral tissues.

Taken together with previous findings, the present results indicate that at the end of the aging process of the nervous system deficits are found in dopamine or neuropeptide synapses with regard to both transmitter store and utilization, to transmitter receptor and turnover and probably also to the transduction mechanism as indicated in studies on cyclic AMP and calcium induced protein phosphorylation. These changes are seen in many neuropeptide systems and some monoamine systems and are also associated with the reduction of receptor-receptor interactions. Thus, plasticity in many neuropeptide and monoamine synapses is lost in the aged brain resulting in a loss of their ability to perform homeostatic and heterostatic responses (Fuxe et al., 1986b; Agnati et al., 1986c).

ACKNOWLEDGMENTS

This work has been supported by a grant from L. Osterman Stiftelse, by a CNR international grant and by a grant (04X-715) from the Swedish Medical Research Council. For excellent secretarial assistance we are grateful to Mrs Monia Särd.

REFERENCES

Agnati LF, Benfenati F, Cortelli P, D'Alessandro R (1978) New methods to quantify catecholamine stores visualized by means of the Falck-Hillarp technique. Neurosci Lett 10:11-17.

Agnati LF, Fuxe K, Benfenati F, Toffano G, Cimino M, Battistini N, Calza L, Merlo Pich E (1984a) Computer assisted morphometry and microdensitometry of transmitter identified neurons with special reference to the mesostriatal dopamine pathway. III. Studies on aging processes. Acta Physiol Scand 532:45-61.

Agnati LF, Fuxe K, Benfenati F, Zini I, Zoli M, Fabbri L, Härfstrand A (1984b) Computer assisted morphometry and microdensitometry of transmitter identified neurons with special reference to the mesostriatal dopamine pathway. I. Methodological aspects. Acta Physiol Scand (Suppl) 532:5-36.

Agnati LF, Fuxe K, Battistini N, Benfenati F (1984c) Aging brain and dopamine receptors: Abnormal regulation by CCK-8 of ^{3}H-spiperone labelled dopamine receptors in striatal membranes. Acta Physiol Scand 120:464-467.

Agnati LF, Fuxe K, Calza L, Giardino L, Zini I, Toffano G, Goldstein M, Marrama P, Gustafsson J-Å, Yu Z-Y, Cuello C, Terenius L, Lang R, Ganten D (1985a) Morphometrical and microdensitometrical studies on monoaminergic and peptidergic neurons in the aging brain. In: Agnati LF, Fuxe K (eds): Quantitative Neuroanatomy in Transmitter Research. MacMillan Press, London, pp. 91-112.

Agnati LF, Fuxe K, Giardino L, Calza L, Zoli M, Battistini N, Benfenati F, Vanderhaeghen JJ, Guidolin D, Ruggeri M, Goldstein M (1985b) Evidence for cholecystokinin-dopamine receptor interactions in the central nervous system of the adult and old rat. Studies on their functional meaning. In: Vanderhaeghen JJ (ed): Neuronal Cholecystokinin, vol. 448. Ann N.Y. Acad Sci, New York, pp. 315-333.

Agnati LF, Fuxe K, Zoli M, Zini I, Toffano G, Ferraguti F (1986a) A correlation analysis of the regional distribution of central enkephalin and β-endorphin immunoreactive terminals and of opiate receptors in adult and old male rats: Evidence for the existence of two main types of communication in the central nervous system: the volume transmission and the wiring transmission. Acta Physiol Scand 128:201-207.

Agnati LF, Fuxe K, Zoli M, Grimaldi R, Bernardi P, Härfstrand A, Zini I, Gavioli G, Goldstein M, Gustafsson J-Å (1986b) Morphofunctional evidence for an alteration in central cardiovascular regulation in aging especially in relation to stress induced alteration in cardiovascular function. In: Vezzadini P, Facchini A, Labò G (eds): Neuroendocrine system and aging. EURAGE, pp. 37-49.

Agnati LF, Fuxe K, Zoli M, Merlo Pich E, Benfenati F, Zini I, Goldstein M (1986c) Aspects on the information handling by the central nervous system: focus on cotransmission in the aged rat brain. In: Hökfelt T, Fuxe K, Pernow B (eds): Progress in Brain Research. Elsevier Science Publ, Amsterdam, pp. 291-301.

Agnati LF, Fuxe K, Zoli M, Zini I, Härfstrand A, Toffano G, Goldstein M (1987) Morphometrical and microdensitometrical studies on phenylethanolamine-N-methyltransferase and neuropeptide Y immunoreactive neurons in the rostral medulla oblongata of the adult and old male rat. Neurosci, in press.

Benfenati F, Cimino M, Agnati LF, Fuxe K (1986) Quantitative autoradiography of central neurotransmitter receptors: methodological and statistical aspects with special reference to computer-assisted image analysis. Acta Physiol Scand 128:129-146.

Cintra A, Fuxe K, Härfstrand A, Agnati LF, Wikström A-C, Okret S, Vale W, Gustafsson J-Å (1987) Presence of glucocorticoid receptor immunoreactivity in corticotrophin releasing factor and in growth hormone releasing factor immunoreactive neurons of the rat di- and telencephalon. Neurosci Lett 77:25-39.

Creese I, Schneider R, Snyder SH (1977) ^{3}H-spiroperidol labels dopamine receptors in pituitary and brain. Eur J Pharmacol 46:377-381.

Esposito E, Petrillo P, Sbacchi M, Tavani A, Samanin R (1987) Dopamine denervation of the nucleus accumbens induces a selective increase in the number of delta opioid binding sites. Brain Res, in press.

Farabegoli C, Merlo Pich E, Cimino M, Agnati LF, Fuxe K (1987) Chronic uridine treatment reduces the level of ^{3}H-spiperone labelled dopamine receptors and enhances their turnover rate in striatum of young rats. Relationship to dopamine dependent behaviours. Acta Physiol Scand, in press.

Fuxe K, Calza L, Benfenati F, Zini I, Agnati LF (1983) Quantitative autoradiographic localization of (^{3}H)imipramine binding sites in the brain of the rat: Relationship to ascending 5-hydroxytryptamine neuron systems. Proc Natl Acad Sci USA 80:3836-3840.

Fuxe K, Agnati LF, Andersson K, Martire M, Ögren S-O, Giardino L, Battistini N, Grimaldi R, Farabegoli C, Härfstrand A, Toffano G (1984) Receptor-receptor interactions in the central nervous system. Evidence for the existence of heterostatic synaptic mechanisms. In: Vizi ES, Magyar K (eds): Regulation of transmitter function: Basic and clinical aspects. Developments in Neurosciences Series, vol 17. Elsevier Science Publisher, pp. 129-140.

Fuxe K, Agnati LF, Härfstrand A, Eneroth P, Kitayama I, Farabegoli C, Tesini M, Toni R, Goldstein M (1986a) New vistas on the morphofunctional organization of the endocrine hypothalamus. Focus on aging induced changes in the arcuate nucleus and in the medianosomes of the rat. In: Vezzadini P, Facchini A, Labò G (eds): Neuroendocrine system and aging. EURAGE, pp. 13-25.

Fuxe K, Agnati LF, Zoli M, Benfenati F, Zini I, Härfstrand A, Eneroth P, Toffano G (1986b) Age induced changes in the trophic signals and information handling in the central nervous system. Focus on peptide transmission. In: Bès A et al. (eds): Senile dementias: early detection. John Libbey Eurotext, pp. 273-280.

Fuxe K, Agnati LF, Härfstrand A, Janson AM, Neumeyer A, Andersson K, Ruggeri M, Zoli M, Goldstein M (1986c) Morphofunctional studies on the neuropeptide Y/adrenaline costoring terminal systems in the dorsal cardiovascular region of the medulla oblongata. Focus on receptor-receptor interactions in cotransmission. In: Hökfelt T, Fuxe K, Pernow B (eds): Progress in Brain Research, vol 68. Elsevier Science Publisher, B.V., pp. 303-320.

Fuxe K, Meller E, Goldstein M, Benfenati F, Agnati LF (1986d) Analysis of (^{3}H)Spiperone binding sites in the rat striatum and frontoparietal cortex by means of quantitative receptor autoradiography after inactivation of dopamine receptors by N-ethoxy-carbonyl-2-ethoxy-1,2-dihydroquinoline in vivo: selective protection by sulpride in the striatum. Neurosci Lett 64:163-168.

Hamblin MW, Creese I (1983) Behavioral and radioligand binding evidence for irreversible dopamine receptor blockade by N-ethoxy-carbonyl-2-ethoxy-1,2-dihydroquinoline. Life Sci 32:2247-2255.

Kalivas PW, Bronson M (1985) Mesolimbic dopamine lesions produce an augmented behavioral response to enkephalin. Neuropharmacology 24:931-936.

Kitayama I, Janson AM, Fuxe K, Agnati LF, Cintra A, Ögren S-O, Härfstrand A, Eneroth P, Tsutsumi T, Jonsson G, Steinbusch HWM, Visser TJ (1987) Effects of acute and chronic treatment with imipramine on 5-hydroxytryptamine nerve cell groups and on bulbospinal 5-hydroxytryptamine/substance P/thyrotropin releasing hormone immunoreactive neurons in the rat. A morphometric and microdensitometric analysis. J Neural Trans 70:251-285.

Langer SZ, Briley M (1981) High affinity ^{3}H-imipramine binding: a new biological tool for studies in depression. Trends in Neurosciences 4:28-31.

Leff SE, Gariano R, Creese I (1984) Dopamine receptor turnover rates in rat striatum are age dependent. Proc Natl Acad Sci USA 81:3910-3914.

McDougal JN, Marques PR, Burks TF (1981) Reduced tolerance to morphine thermoregulatory effects in senescent rats. Life Sci 28:137-145.

Meller E, Bohmaker K, Goldstein M, Friedhoff AJ (1985) Inactivation of D1 and D2 dopamine receptors by N-ethoxy-carbonyl-2-ethoxy-1,2-dihydroquiniline in vivo: selective protection by neuroleptics. J Pharmacol Exp Ther 233:656-662.

Roth GS (1983) Brain dopaminergic and opiate receptors and responsiveness during aging. In: Agnoli A, Crepaldi G, Spano PF, Trabucchi M (eds): Aging brain and ergot alkaloids. Raven Press, New York.

Rouot B, Snyder SH (1979) ^{3}H-para-aminoclonidine: A novel ligand which binds with high affinity to α-adrenergic receptors. Life Sci 25:769-774.

Schoffelmeer ANM, Hansen HA, Stoof JC, Mulder AH (1986) Blockade of D-2 dopamine receptors strongly enhances the potency of enkephalins to inhibit dopamine-sensitive adenylate cyclase in rat neostriatum: involvement of δ- and μ-opioid receptors. J Neurosci 6:2235-2239.

Stinus L, Winnock M, Kelley AE (1985) Chronic neuroleptic treatment and mesolimbic dopamine denervation induce behavioural supersensitivity to opiates. Psychopharmacology 85:323-328.

Zoli M, Agnati LF, Fuxe K, Zini I, Merlo Pich E, Grimaldi R, Härfstrand A, Goldstein M, Wikström A-C, Gustafsson J-Å (1987) Morphometrical and microdensitometrical studies on phenylethanol-amine-N-methyltransferase and neuropeptide Y immunoreactive nerve terminals and on glucocorticoid receptor immunoreactive nerve cell nuclei in the paraventricular hypothalamic nucleus in adult and old male rats. Neurosci, in press.

New Trends in Aging Research
G. Pepeu, B. Tomlinson, C.M. Wischik (eds)
Fidia Research Series, vol. 15
Liviana Press, Padova © 1988

CHANGES OF NEUROTRANSMITTER RELEASE IN THE OLD RAT BRAIN AND EFFECTS OF PHOSPHATIDYLSERINE TREATMENT

Maurizio Raiteri, Anna Maria Caviglia, Mario Marchi, Guido Maura and Anna Pittaluga

Istituto di Farmacologia e Farmacognosia, Università di Genova,
Viale Cembrano 4, 16148 Genova, Italy

INTRODUCTION

It is well known that several neurotransmitter systems undergo changes with advanced age in the CNS. Results from pharmacological and morphological investigations indicate that functional modifications may occur at different levels. At the presynaptic level changes may occur during aging in several neurochemical parameters such as uptake, synthesis and compartmentation of neurotransmitters (for reviews see: Bartus et al., 1982; Hardy et al., 1985). The alteration of these neuronal activities is likely to lead to changes in the release of neurotransmitters. However, the literature contains scarce information on this important functional parameter in the CNS during aging.

We have previously reported that selective changes occur at the presynaptic level in the central cholinergic system. Our results using superfused nerve endings prepared from different brain areas have shown alterations of several parameters including ^{3}H-ACh release (Marchi et al., 1983). A decrease in endogenous ACh release has also been observed using electrically stimulated cortical slices (Pedata et al., 1983).

Abbreviations: BC-PS, phosphatidylserine; DA, dopamine; NA, noradrenaline, HPLC, high performance liquid chromatography.

Recently Pedata et al. (1985) reported that prolonged administration of phosphatidylserine (BC-PS) to 24 month old rats restored the age-dependent impairment of ACh release. Behavioral effects of BC-PS, including changes of some performances, have also been observed (Drago et al., 1981; Corwin et al., 1985) suggesting the possibility of a pharmacological approach to ameliorate a cognitive impairment possibly related to a cholinergic deficit.

In the present investigation we have extendend our previous findings and compared in adult and old rats the release of dopamine (DA) and noradrenaline (NA) using superfused nerve terminals. We have also examined the effect of a chronic treatment with BC-PS on the release of these catecholamines in adult and old animals.

MATERIALS AND METHODS

Male Sprague Dawley rats were used for this study. Adult (3-4 months) and aged (22-24 months) animals were treated for one month with BC-PS (15 mg/kg; i.p.; daily) or with saline. The animals were killed by decapitation 24 hours after the last injection and the brain was dissected out immediately. Crude synaptosomal fractions (P_2) were prepared from different brain areas. The release of neurotransmitters was studied in superfusion as previously described (Raiteri et al., 1974). Endogenous DA was determined by HPLC, with dual-cell coulometric detection, essentially according to Achilli et al. (1985).

RESULTS AND DISCUSSION

The releases of ^{3}H-DA and ^{3}H-NA were studied in synaptosomes prepared from frontal and occipital cortex, respectively (Fig. 1). The nerve endings were superfused with Krebs-bicarbonate medium containing varying concentration of Ca^{2+} ions and depolarized with 15 mM KCl. The release of ^{3}H-DA elicited by high-K^+ in a medium containing from 0.2 to 1.2 mM Ca^{2+} was lower in old rats than in adult animals (Fig. 1A); however, the extent of this decrease depended upon the Ca^{2+} concentration in the medium: it was percentually more pronounced when the Ca^{2+} concentration was low (0.2 mM). Interestingly, no significant difference between adult and aged rats could be detected when the Ca^{2+} concentration was raised to 3.6 mM (Fig. 1A). Also the depolarization-evoked release of ^{3}H-NA was significantly decreased in the aged animals (Fig. 1B). However, the changes observed do not appear to be dependent upon the concentration of Ca^{2+} in the medium (Fig. 1B).

Besides that of ^{3}H-DA, also the release of endogenous DA was studied in nerve endings prepared from corpus striatum of adult and old rats (Table 1). The K^+-evoked release of endogenous DA from striatal synaptosomes was significantly lower in the old

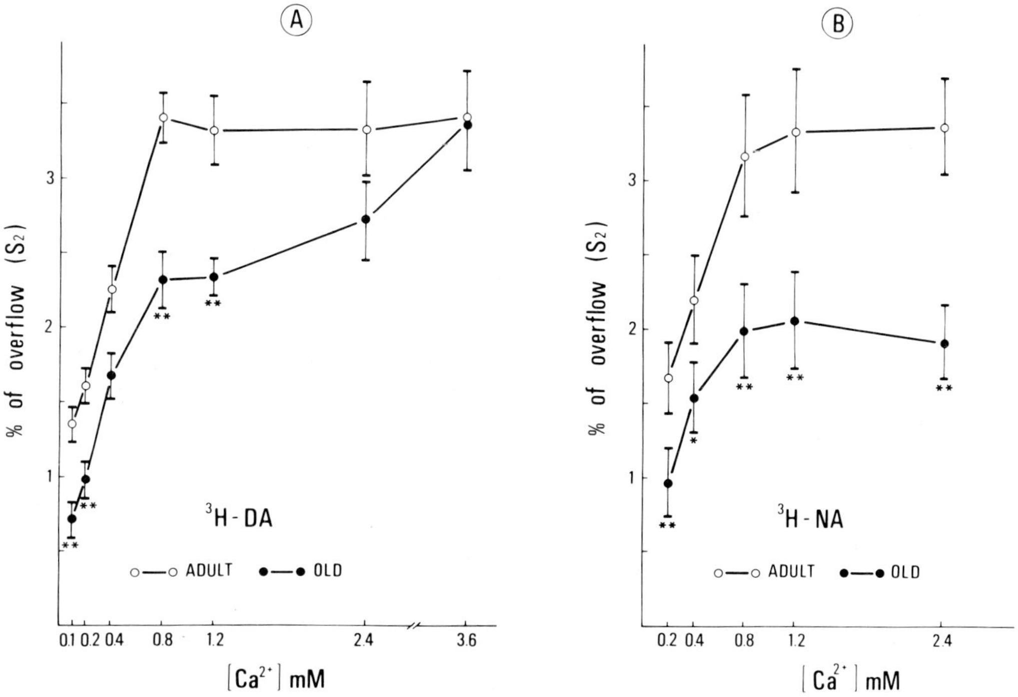

Figure 1. Ca^{2+}-dependency of the K^+-evoked release of ^{3}H-DA (panel A) and ^{3}H-NA (panel B) from superfused synaptosomes in adult and aged rats. ^{3}H-DA release was studied in the frontal cortex and ^{3}H-NA release in the occipital cortex. Results are expressed as a percentage of the tritium content of the synaptosomes at the onset of the respective collection period. To evaluate the stimulation-evoked release the evoked overflow was calculated by subtraction of the estimated basal output.

compared to the adult animals. No significant differences were detected in the basal release (Table 1).

Figure 2 shows the effect of the chronic treatment with BC-PS on DA release. In the old rats treated with BC-PS the K^+-evoked release of endogenous DA from striatal

Table 1. *Endogenous dopamine release*

	Adult	Old	% of adult
Basal*	3.21 ± 0.38 (23)	3.30 ± 0.18 (23)	+2.8
K^+-evoked*	7.02 ± 0.45 (23)	5.08 ± 0.29** (23)	−28

* pmoles/mg prot/6 min; ** $P < 0.01$ versus adult.

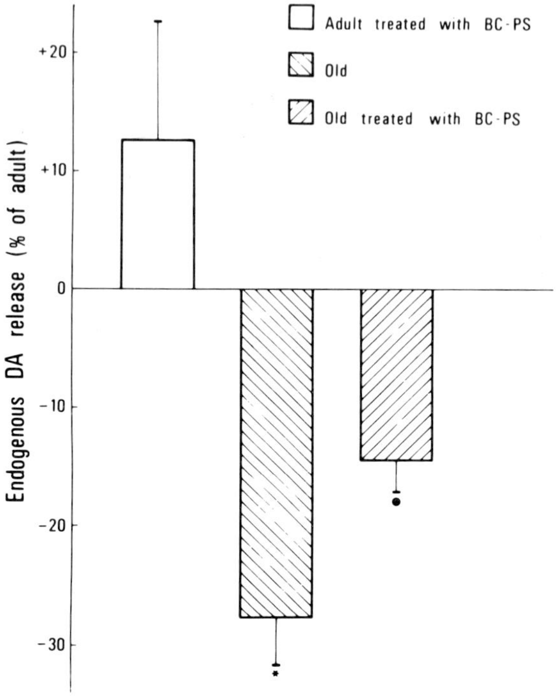

Figure 2. Effect of chronic treatment with BC-PS on endogenous DA release from striatal synaptosomes. Values are presented as percent ± S.E.M. of untreated adult levels. * $P<0.01$ vs. adult; ● $P<0.01$ vs. old.

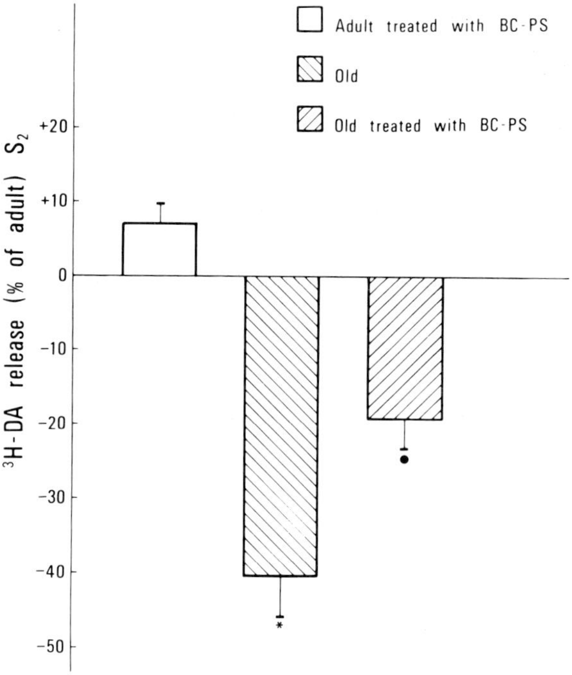

Figure 3. Effect of chronic treatment with BC-PS on ^{3}H-DA release from synaptosomes prepared from the frontal cortex. Values are presented as percentage (±S.E.M.) of untreated adult levels. * $P<0.01$ vs. adult; ● $P<0.01$ vs. old.

nerve endings was significantly increased compared to the untreated aged controls. The chronic treatment with BC-PS did not alter the basal release of DA both in the adult and in the old animals (not shown).

Also the depolarization-evoked release of ^{3}H-DA from frontal cortex synaptosomes was significantly increased in the old rats following the chronic treatment with BC-PS (Fig. 3). Interestingly, the treatment with BC-PS did not affect the K^+-evoked release of ^{3}H-NA in nerve endings prepared from the occipital cortex of old animals (Fig. 4).

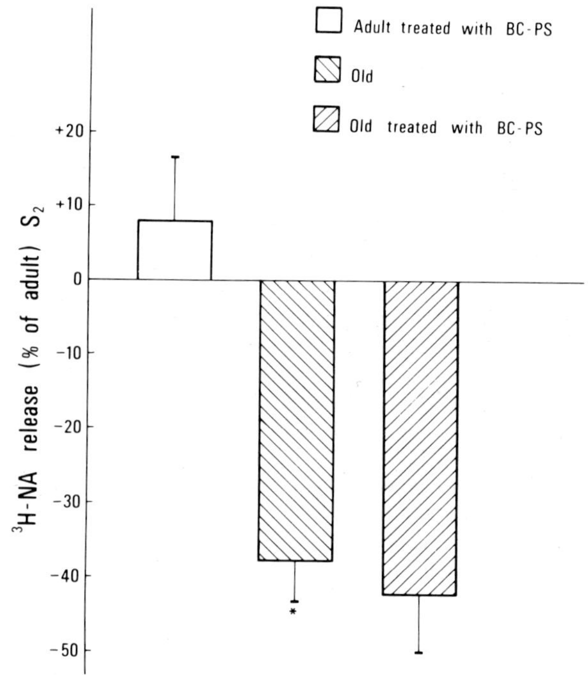

Figure 4. Effect of chronic treatment with BC-PS on ^{3}H-NA release from synaptosomes prepared from the occipital cortex. Values are presented as percentage ± S.E.M. of untreated adult levels. * $P < 0.01$ vs. adult.

CONCLUSIONS

1. Our results show marked age-dependent changes in the K^+-evoked release of DA and NA in some brain areas.

2. Dopaminergic and noradrenergic nerve terminals do not seem to be equally susceptible to changes of Ca^{2+} concentration in the external medium.

3. The chronic treatment with BC-PS increased in the old animals the K^+-evoked release of DA both in the corpus striatum and in the cerebral cortex. This effect seems to be selective since NA release in the occipital cortex was not affected.

ACKNOWLEDGMENTS

This work was supported by Grants from the Italian Ministry of Education and from the Italian C.N.R. The aged rats were kindly supplied by the Italian Study Group on Brain Aging. Phosphatidylserine was kindly supplied by FIDIA Research Laboratories, Abano Terme, PD, Italy. The authors wish to thank Dr. Paola Bocchieri, Dr. Lucia Garbarino and Mr. Marco Ferlito for their skilful technical assistance.

REFERENCES

Achilli G, Perego C, Ponzio F (1985) Application of the dual-cell coulometric detector: a method for assaying monoamines and their metabolites. Anal Biochem 148:1-9.

Bartus RT, Dean III RL, Beer B, Lippa AS (1982) The cholinergic hypothesis of geriatric memory dysfunction. Science 217:408-417.

Corwin J, Dean III RL, Bartus RT, Rotrosen J, Watkins DL (1985) Behavioral effects of phosphatidylserine in the aged Fischer 344 rat: amelioration of passive avoidance deficits without changes in psychomotor task performance. Neurobiol Aging 6:11-15.

Drago F, Canonico PL, Scapagnini U (1981) Behavioral effects of phosphatidylserine in aged rats. Neurobiol Aging 2:209-213.

Hardy J, Adolfsson R, Alafuzoff I, Bucht G, Marcusson J, Nyberg P, Perdahl E, Wester P, Winblad B (1985) Transmitter deficits in Alzheimer's disease. Neurochem Int 7:545-563.

Marchi M, Paudice P, Raiteri M (1983) Choline uptake, acetylcholine synthesis, and regulation of acetylcholine release through autoreceptors in the aging rat cortex. In: Samuel D, Algeri S, Gershon S, Grimm VE, Toffano G (eds): Aging of the Brain. Raven Press, New York, pp. 191-195.

Pedata F, Slavikova J, Kotas A, Pepeu G (1983) Acetylcholine release from rat cortical slices during postnatal development and aging. Neurobiol Aging 4:31-35.

Pedata F, Giovannelli L, Spignoli G, Giovannini MG, Pepeu G (1985) Phosphatidylserine increases acetylcholine release from cortical slices in aged rats. Neurobiol Aging 6:337.

Raiteri M, Angelini F, Levi G (1974) A simple apparatus for studying the release of neurotransmitters from synaptosomes. Eur J Pharmacol 25:411-414.

New Trends in Aging Research
G. Pepeu, B. Tomlinson, C.M. Wischik (eds)
Fidia Research Series, vol. 15
Liviana Press, Padova © 1988

NICOTINIC AND MUSCARINIC CHOLINERGIC RECEPTOR HETEROGENEITY IN THE HUMAN BRAIN AT NORMAL AGING AND DEMENTIA OF ALZHEIMER TYPE

Agneta Nordberg, Abdu Adem, Lena Nilsson and Bengt Winblad[1]

Department of Pharmacology, University of Uppsala, Uppsala, and
[1]Department of Geriatric Medicine, Karolinska Institute,
Huddinge Hospital, Sweden

INTRODUCTION

The cholinergic receptors in the brain are classically divided into two types, the muscarinic and nicotinic. That the former type exists has been well established for several years; it has been well characterized in the rodent brain, while our knowledge concerning the nicotinic receptors in the brain has only been improved upon recent years.

Subtypes of the muscarinic and nicotinic receptors have been characterized in the rodent brain. Based on agonist binding, Birdsall et al. (1978; 1980) suggested that there were three different agonist binding sites (superhigh, high and low affinity). Moreover, muscarinic receptors were subclassified into M1 and M2 sites based on antagonist binding (Goyal and Rattan, 1978; Hammer et al., 1980; 1982). Recently a new antagonist, AF-DX-116A, was used for further subdivision of M2 sites (Hammer et al., 1986).

Abbreviations: ^{3}H-ACh, ^{3}H-acetylcholine; AD/SDAT, Alzheimer's disease, senile dementia of Alzheimer type; Atr, Atropine; AV, Anteroventral nucleus of thalamus; DM, Dorsomedial nucleus of thalamus; MID, Multi-infarct dementia; Phys, Physostigmine; PL, Posterolateral nucleus of thalamus; PLV, Posterolateral ventral nucleus of thalamus; ^{3}H-TC, ^{3}H-tubocurarine; THA, 9-amino-1.2.3.4-tetrahydroacridine.

The presence of at least three nicotinic binding sites can be detected in the rodent brain using labelled ligands such as acetylcholine (ACh) (high affinity), nicotine (high affinity, low affinity) and α-bungarotoxin (neuromuscular type) (for reviews see Larsson et al., 1985; Adem, 1987).

We here describe the heterogeneity of cholinergic receptor subtypes in the human brain. An understanding of receptor changes in the normal aging processes is fundamental to any evaluation of findings from pathological brains with, for example, dementia.

SUBTYPES OF MUSCARINIC RECEPTORS IN NORMAL AGING

A similarity seems to exist between the rodent (Birdsall et al. 1978) and the human brain concerning number and affinity of muscarinic receptors and subtypes (Nordberg and Winblad, 1981; Undén et al., 1983; Caulfield et al., 1983; Garvey et al., 1983; Cortes et al., 1986; Nordberg et al., 1986; Adem et al., 1988a). The muscarinic receptors are mainly the M1 type in the human cerebral cortex, hippocampus (Cortes et al. 1986, Adem et al. 1988a), while the M2 type in the thalamus and brain stem (Cortes et al., 1987). It has been reported that during normal aging the number of muscarinic receptors are reduced (White et al., 1977; Perry, 1980; Nordberg and Winblad, 1981; Rinne, 1987), unchanged (Davies and Verth, 1978; Allen et al., 1983) or increased (Nordberg and Winblad, 1986a). In some studies the brain material was obtained from individuals over 50 years, younger individuals being excluded, and this may have contributed to the discrepancies in the results reported. A more important explanation may, however, be that different patterns of age-related muscarinic receptor changes can be observed in different areas of the brain. Thus, a decrease in number of muscarinic receptors has been reported for various regions of the cortex (White et al., 1977; Perry, 1980; Rinne, 1987) and hippocampus (Nordberg and Winblad, 1981; Nordberg et al., 1982) while an increased number of receptor binding sites was obtained in the thalamus (Nordberg and Winblad, 1986a). Allen et al. (1983) found no change in caudate nucleus of brains of 50 to 90 years of age while Rinne (1987) recently reported a significant decrease in the caudate nucleus of brains of 4 to 93 years of age.

Table 1. *Effect of normal aging on subtypes of muscarinic receptors in human cerebral cortex and thalamus*

	^{3}H-QNB	M_1	M_2
Cortex	↓ **	↓ *	→
Thalamus	↑ ***	↑ **	↑ ***

Number of muscarinic receptors was measured using ^{3}H-QNB (0.2nM). To differentiate between M_1 and M_2 binding sites, the ^{3}H-QNB binding was performed in the presence of carbachol 10^{-4} M and pirenzepine 300 nM respectively (Nordberg et al., in preparation). The arrows in the table indicate increased (↑), decreased (↓) and unchanged (→) number of receptors at normal aging.

To further evaluate these observations, the effect of aging on the muscarinic M1 and M2 subtypes was studied in different brain regions. In the cortex of seven to eighty-year-old individual, a significantly lower ($p<0.05$) number of M1 sites were observed while in the aged no significant changes were found in the number of M2 sites. Furthermore, in the thalamus there was a significant increase in both M2 and M1 subtypes with age. Between the age of 10 and 80 years the number of M2 sites increased by about 100% ($p<0.001$) while the M1 sites increased by about 50% ($p<0.01$). The thalamus is a region of the brain that is known not to project cholinergic axons but to be a target of cholinergic innervation.

These findings suggest that muscarinic receptor subtypes can change in different directions in various areas of the brain in normal aging.

SUBTYPES OF MUSCARINIC RECEPTORS IN DEMENTIA

In senile dementia of the Alzheimer type (AD/SDAT) the number of muscarinic receptors in brain have been reported by most authors to be either unchanged (for a review see Nordberg and Winblad, 1986a) or increased (Nordberg and Winblad, 1986b; Nordberg et al., 1987b; London and Waller, 1986). These findings indicate a possible upregulation of the muscarinic receptors as a response to the loss of presynaptic terminals (low choline acetyltransferase activity) (Nordberg et al., 1983). A few authors have however observed a decrease in the number of muscarinic receptors in AD/SDAT (Reisine et al., 1978; Rinne et al., 1985). This might be the consequence of non-specific neuronal loss (Palacios et al., 1986). Recently Mash et al. (1985) reported a selective loss of M2 receptors in the cortex of AD/SDAT patients. This observation has not been confirmed by other investigators (Caulfield et al., 1983; Gulya et al., 1986; Nordberg et al., 1986). The discrepancy in findings might be explained by the different criteria used for the histopathological classifications. In multi-infarct dementia (MID) and "mixed" AD/MID a decrease in the number of muscarinic receptor binding sites has been found in some brain regions (Nordberg et al., 1982; Jenni-Eiermann et al., 1984; Rinne et al., 1985). When changes in subtypes of muscarinic receptors were analysed, a lower proportion of superhigh affinity muscarinic binding sites was observed in the hippocampus at AD/MID (Nordberg et al., 1986). In the thalamus of both AD/SDAT and MID patients, no increase with age in the number of muscarinic receptors was noticed (Nordberg and Winblad, 1986a). This observation indicates a disturbance of the normal aging process in individuals with dementia.

An in vitro model, using postmortem brain slices obtained with short postmortem delay, can be used to study the regulatory function of cholinergic receptors on brain ^{3}H-ACh release (Nilsson et al., 1986). After preloading with labelled choline the potassium evoked release of ^{3}H-ACh is measured. As shown in Figure 1 physostigmine (10^{-4}M) significantly decreases while atropine (10^{-5}M) increases the potassium evoked release in human control cortical tissue. These effects on control tissue are elicited by negative and positive feedback mechanisms respectively via presynaptic muscarinic autoreceptors. In AD/SDAT cortical tissue, atropine also enhances ^{3}H-ACh release (Fig. 1) indicating a preservation of functionally active muscarinic autoreceptors. Unlike control tissue, physostigmine in AD/SDAT tissue induces an increased ^{3}H-ACh release (for further discussion see below).

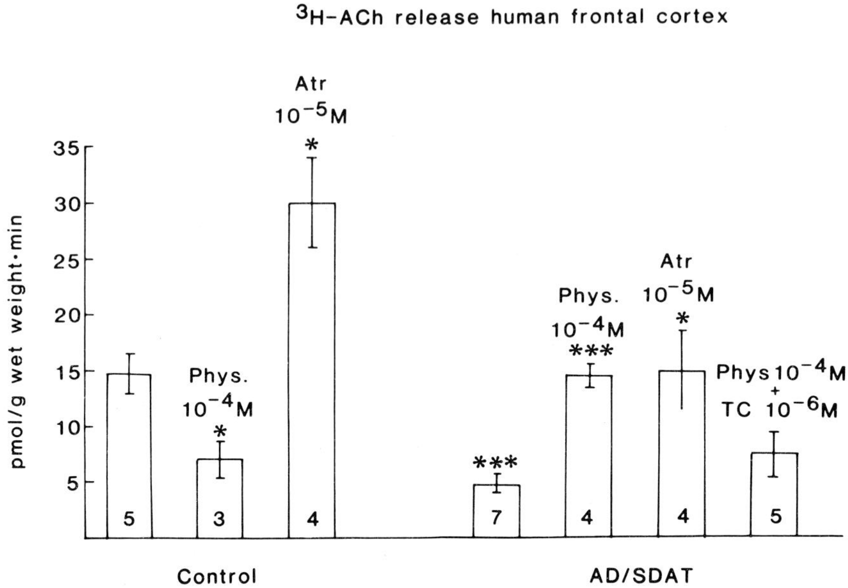

Figure 1. Effect of physostigmine (Phys), Atropine (Atr) and Phys + Tubocurarine (TC) on the evoked release of ^{3}H-acetylcholine (^{3}H-ACh) in frontal cortex of control and Alzheimer brains. Mean value ± S.E.. Numbers within columns indicate number of experiments.

SUBTYPES OF NICOTINIC RECEPTORS IN NORMAL AGING

Relatively few reports on nicotinic receptors in human brain are available. In the studies, radioactive ligands such as tubocurarine (Nordberg and Winblad, 1981), α-bungarotoxin (Volpe et al., 1979; Davies and Feisullin, 1981; Nordberg et al., 1982), nicotine (Nordberg et al., 1985; Shimohama et al., 1985; Whitehouse et al., 1986; Nordberg and Winblad, 1986b; Flynn and Mash, 1986) and ACh (Larsson et al., 1987; Nordberg and Winblad, 1986b; Whitehouse et al., 1986) have been used. For some of the ligands such as nicotine (Shimohama et al., 1985; Adem et al., 1988b) and ACh (Larsson et al., 1987; Adem et al., 1987) multiple binding sites have been observed in the human brain.

In the human brain the high affinity nicotinic receptors are distributed differently (Table 2). The binding of ^{3}H-nicotine and ^{3}H-ACh (in the presence of atropine) is highest in the thalamus, putamen, caudate nucleus, intermediate in the cortex, hypothalamus and low in the hippocampus, globus pallidus (Table 2). A similar regional distribution was reported by Shimohama et al. (1985) using ^{3}H-nicotine.

Receptor autoradiography also indicates a high labelling of ^{3}H-ACh and ^{3}H-nicotine in the human thalamus (Adem et al., 1988b). A high labelling of ^{3}H-ACh has been observed in the anteroventral nucleus and dorsomedial nucleus of the thalamus while a lower labelling was found in the posterolateral nucleus and the posterolateral ventral nucleus of the thalamus (Fig. 2).

Table 2. *Distribution of high affinity nicotinic receptors in discrete areas of human brain as measured by ^{3}H-ACh (10 nM) and ^{3}H-nicotine (5 nM)*

Brain region	pmol/g protein	
	^{3}H-ACh (10 nM)	^{3}H-nicotine (5nM)
Thalamus	14.2 ± 2.2	24.0 ± 1.9
Caudate nucleus	6.9 ± 0.8	18.9 ± 1.6
Putamen	6.2 ± 0.9	18.7 ± 1.5
Substantia nigra	5.5 ± 1.2	17.3 ± 2.2
Cortex cinguli	4.8 ± 0.6	14.1 ± 2.7
Hypothalamus	4.5 ± 1.0	13.6 ± 1.8
Olfactory bulb	2.7 ± 0.5	13.0 ± 0.7
Hippocampus	2.4 ± 0.6	8.4 ± 1.6
Globus pallidus	2.6 ± 1.3	3.8 ± 0.8

Mean values ± S.E. for 3 to 5 individuals are given (data taken from Adem et al., 1987; Nordberg et al., in preparation).

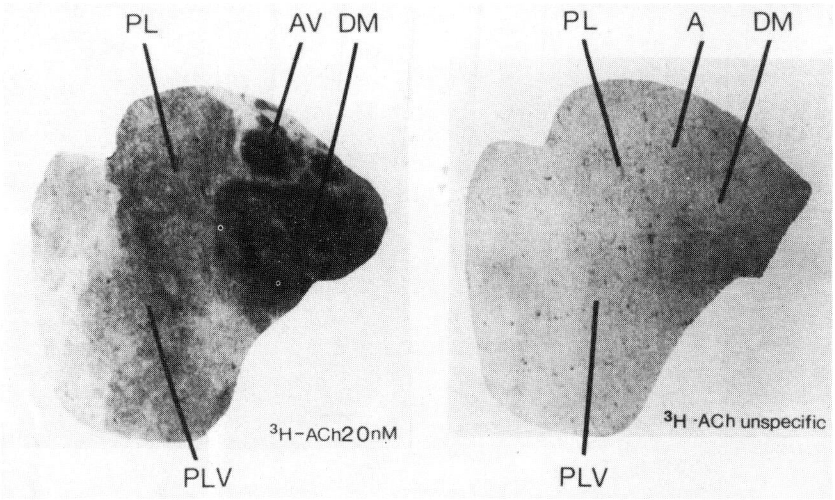

Figure 2. Autoradiographical localization of ^{3}H-ACh binding sites in 14 μm coronal sections of thalamus from a 65-year-old male A. Total ^{3}H-ACh binding. B. Unspecific ^{3}H-ACh binding in the presence of unlabelled nicotine 10^{-4}M. AV = Anteroventral nucleus of thalamus; DM = Dorsomedial nucleus of thalamus; PL = Posterolateral nucleus of thalamus; PLV = Posterolateral ventral nucleus of thalamus.

Competition studies with nicotine versus ^{3}H-nicotine indicate a complexity in subsites (Table 3). As shown in Table 3, a Hill coefficient of less than one is obtained in the cortex, thalamus and hippocampus. In all three brain areas ^{3}H-nicotine seems to preferentially label a high affinity site with an affinity constant in a nanomolar range (about 80% of the total number of binding sites). In the thalamus and hippocampus an additional superhigh affinity binding site is observed (about 15%) while in the cortex

Table 3. *Proportion of subtypes of nicotinic receptors in the human thalamus, hippocampus and temporal cortex obtained by competition studies using ^{3}H-nicotine (5nM) and unlabelled nicotine (10^{-11} - 10^{-4} M)*

	Thalamus	Hippocampus	Cortex
n^a_H	0.64	0.48	0.59
K_{SH}	0.2×10^{-9}	0.5×10^{-9}	—
K_H	14×10^{-9}	70×10^{-9}	5×10^{-9}
K_L	—	—	4×10^{-7}
% V_{SH}	15	14	—
% V_H	78	85	82
% V_L	—	—	18

a = Hill coefficient; super high (K_{SH}), high (K_H) and low (K_L) affinity constants; % fraction of sites with super high (% V_{SH}), high (% V_H) and low (% V_L) affinity.

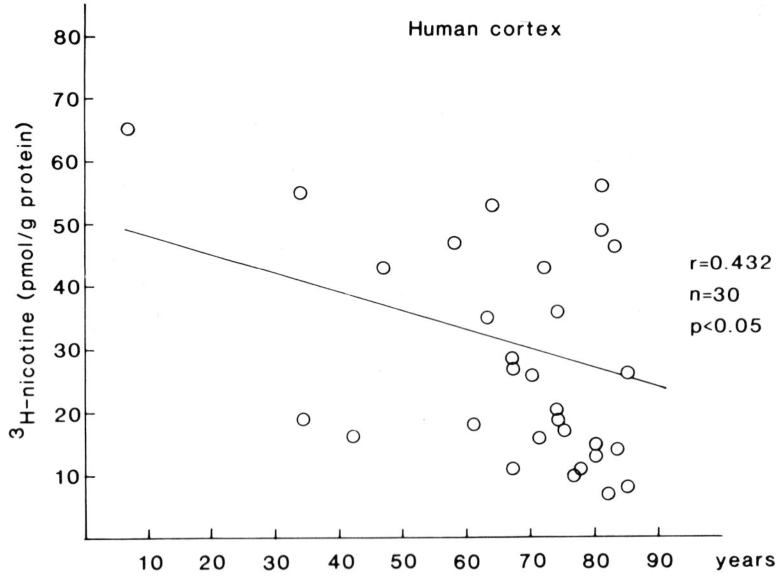

Figure 3. Specific ^{3}H-nicotine (5 nM) (pmol/g protein) binding in human frontal cortex at normal aging (7-90 years). Each point represents data from one individual.

an additional site (about 18%) with a low affinity is found. (Nordberg et al., in preparation). These findings support the hypothesis that there are multiple subtypes of nicotinic binding sites in the human brain (Adem et al., 1988b; 1987).

The different regional distribution of the nicotinic subsites might explain the finding that a significant decrease in ^{3}H-nicotine binding is observed in the frontal cortex in normal aging (Fig. 3), while there is a significant increase with age in the thalamus (Fig. 4) (Nordberg et al., in preparation). Other nicotinic ligands such as ^{3}H-α-bungarotoxin and ^{3}H-tubocurarine binding have shown changes that vary depending on the different brain areas during normal aging (Nordberg and Winblad, 1986a). These varying changes in the nicotinic receptor subtypes in normal aging may be due to different synaptic localizations (pre and/or postsynaptic) of the subtypes in discrete brain areas.

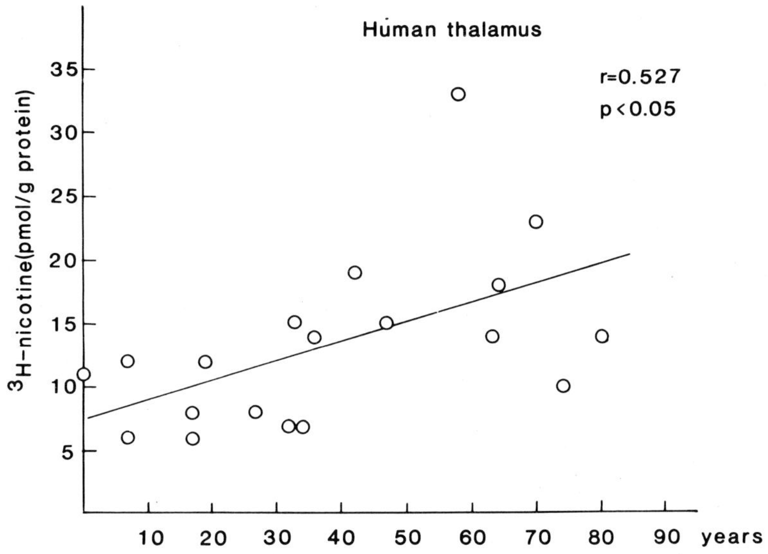

Figure 4. Specific ^{3}H-nicotine (5 nM) (pmol/g protein) binding in human thalamus at normal aging (0-80 years). Each point represents data from one individual.

SUBTYPES OF NICOTINIC RECEPTORS IN DEMENTIA

Recently a decrease in the number of high affinity nicotinic receptors in cortical areas of AD/SDAT brains have been reported independently by three research groups (Whitehouse et al., 1986; Nordberg and Winblad, 1986b; Flynn and Mash, 1986). No change in the affinity of the high affinity nicotinic binding sites was observed (Whitehouse et al., 1986). The reduction in the number of high affinity nicotinic binding sites was consistent with the reduction in both the choline acetyltransferase activity and the in vitro potassium evoked release of ^{3}H-ACh (Nordberg et al., 1987a). This observation might indicate that the high affinity nicotinic receptors are predominantly presynaptically located.

As pointed out earlier in Figure 1, physostigmine (10^{-4}M) enhances the evoked release of ^{3}H-ACh in AD/SDAT cortical tissue to the control level (Nilsson et al., 1986). A similar effect is also obtained with the ACh-esterase inhibitor 9-amino-1,2,3,4-tetrahydroacridine (THA) (data not shown) (Nilsson et al., 1987). Since the effect can be partially blocked in the presence of the nicotinic antagonist tubocurarine (TC) (Fig. 1), nicotinic receptors might influence the ACh release in AD/SDAT brain tissue. We recently observed a 100-fold reduction in the affinity of the low affinity nicotinic binding sites in AD/SDAT cortex (Nordberg et al., 1988). Although physostigmine and THA in AD/SDAT tissue cause an increase in junctional ACh content via ACh-esterase inhibition, this increase in ACh with respect to control tissue might not be sufficient to induce desensitization of the nicotinic receptors. These phenomena, combined with a change (decrease) in the affinity of some of the nicotinic receptors, might explain the mechanism of action of physostigmine and THA in AD/SDAT cortical tissue. However, an additional direct action of these substances on the nicotinic and muscarinic receptors cannot be ruled out and is currently under investigation in our laboratory.

ACKNOWLEDGEMENT

The financial support from the Swedish Medical Research Council, the Swedish Tobacco Company, "Stiftelsen för gamla tjänarinnor" and the Hånell Family, Gävle, Sweden is gratefully acknowledged.

REFERENCES

Adem A (1987) Characterization of muscarinic and nicotinic receptors in neural and non-neural tissue: Changes in Alzheimer's disease. Acta Universitas Upsaliensis 32:4-61.

Adem A, Synnergren B, Botros M, Öhman B, Winblad B, Nordberg A (1987) ^{3}H-acetylcholine nicotinic recognition sites in human brain: characterization of agonist binding. Neurosci Letters 83:298-302.

Adem A, Romanelli L, Sara V, Winblad B, Nordberg A (1988a) Multiple muscarinic receptor subtypes in foetal and adult human brain: comparison of ^{3}H-pirenzepine and ^{3}H-quinuclidinyl benzilate binding. In manuscript.

Adem A, Sing Jossan S, Brandt I, Winblad B, Nordberg A (1988b) Distribution of nicotinic receptors in human thalamus as visualized by ^{3}H-nicotine and ^{3}H-acetylcholine receptor autoradiography. J Neural Transm, in press.

Allen SJ, Benton JS, Goodhart MJ, Haan EA, Sims NR, Smith CCT, Spillane JA, Bowen DM, Davison AN (1983) Biochemical evidence of selective nerve cell changes in the normal ageing human and rat brain. J Neurochem 41:256-265.

Birdsall NJM, Burgen ASV, Hulme EC (1978) The binding of agonists to brain muscarinic receptors. Mol Pharmacol 14:723-736.

Birdsall NJM, Hulme EC, Burgen ASV (1980) The character of the muscarinic receptors in different regions of the rat brain. Proc R Soc Lond Ser B Biol Sci 207:1-12.

Caulfield MP, Straughan DW, Cross AJ, Cron T, Birdsall NJM (1982) Cortical muscarinic receptor subtypes and Alzheimer's disease Lancet 11:1277.

Cortés R, Probst A, Palacios JM (1987) Quantitative light microscopic autoradiographic localization of cholinergic muscarinic receptors in the human brain: forebrain. Neurosci 1:65-107.

Cortés R, Probst A, Tobler HJ, Palacios JM (1986) Muscarinic cholinergic receptor subtypes in the human brain. II. Quantitative autoradiographic studies. Brain Res 362:239-253.

Davies P, Feisullin S (1981) Postmortem stability of α-bungarotoxin binding sites in mouse and human brain. Brain Res 216:449-454.

Davies P, Verth A (1978) Regional distribution of muscarinic acetylcholine receptors in normal and Alzheimer's type dementia brains. Brain Res 138:385-392.

Flynn DD, Mash DC (1986) Characterization of L-(^{3}H) Nicotine binding in human cerebral cortex: comparison between Alzheimer's disease and the normal. J Neurochem 47:1948-1954.

Garvey JM, Rossor M, Iversen LL (1984) Evidence for multiple muscarinic receptor subtypes in human brain. J Neurochem 43:299-302.

Goyal RK, Rattan S (1978) Neurohumoral, hormonal and drug receptors for the lower esophageal sphincter. Gastroenterology 74:598-618.

Gulya K, Watson M, Vickroy TW, Roeske WR, Perry R, Perry E, Duckles SP, Yamamura HI (1986) Examination of cholinergic and neuropeptide receptor alterations in senile dementia of the Alzheimer's type (SDAT). In: Fisher A, Hanin I, Lachman C (eds): Alzheimer's and Parkinson's diseases. Plenum Press, NY, pp. 109-116.

Hammer R, Berrie CP, Birdsall NJM, Burgen ASV, Hulme EC (1980) Pirenzepine distinguishes between different subclasses of muscarinic receptors. Nature 283:90-92.

Hammer R, Giachetti A (1982) Muscarinic receptor subtypes: M1 and M2, biochemical and functional characterization. Life Sci 31:2991-2998.

Hammer R, Giraldo E, Schiari GB, Monferini E, Ladinisky H (1986) Binding profile of a novel cardioselective muscarine receptor antagonist, AF-DX 116, to membranes of peripheral tissues and brain in the rat. Life Sci 38:1653-1662.

Jenni-Eiermann S, von Hahn HP, Honegger CG, Ulrich J (1984) Studies on neurotransmitter binding in senile dementia-comparison of Alzheimer's and mixed vascular-Alzheimer's dementias. Gerontology 30:350-358.

Larsson C (1985) Nicotinic receptors in the central nervous system: Methodological and functional aspects. Acta Universitas Upsaliensis 104:4-45.

London ED, Waller SB (1986) Relationships between choline acetyltransferase and muscarinic binding in aging rodent brain and in Alzheimer brains. In: Hanin I (ed): Dynamic of cholinergic function. Advances in Behavioral Biology, vol 30. Plenum Press, NY, pp. 215-224.

Larsson C, Lundberg P-Å, Halén A, Adem A, Nordberg A (1987) In vitro binding of ^{3}H-acetylcholine to nicotinic receptors in rodent and human brain. J Neural Transm 69:3-18.

Mash DC, Flynn DD, Potter LT (1985) Loss of M2 muscarine receptors in the cerebral cortex in Alzheimer's disease and experimental denervation. Science 228:1115-1117.

Nilsson L, Adem A, Hardy J, Winblad B, Nordberg A (1987) Do tetrahyderaminoacridine (THA) and physostigmine restore acetylcholine release in Alzheimer brains via nicotinic receptors? J Neural Transm 70: 357-368.

Nilsson L, Nordberg A, Hardy J, Wester P, Winblad B (1986) Physostigmine restores ^{3}H-acetylcholine efflux from Alzheimer brain slices to normal level. J Neural Transm 67:275-285.

Nordberg A, Adem A, Hardy J, Winblad B (1988) Changes in nicotinic receptor subtypes in temporal cortex of Alzheimer brains. Neurosci Letters 86:317-321.

Nordberg A, Adem A, Nilsson L, Winblad B (1987a) Cholinergic deficits in CNS and peripheral non-neuronal tissue in Alzheimer dementia. In: Dowdall M, Hawthorne J (eds): Cellular and Molecular Basis of Cholinergic Function. Ellis-Horwood, Chichester, Sussex, pp. 858-868.

Nordberg A, Adolfsson R, Marcusson J, Winblad B (1982) Cholinergic receptors in the hippocampus in normal aging and dementia of Alzheimer type. In: Giacobini E, Filogamo G, Giacobini G, Vernadakis A (eds): The Aging brain: Cellular and Molecular Mechanisms of Aging in the Nervous System. Raven Press, NY, pp. 231-246.

Nordberg A, Alafuzoff I, Winblad B (1986) Muscarinic receptor subtypes in hippocampus in Alzheimer's disease and mixed dementia type. Neurosci Letters 70:160-164.

Nordberg A, Larsson C, Adolfsson R, Alafuzoff I, Winblad B (1983) Muscarinic receptor compensation in hippocampus of Alzheimer patients. J Neural Transm 56:13-19.

Nordberg A, Nyberg P, Adolfsson R, Winblad B (1987b) Cholinergic topography in Alzheimer brains: A comparison with changes in the monoaminergic profile. J Neural Transm 69:19-32.

Nordberg A, Nyberg P, Winblad B (1985) Topographic distribution of choline acetyltransferase activity, muscarinic and nicotinic receptors in Parkinson brains. Neurochem Pathol 3:223-236.

Nordberg A, Winblad B (1981) Cholinergic receptors in human hippocampus-regional distribution and variance with age. Life Sci 29:1937-1944.

Nordberg A, Winblad B (1986a) Brain nicotinic and muscarinic receptors in normal aging and dementia. In: Fisher A, Hanin I, Lachman C (eds): Alzheimer's and Parkinson's disease. Plenum Press, NY, pp. 95-108.

Nordberg A, Winblad B (1986b) Reduced number of ^{3}H-nicotine and ^{3}H-acetylcholine binding sites in the frontal cortex of Alzheimer brains. Neurosci Letters 72:115-119.

Palacios JM, Cortés R, Probst A, Karobath M (1986) Mapping of subtypes of muscarinic receptors in the human brain with receptor autoradiographic techniques. Trends in Neurosci (suppl. 11):56-60.

Perry E (1980) The cholinergic system in old age and Alzheimer's disease. Age and Aging 9:1-8.

Reisine TD, Yamamura HI, Bird ED, Spoke E, Enna E (1978) Pre and postsynaptic neurochemical alterations in Alzheimer's disease. Brain Res 159:477-480.

Rinne JO (1987) Muscarinic and dopaminergic receptors in the aging human brain. Brain Res 404:162-168.

Rinne JO, Laakso K, Lönnberg P, Mölsä P, Paljarvi L, Rinne JK, Säkö E, Rinne UK (1985) Brain muscarinic receptors in senile dementia. Brain Res 336:19-25.

Shimohama S, Taniguchi T, Fujiwara M, Kameyama M (1986) Changes in nicotinic and muscarinic cholinergic receptors in Alzheimer type dementia. J Neurochem 3:288-293.

Undén A, Meyersson B, Winblad B, Sachs C, Bartfai T (1983) Postmortem changes in binding to the muscarinic receptor from human cerebral cortex. J Neurochem 41:102-106.

Volpe BT, Francis A, Gazzaniga MS, Schechter N (1979) Regional concentration of putative nicotinic-cholinergic receptor sites in human brain. Exp Neurol 66:737-744.

White P, Goodhart MJ, Keet J, Hiley CR, Carrasco LH, Williams IEI (1977) Neocortical cholinergic neurons in elderly people. Lancet 1:668-670.

Whitehouse P, Martino AM, Antuono PG, Lowenstein PR, Coyle JT, Price DL, Kellar KJ (1986) Nicotinic acetylcholine binding sites in Alzheimer's disease. Brain Res 371:146-151.

New Trends in Aging Research
G. Pepeu, B. Tomlinson, C.M. Wischik (eds)
Fidia Research Series, vol. 15
Liviana Press, Padova © 1988

D-1 DOPAMINE RECEPTORS IN THE BRAIN AND RETINA OF AGED RATS: EFFECT OF CHRONIC BLOCKADE BY SCH 23390

O. Giorgi, M.L. Porceddu, G. De Montis[1], G. Toffano[2] and G. Biggio

Department of Experimental Biology, Chair of Pharmacology, and
[1]Institute of Biochemical Pharmacology and Pathology,
University of Cagliari; and [2]FIDIA Research Laboratories,
Department of Biochemistry, Abano Terme, Italy

INTRODUCTION

Two subtypes of dopamine (DA) receptors, termed D-1 and D-2, are present in the central nervous system. D-1 receptors increase the activity of adenylate cyclase (AC) upon stimulation, whereas D-2 receptors either decrease or have no effect on cyclic AMP synthesis (Kebabian and Calne, 1979; Stoof and Kebabian, 1981).

Age-related differences in therapeutic dosages and extrapyramidal side effects have been reported for the clinical use of antipsychotic drugs (Ayd, 1961). Since these agents are believed to exert their therapeutic as well as extrapyramidal side effects by blocking DA receptors in the brain, one might expect age-correlated alterations in DA receptor binding activity and function. Indeed, different laboratories have reported age-related decreases in the density of striatal D-2 receptors (Morgan et al., 1984; Norman et al., 1985; O'Boyle and Waddington, 1984b) and in the responsiveness to DA of striatal AC (Govoni et al., 1977; Schmidt and Thornberry, 1978; Giorgi et al., 1987b). Therefore, a concomitant reduction in the density of D-1 receptors can be expected to occur in the striatum of senescent rats. However, contradictory age-related changes in D-1 receptors have been observed in the basal ganglia of different animal species. Thus, D-1 receptors have been reported to increase in the human caudate nucleus and putamen during normal aging (Morgan et al., 1984) and to decrease (Norman et al., 1985) or remain unaltered (O'Boyle and Waddington, 1984b) in the striatum of aged rats. In these studies, antagonist ligands, like ^{3}H-piflutixol and ^{3}H-fluphenazine, which bind with similar affinity to D-2 and D-1 receptors (Billard et al., 1984) were used to label D-1 receptors.

The recent availability of ^{3}H-SCH 23390, the radiolabelled form of the most selective D-1 antagonist known at present (Iorio et al., 1983), prompted us to use this compound as a selective probe to establish if changes in the density and/or affinity of D-1 receptors indeed occur in the striatum, substantia nigra (s. nigra), prefrontal cortex and in the retina of senescent rats. In adult rats, the binding parameters of different neurotransmitter receptors, including D-2 DA receptors and the biological responses induced by their activation, can be modified in response to long term treatment with selective antagonists. Thus, the interruption of striatal DAergic transmission elicited by chronic blockade of DA receptors results in a behavioral supersensitivity to DA receptor agonists and in an enhanced binding of different DA receptor ligands (Burt et al., 1977; Creese et al., 1977; Staunton et al., 1982). In aged rodents, relative deficits in the ability of D-2 receptors to exhibit up-regulation in response to chronic DA receptor antagonist drug treatment have been described (Randall et al., 1981). D-1 receptor up-regulation has been observed in the striatum, s. nigra and retina of adult rats following chronic treatment with the selective antagonist SCH 23390 (Porceddu et al., 1985; Porceddu et al., 1986b; Porceddu et al., 1987a). Here we report aging-related impairments in the ability of D-1 receptors in the rat brain and retina to exhibit up-regulation in response to repeated SCH 23390 administration.

These findings are discussed in terms of previously reported age-related declines in other biochemical parameters of DA receptor function and in relation to the emergence of extrapyramidal side effects with antipsychotic treatment.

METHODS

Animals

Male Sprague-Dawley rats aged 3, 14, 21 and 26 months were provided by the Italian Study Group on Brain Aging. The animals were housed in our animal care facilities under 12 h light-dark cycles (lights on 8.00 a.m. - 8.00 p.m.) at 23 ± 2°C with food and water freely available.

Chronic Treatments

Adult (3-month-old) and aged (21-month-old) rats were treated three times daily (at 8.00 a.m., 4.00 p.m. and 10.00 p.m.) for 12 consecutive days with SCH 23390 (Shering-Plough, USA) at a dose of 0.03 mg/kg, s.c. Control rats were injected with an equal volume of the vehicle (1 ml/kg, s.c.). Three days after the last injection, rats were decapitated and the striata, s. nigrae, prefrontal cortices and retinae were rapidly dissected out and stored at -80°C.

^{3}H-SCH 23390 Binding

Tissues were homogenized in 100 volumes of ice-cold 50 mM Tris-HCl buffer, pH 7.4 and centrifuged for 10 min. at 48,000 × g. The pellet was washed once by resuspension and recentrifugation in 100 volumes of the same buffer. The final pellet was resuspended in 200 volumes of 50 mM Tris-HCl buffer, pH 7.4, containing 120 mM NaCl, 5 mM KCl, 2 mM $CaCl_2$ and 1 mM $MgCl_2$. Binding assays were performed according to Billard et al. (1985) with minor modifications (Giorgi et al., 1987 a). Binding assays in the prefrontal cortex were carried out in the presence of 100 nM ketanserin to prevent the binding of ^{3}H-SCH 23390 to 5 HT_2 receptors. The maximum number of binding sites (Bmax) and the apparent dissociation constant (K_D) were calculated by linear regression analysis of Scatchard plots of specific ^{3}H-SCH 23390 binding isotherms. Protein was measured after Lowry et al. (1951), using bovine serum albumin as a standard.

RESULTS

Distinct changes in D-1 receptors were observed in different neural tissues of senescent rats. An age-related decrease in the density (Bmax) of D-1 receptors was detected in the striatum (-24% and -45% for 21 and 26-month-old rats, respectively) and in the s. nigra (-23%), whereas the affinity (K_D) of D-1 receptors for ^{3}H-SCH 23390 was unchanged in senescent rats (Fig. 1 and Tables 1 and 2).

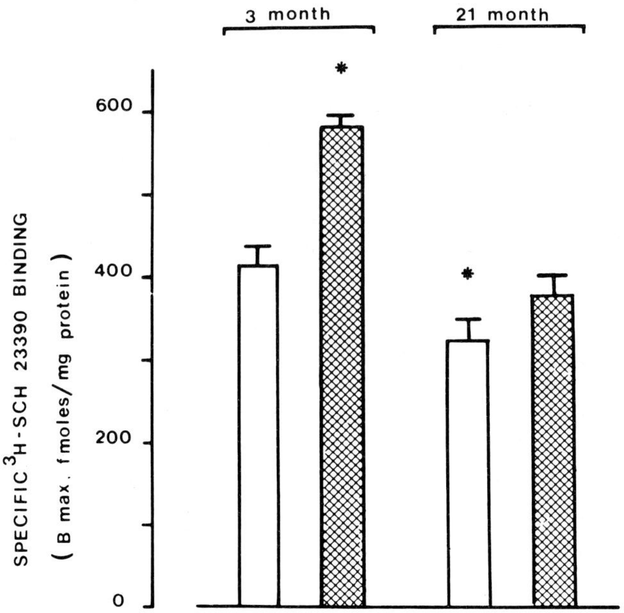

Figure 1. Effect of chronic treatment with SCH 23390 on the density of D-1 DA receptors in the s. nigra of adult and aged rats. Drugs were administered as described in "Methods" and rats were sacrificed 3 days after the last injection. Values are the mean ± S.E.M. of 3 independent experiments each run in triplicate. White columns, solvent; hatched columns, SCH 23390. The apparent dissociation constant (K_D) values (nM) for each experimental group were: 3 month control, 0.36 ± 0.02; 3 month SCH 23390, 0.31 ± 0.04; 21 month control, 0.34 ± 0.05; 21 month SCH 23390, 0.30 ± 0.06. *$p < 0.05$ vs. the 3-month-old control group.

Table 1. *Decrease in the density of ^{3}H-SCH 23390 binding sites in the striatum of senescent rats*

Age (months)	Specifically bound ^{3}H-SCH 23390	
	Bmax (fmoles/mg protein)	K_D (nM)
3	1053 ± 89	0.49 ± 0.09
14	854 ± 31	0.48 ± 0.07
26	573 ± 71*	0.61 ± 0.10

The total number of binding sites (Bmax) and the apparent dissociation constant (K_D) were determined by linear regression analysis of Scatchard plots from ^{3}H-SCH 23390 binding isotherms. Shown are the mean ± S.E.M. of 8 separate experiments, each run in triplicate.
* $p < 0.05$ vs 3-month-old rats (analysis of variance followed by Student's t test).

Table 2. *^{3}H-SCH 23390 binding in the striatum of adult and aged rats chronically treated with SCH 23390*

Experimental group	Specifically bound ^{3}H-SCH 23390	
	Bmax (fmoles/mg protein)	K_D (nM)
3 month, solvent	1081 ± 76	0.57 ± 0.06
3 month, SCH 23390	1490 ± 134*	0.53 ± 0.03
21 month, solvent	820 ± 34*	0.43 ± 0.07
21 month, SCH 23390	890 ± 30*	0.51 ± 0.05

Rats were treated and ^{3}H-SCH 23390 binding assays were carried out as described in "Methods". Shown are the mean ± S.E.M. of five independent experiments, each run in triplicate.
* $p < 0.05$ vs the 3-month-old control group.

In contrast, the density of D-1 receptors was significantly increased in the retina of aged rats (+44%) as compared with 3-month-old controls (Fig. 2), whilst no age-related changes in the density or in the affinity of D-1 receptors were detected in the prefrontal cortex (Table 3).

As previously reported, chronic treatment with SCH 23390 increased the number of ^{3}H-SCH 23390 binding sites in the striatum (+38%) and in the s. nigra (+39%) of adult rats (Porceddu et al., 1985; Porceddu et al., 1986b), but did not alter the Bmax of D-1 receptors in the nigrostriatal system of 21-month-old rats (Table 2 and Fig. 1). The K_D of nigral and striatal D-1 receptors of adult and senescent rats did not change in response to repeated administration of SCH 23390 (Table 2 and Fig. 1). On the other hand, cortical D-1 receptors were not affected by the repeated administration of SCH 23390 to adult and aged rats (Table 3).

Finally, a significant up-regulation of retinal D-1 receptors was induced by chronic treatment with SCH 23390 to adult rats, whereas no significant changes in retinal D-1 receptors were induced by the same treatment in aged rats (Fig. 2).

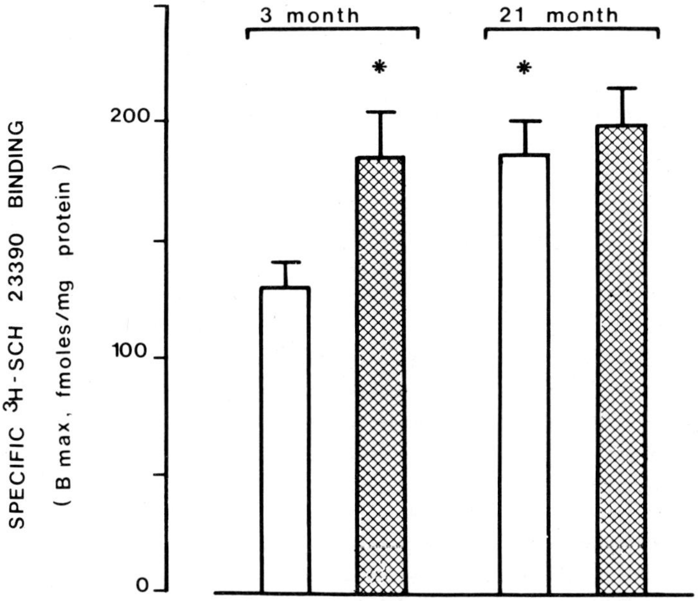

Figure 2. Effect of chronic treatment with SCH 23390 on the density of D-1 DA receptors in the retina of adult and aged rats. SCH 23390 was injected as described in "Methods" and animals were killed 3 days after the last administration. Shown are the mean ± S.E.M. of 3 independent experiments, each run in triplicate. White columns, solvent; hatched columns, SCH 23390. The K_D values (nM) for each group were as follows: 3 month control, 0.46 ± 0.02; 3 month SCH 23390, 0.43 ± 0.04; 21 month control, 0.43 ± 0.02; 21 month SCH 23390, 0.40 ± 0.03. *$p < 0.05$ vs the 3-month-old control group.

Table 3. *D-1 Dopamine receptors in the prefrontal cortex are not affected by age or chronic treatment with SCH 23390*

Experimental group	Specifically bound ³H-SCH 23390	
	Bmax (fmoles/mg protein)	K_D (nM)
3 month, solvent	65 ± 8	0.45 ± 0.04
3 month, SCH 23390	79 ± 5	0.46 ± 0.04
21 month, solvent	69 ± 5	0.53 ± 0.03
21 month, SCH 23390	82 ± 4	0.49 ± 0.05

³H-SCH 23390 binding assays were carried out in the presence of 100 nM ketanserin. Shown are the mean ± S.E.M. of three independent experiments, each run in triplicate.

DISCUSSION

In agreement with previous reports indicating a progressive decline in DA-stimulated AC activity in the striatum of aged rats (Govoni et al., 1977; Schmidt and Thornberry, 1978; Giorgi et al., 1987b) we have shown that striatal D-1 receptors labelled with ^{3}H-SCH 23390 undergo age-related changes. However, contradictory alterations in the density of striatal D-1 receptors have been reported to occur with advancing age. Thus, in line with our results, Norman et al. (1985) observed a decrease in the density of D-1 receptors in the striatum of aged rats. In contrast, it has been reported that D-1 receptors labelled with ^{3}H-piflutixol are unchanged in the striatum of senescent rats (O'Boyle and Waddington, 1984b). Since the Hill coefficient for displacement of ^{3}H-piflutixol by SCH 23390 is less than unity (O'Boyle and Waddington, 1984a), whereas the Hill coefficient for displacement of ^{3}H-SCH 23390 by various DA receptor antagonists is indistinguishable from unity (Hess et al., 1986), the results of binding studies using ^{3}H-SCH 23390 or ^{3}H-piflutixol are not necessarily equivalent.

The large increment in the density of D-1 receptors observed in the caudate nucleus and putamen of the aging human brain (Morgan et al., 1984) indicates that these receptors may undergo opposite changes in different animal species, although the cause of this species-related difference is still unclear.

In rodents, the loss of striatal DA-sensitive AC and ^{3}H-SCH 23390 binding sites precedes by 6 to 12 months smaller reductions of DA levels and turnover (Finch et al., 1981; Giorgi et al., 1987b). Therefore, the striatal D-1 receptors lost with age are probably not located on the nerve endings of nigrostriatal DAergic fibers. Accordingly, striatal lesions induced by the neurotoxins kainic acid or quisqualic acid induce a nearly complete loss of DA-stimulated AC activity (Schwarcz et al., 1978) and D-1 receptors in this brain area (Porceddu et al., 1986a; Altar et al., 1987), indicating that striatal D-1 receptors lost with age are predominantly located on the cell bodies of intrinsic neurons.

Our finding that the density of ^{3}H-SCH 23390 binding sites is reduced in the s. nigra of senescent rats is in line with a previous report on the age-related decrease in nigral DA-stimulated AC activity (Govoni et al., 1977). It is unclear at present whether nigral D-1 receptors lost with age are located on cell bodies or on nerve endings. In fact, there is experimental evidence that a major fraction of nigral D-1 receptors is located on the nerve endings of striatonigral afferent fibers (Spano et al., 1977; Porceddu et al., 1986b), whereas a smaller fraction is located on the cell bodies of DAergic nigrostriatal neurons (Savasta et al., 1986; Porceddu et al., 1987b).

The loss of D-1 receptors in the nigrostriatal system of aged rats may be relevant in view of the recently evidenced behavioral effects mediated by these receptors. Thus, it has been shown that the selective stimulation of D-1 receptors elicits rotation in rats with 6-OH-DA induced unilateral lesions of the nigrostriatal DAergic pathway (Arnt and Hyttel, 1984). In addition, certain forms of stereotypy and grooming are mediated by D-1 receptors (Molloy and Waddington, 1984; Molloy and Waddington, 1985). Hence, it is tempting to speculate that neuronal systems dependent on D-1 receptor mediated mechanisms become dysfunctional below a critical extent of receptor loss with age, thereby contributing to some of the alterations in DAergic functions observed in aged rodents (Finch et al., 1981; Randall et al., 1981).

It is well known that the biochemical properties of neurotransmitter receptors may be altered by chronic blockade with selective antagonists. Accordingly, the repeated administration of SCH 23390 to adult rats induces a significant increase in the Bmax of striatal, nigral and retinal D-1 receptors (Porceddu et al., 1985; Porceddu et al., 1986b; Porceddu et al., 1987a). Our data suggest that in old rats the up-regulation of D-1 DA receptors in response to long term treatment with SCH 23390 is impaired, although age-related alterations in the threshold for supersensitivity cannot be ruled out. It is worth noting that at the dose used in the chronic treatment experiments (0.03 mg/kg, s.c.), SCH 23390 can prevent the stereotyped behavior induced by apomorphine in adult and aged rats (not shown), indicating that metabolic or pharmacokinetic factors are not involved in the lack of D-1 receptor up-regulation following chronic neuroleptic blockade in aged rats.

The development of DA receptor supersensitivity after chronic blockade in adult rats does not seem to be a generalized phenomenon, since D-1 receptors in the prefrontal cortex were not affected by drug treatment.

Long-term treatment with neuroleptic agents results in tolerance to the increase in DA turnover and activation of tyrosine hydroxylase observed after a single injection of these drugs in the striatum (Lerner and Nosè, 1977). In contrast, tolerance does not develop to the increase in DA synthesis and turnover induced by a single dose of neuroleptics in cortical areas (Scatton et al., 1976). This lack of tolerance to the increased DA turnover in cortical regions may be related to both, the lack of receptor up-regulation after long-term treatment with neuroleptics and the antipsychotic effects of these agents. Taken together, these results suggest that the neurochemical adaptation to the chronic effects of selective DA receptor antagonists is differentially regulated in nigrostriatal and mesocortical DAergic pathways. This differential regulation may play a role in the therapeutic and extrapyramidal side effects of antipsychotic drugs. Thus, during chronic administration of neuroleptics in man, extrapyramidal side-effects show a tendency to diminish (Hollister, 1972) whilst tolerance to the antipsychotic effects of these agents is not observed (Levine et al., 1980). Moreover, our findings are in line with clinical observations that older patients exhibit a higher tendency to develop extrapyramidal side-effects (Ayd, 1961). These observations suggest that aging reduces the capacity for functional adaptation of central DAergic mechanisms.

It is now well established that light exposure enhances, whereas dark exposure inhibits, the activity of retinal DAergic neurons (Iuvone et al., 1978). Moreover, retinal D-1 receptors undergo rapid plastic adaptations in response to physiological changes in the activity of DAergic neurons. In fact, D-1 receptors are decreased in the retina of light-exposed rats (Porceddu et al., 1987a). Hence, it may be speculated that the increased density of D-1 receptors in the retina of senescent rats may result from a decreased activation of DAergic neurons in response to light exposure. It should be pointed out, however, that light exposure activates to the same extent retinal DAergic neurons of adult and aged rats as reflected by the increase in DOPAC content and in the DOPAC/DA ratio (not shown). Therefore, the age related increase in the density of retinal D-1 receptors probably results from postsynaptic rather than presynaptic mechanisms.

Finally, the neurochemical adaptation of retinal DA receptors is altered by aging, as indicated by our finding that chronic treatment with SCH 23390 increases the density of

D-1 receptors of adult rats by 43%, but does not alter the Bmax of ^{3}H-SCH 23390 binding sites in the retina of aged rats.

REFERENCES

Altar CA, Marien MR (1987) Picomolar affinity of ^{125}I-SCH 23982 for D-1 receptors in brain demonstrated with digital substraction autoradiography. J of Neurosci 7:213-222.

Arnt J, Hyttel J (1984) Differential inhibition by dopamine D-1 and D-2 antagonists of circling behaviour induced by dopamine agonists in rats with unilateral 6-hydroxydopamine lesions. Eur J Pharmacol 102:349-354.

Ayd FJ (1961) A survey of drug induced extrapyramidal reactions. JAMA 175:1054-1060.

Billard W, Ruperto V, Crosby G, Iorio LC, Barnett A (1984) Characterization of the binding of ^{3}H-SCH 23390, a selective D-1 receptor antagonist ligand, in rat striatum. Life Sci 35: 1885-1893.

Burt DR, Creese I, Snyder SH (1977) Antischizophrenic drugs: chronic treatment elevates dopamine receptor binding in brain. Science 196:326-328.

Creese I, Burt DR, Snyder SH (1977) Dopamine receptor binding enhancement accompanies lesion-induced behavioral supersensitivity. Science 197:596-598.

Finch CE, Marshall JF, Randall PK (1981) Aging and basal ganglia functions. Ann Rev Gerontol Geriatr 2:49-87.

Giorgi O, Calderini G, Toffano G, Biggio G (1987a) D-1 dopamine receptors labelled with ^{3}H-SCH 23390: decrease in the striatum of aged rats. Neurobiology of Aging 8:51-54.

Giorgi O, De Montis G, Porceddu ML, Mele S, Biggio G (1987b) Developmental and age-related changes in D-1 dopamine receptors and dopamine content in the rat striatum. Dev Brain Res 35:283-290.

Govoni S, Loddo P, Spano PF, Trabucchi M (1977) Dopamine receptor sensitivity in brain and retina of rats during aging. Brain Res 138:565-570.

Hess EJ, Battaglia G, Norman AB, Iorio LC, Creese I (1986) Guanine nucleotide regulations of agonist interactions at ^{3}H-SCH 23390-labelled D-1 dopamine receptors in rat striatum. Eur J Pharmacol 121:31-38.

Hollister LE (1972) Mental disorders-antipsychotic and antimanic drugs. New England Journal of Medicine 286:984-987.

Iorio LC, Barnett A, Leitz FH, Houser VP, Korduba CA (1983) SCH 23390, a potential benzazepine antipsychotic with unique interactions on dopaminergic systems. J Pharm Exp Ther 226:462-468.

Iuvone PM, Galli CL, Garrison-Gund CK, Neff NH (1978) Light stimulates tyrosine hydroxylase activity and dopamine synthesis in retinal amacrine neurons. Science 202:901-902.

Kebabian JW, Calne DB (1979) Multiple receptors for dopamine. Nature (London) 277:93-96.

Lerner P, Nosè P (1977) Haloperidol: effect of long-term treatment on rat striatal dopamine synthesis and turnover. Science 197:181-183.

Levine I, Schooler NR, Severe J, Escobar J, Gelenberg A, Mandel M, Sovner R, Steinbook R (1980) Discontinuation of oral and depot fluphenazine in schizophrenic patients after one year of continuous medication: a controlled study. In: Cattabeni F, Racagni G, Spano PF, Costa E (eds): Long-term effects of neuroleptics. Adv Biochem Pharmacol, Vol. 24, pp. 483-493.

Lowry OH, Rosebrough NJ, Farr AL, Randall RJ (1951) Protein measurement with the Folin phenol reagent. J Biol Chem 193:265-275.

Molloy AG, Waddington JL (1984) Dopaminergic behaviour stereospecifically promoted by the D-1 agonist R-SKF 38393 and selectively blocked by the D-1 antagonist SCH 23390. Psychopharmacology 82:409-410.

Molloy AG, Waddington JL (1985) Sniffing, rearing and locomotor responses to the D-1 dopamine agonist R-SKF 38393 and to apomorphine: differential interactions with the selective D-1 and D-2 antagonists SCH 23390 and metoclopramide. Eur J Pharmacol 108:305-308.

Morgan DC, Marcusson JD, Winblad B, Finch CE (1984) Reciprocal changes in D_1 and D_2 dopamine binding sites in human caudate nucleus and putamen during normal aging, ^{3}H-fluphenazine as a dopamine receptor ligand. Soc Neurosci Abstr 10:445.

Norman AB, Battaglia G, Creese I (1985) Differential recovery rates of D-1 and D-2 dopamine receptors in rat striatum as a function of aging and chronic drug treatments. Soc Neurosci Abstr 11:456.

O'Boyle KM, Waddington JL (1984a) Selective and stereospecific interactions of R-SK&F 38393 with ^{3}H-piflutixol but not ^{3}H-spipirone binding to striatal D-1 and D-2 dopamine receptors: comparison with SCH 23390. Eur J Pharmacol 98:433-436.

O'Boyle KM, Waddington JL (1984b) Loss of rat striatal dopamine receptors with aging is selective for D-2 but not D-1 sites: association with increased non-specific binding in the D-1 ligand ^{3}H-piflutixol. Eur J Pharmacol 105:171-174.

Porceddu ML, Ongini E, Biggio G (1985) ^{3}H-SCH 23390 binding sites increase after chronic blockade of D-1 dopamine receptors. Eur J Pharmacol 118:367-370.

Porceddu ML, Ongini E, Biggio G (1986a) ^{3}H-SCH 23390 binding in striatum and substantia nigra: localization and functional changes. In: Biggio G, Spano PF, Toffano G, Gessa GL (eds): Modulation of Central and Peripheral Transmitter Function. Springer, Berlin, pp. 473-480.

Porceddu ML, Giorgi O, Ongini E, Mele S, Biggio G (1986b) ^{3}H-SCH 23390 binding sites in the rat substantia nigra: evidence for a presynaptic localization and innervation by dopamine. Life Sci 39:321-328.

Porceddu ML, De Montis G, Mele S, Ongini E, Biggio G (1987a) D-1 dopamine receptors in the rat retina: effect of dark adaptation and chronic blockade by SCH 23390. Brain Res 424:264-271.

Porceddu ML, Giorgi O, De Montis G, Mele S, Cocco L, Ongini E, Biggio G (1987b) 6-hydroxydopamine-induced degeneration of nigral dopamine neurons: differential effect on nigral and striatal D-1 dopamine receptors. Life Sci 41:697-706.

Randall PK, Severson JA, Finch CE (1981) Aging and the regulation of striatal dopaminergic mechanisms in mice. J Pharmacol Exp Ther 219:695-700.

Savasta M, Dubois A, Benavides J, Scatton B (1986) Different neuronal location of ^{3}H-SCH 23390 binding sites in pars reticulata and pars compacta of the substantia nigra in the rat. Neurosci Lett 72:265-271.

Scatton B, Glowinski J, Julou L (1976) Dopamine metabolism in the mesolimbic and mesocortical dopaminergic systems after single or repeated administrations of neuroleptics. Brain Res 109:184-189.

Schmidt MJ, Thornberry JF (1978) Cyclic AMP and cyclic GMP accumulation in vitro in brain regions of young, old and aged rats. Brain Res 139:169-177.

Schwarcz R, Creese I, Coyle JT, Snyder SH (1978) Dopamine receptors localized on cerebral cortical afferents to rat corpus striatum. Nature (London) 271:766-768.

Spano PF, Trabucchi M, Di Chiara G (1977) Localization of nigral dopamine-sensitive adenylate cyclase on neurons originating from corpus striatum. Science 196:1343-1345.

Staunton DA, Magistretti PJ, Koob GF, Shoemaker WJ, Bloom FE (1982) Dopaminergic supersensitivity induced by denervation and chronic receptor blockade is additive. Nature 299:72-74.

Stoof JC, Kebabian JW (1981) Opposing roles for D-1 and D-2 dopamine receptors on efflux of cyclic AMP from rat neostriatum. Nature (London) 294:366-368.

New Trends in Aging Research
G. Pepeu, B. Tomlinson, C.M. Wischik (eds)
Fidia Research Series, vol. 15
Liviana Press, Padova © 1988

DELAYED POSTISCHEMIC ENERGY FAILURE IN BRAIN CORTEX OF AGED RATS

Siegfried Hoyer

Department of Pathochemistry and General Neurochemistry
University of Heidelberg, FRG

INTRODUCTION

In the year 2000 people aged 60 years and over will account for about 10% of the world's population. This is due to increased life expectancy (WHO, 1972). The proportion of aged individuals in relation to the total population has increased mainly because mortality has decreased (Rosenwaike et al., 1980).

The most common brain disorders in the middle-aged and the elderly are degenerative brain disorders, such as Alzheimer's and Parkinson's diseases (Price et al., 1986), and ischemic tissue damage following to cessation of blood flow and critically low hypoperfusion which respectively cause long lasting psychological and/or neurological deficits. Concerning ischemia, age was found to be one of the most important risk factors for brain infarction and mortality from it (Fuller et al., 1983; Hubert et al., 1983).

Smooth working of the mind depends on both a sufficient supply of substrates to, and the availability of energy rich compounds in the brain, the latter being fundamental to, for example, cell integrity, maintainance of ion homeostasis, information transmission and transportation processes (Siesjö, 1984).

Abbreviations: cci, complete cerebral ischemia; MABP, mean arterial blood pressure; Hb, hemoglobin; Hc, hematocrit; spr, spontaneous recovery; Glu, glucose; Lact, lactate; TCAC, tricarbocylic acid cycle; ATP, adenosine triphosphate; ADP, adenosine diphosphate; AMP, adenosine monophosphate; CrP, creatine phosphate; AN, adenine nucleotide; ECP, energy charge potential; C-skel, carbon skeleton; SEM, standard error of mean.

The aim of the present study was to evaluate the effect of ischemia-induced lesions on glucose and energy metabolism in the brain cortex of aged rats, and to investigate the way in which ischemic metabolic abnormalities recover.

MATERIAL AND METHODS

The study was carried out on 2-year-old male Wistar rats. In general, rats may be considered aged when their strain has a 50% survival rate and when their survival curve is more or less rectangular. In particular, in male Wistar rats, this deflection point was found to occur at the age of 24 months (Hollander et al., 1983).

Complete cerebral ischemia (cci) of 15-minute duration was induced by four-vessel occlusion and hypovolemic hypotension of 30 to 40 mmHg mean arterial blood pressure (MABP). A more detailed account of the operative procedure and the biochemical analysis of brain tissue are reported elsewhere (Hoyer and Krier, 1986). In the fronto-parieto-temporal brain cortex, the concentrations of glucose, lactate, adenine nucleotides and creatine phosphate were determined and the sum of carbon skeletons of tricarboxylic acid cycle (TCAC) intermediates was calculated during cci and in the recovery period of 60 minutes, 24, 48, 72 and 96 hours, respectively.

RESULTS

In arterial blood, a 15 min cci produced a significant increase in glucose concentration; it was still elevated after a 60-min recirculation, returning to normal ranges at 24 h recirculation until the end of the experiment. Likewise, there was a significant increase in the lactate concentration during the 15 min cci; this slowly decreased during recirculation showing abnormally high values until 72 h after the ischemic insult. Further changes were found in the hemoglobin and hematocrit concentrations, both were reduced after 24 h recirculation to the end of the experiment (Table 1).

In the fronto-parieto-temporal brain cortex, the concentrations of glucose, the sum of C-skeletons in TCAC, ATP, the sum of adenine nucleotides, energy charge potential and creatine phosphate dropped significantly whereas lactate, ADP and AMP increased significantly during ischemia. The results are shown in Table 2.

After 60-min recirculation, glucose and the sum of C-skeletons of TCAC intermediates were found to be higher than those observed in control conditions. Both these parameters changed along with ATP, creatine phosphate, the sum of adenine nucleotides, and energy charge potential (high), and lactate (low), as compared to the ischemic period.

After 24 h recirculation, ATP, creatine phosphate, the sum of adenine nucleotides, and energy charge potential were elevated and the sum of C-skeletons of TCAC compounds was reduced with respect to control values. Values for glucose and the sum of C-skeletons (lower), ATP and the sum of adenine nucleotides (higher) were different from those found in the previous investigation using a 60-minute recirculation period.

Table 1. *Steady state parameters*

	MABP	$paCO_2$	paO_2	pH	t	Hb	Hc	Glu	Lact
			mmHg		°C	g/100ml	%	mmol/l	
C	107±7	38±8	159±37	7.44±0.04	37.1±0.2	13.8±1.2	38.3±2.4	7.33±0.85	0.707±0.201
15'cci	37±5 a	37±4	152±35	7.40±0.03	37.1±0.2	12.5±1.4	35.2±5.9	13.51±2.93 a	4.052±1.326 a
15'cci+ 60'spr	105±5	39±3	170±43	7.42±0.05	37.2±0.1	12.5±1.6	35.4±4.3	10.63±3.74 a	2.024±1.015 a
15'cci 24h spr	101±5	39±3	163±27	7.41±0.04	37.2±0.1	10.5±1.7 a	28.8±6.6 a	5.74±1.93	1.525±0.888 a
15'cci+ 48h spr	103±6	39±3	164±29	7.42±0.05	37.2±0.1	10.5±2.1 a	29.8±5.3 a	6.20±2.13	1.912±1.028 a
15'cci+ 72h spr	107±5	39±3	153±20	7.39±0.03	37.0±0.1	11.7±2.8 a	32.4±4.6 a	6.40±1.31	1.407±0.920 a
15'cci+ 96h spr	105±6	39±2	137±28	7.41±0.04	37.0±0.1	11.9±1.5 a	33.2±4.6 a	6.70±1.34	1.059±0.852

Mean values and standard deviations in the steady state parameters mean arterial blood flow (MBAP), pa CO_2, pa 0_2, pH and body temperature t, and of the arterial blood constituents hemoglobin, hematocrit, glucose and lactate under control conditions (C), during a 15 min cci, and during recirculation. a: statistically significantly different from C; $2\alpha \leq 0.05$.

Table 2. *Metabolite concentrations in brain cortex*

	C	15'cci	15'cci +60'spr	15'cci +24h spr	15'cci +48h spr	15'cci +72 spr	15'cci +96h spr
Glu	2.01± 0.11	0.284± 0.037 a	5.03± 0.55 a b	2.29± 0.36 b	2.50± 0.31	3.45± 0.21 a b c	3.21± 0.13 a
Lact	1.39± 0.11	23.97± 1.51 a	1.82± 0.022 b	1.36± 0.19	1.69± 0.13	1.84± 0.08 a	1.60± 0.07
ΣC-Skel	0.355± 0.009	0.293± 0.007 a	0.397± 0.008 a b	0.328± 0.006 a b	0.452± 0.008 a b	0.473± 0.013 a c	0.343± 0.008 b
ATP	2.31± 0.03	0.216± 0.040 a	2.24± 0.06 b	2.56± 0.06 a b	2.05± 0.11 a b	2.09± 0.07 a c	2.31± 0.07 c
ADP	0.258± 0.007	0.406± 0.028 a	0.240± 0.010	0.248± 0.008	0.285± 0.032	0.315± 0.008 a c	0.236± 0.088
AMP	0.038± 0.002	1.168± 0.096 a	0.041± 0.005	0.034± 0.005	0.105± 0.027 a b	0.054± 0.004	0.043± 0.005
CrP	3.41± 0.09	0.519± 0.047 a	3.61± 0.17 b	3.80± 0.06 a	3.23± 0.12 b	3.54± 0.11	3.80± 0.07 a
ΣAN	2.609± 0.033	1.732± 0.120 a	2.518± 0.056 b	2.840± 0.062 a b	2.437± 0.099 b	2.459± 0.073 c	2.584± 0.071 c
ECP	0.936± 0.001	0.252± 0.034 a	0.929± 0.005 b	0.944± 0.003 a	0.897± 0.017 a b	0.914± 0.009 a c	0.937± 0.002 b

Mean values and standard error of means in mol/g wet weight of concentrations of glucose, lactate, sum of C-skeletons in tricarboxylic acid cycle, adenosinphosphates, creatine phosphate, sum of adenine nucleotides, and energy charge potential in brain cortex of 2yr-old rats under control conditions (C), during a 15 min cci, and during different recirculation times.
a: $2\alpha \leq 0.05$ vs C; b: $2\alpha \leq 0.05$ vs preceding investigation; c: $2\alpha \leq 0.05$ 72 h spr and 96 h spr, respectively, vs 24 h spr.

After 48 h recirculation, ATP and energy charge potential were lower than, and the sum of C-skeletons of TCAC metabolites and AMP were higher than those of the controls. ATP, creatine phospate and the sum of adenine nucleotides were reduced, the sum of C-skeletons and AMP were increased with respect to values found in the previous investigation using a 24-h recirculation period.

After 72 h recirculation, the concentrations of glucose, lactate, the sum of C-skeletons of TCAC intermediates and ADP had increased, and the ATP and energy charge potential were lower than those of controls. Glucose values were higher than those found in the previous investigation at 48-h recirculation. The differences to the 24-h recirculation investigation became evident in the glucose concentration, the sum of C-skeletons, ADP (higher), ATP, and the sum of adenine nucleotides and the energy charge potential (lower).

After 96 h recirculation, glucose and creatine phosphate values were higher than those observed in control conditions. The energy charge potential was higher than that observed in the prior 72 h recirculation period, whereas the sum of C-skeletons of TCAC metabolites was lower. The ATP and the sum of adenine nucleotides in the 96-h recirculation period are lower than those observed in the 24-h recirculation.

DISCUSSION

In arterial blood, the stress-induced increase in glucose rapidly normalized in the postischemic recovery period. On the other hand, lactate levels dropped much slower and remained elevated throughout the experimental period. From the other steady state parameters, the decreases in both hemoglobin and hematocrit are remarkable if a comparison is made with the values obtained in control conditions. They were most varied at 24 h recirculation and showed steady improvements towards the end of the experiment. A slight increase in cerebral blood flow but no changes in cerebral oxygen consumption may be expected at a hemoglobin concentration of 10 g/100 ml as has been demonstrated in normovolemic anemia (Borgström et al., 1975). Thus, the changes in tissue metabolism may not have been influenced by these blood constituents.

The main biochemical event in ischemia is the cessation of oxidative and energy producing processes. As a consequence, creatine phospate and ATP concentrations decrease whereas ADP and AMP increase as an expression of energy utilization. There is a reduction in the amounts of oxidizable substrates in TCA cycle, of adenine nucleotides and energy charge potential. These findings, reported repeatedly (Ljunggren et al. 1974; Siesjö and Wieloch, 1985) were found to be aggravated by age (Hoyer and Krier, 1986).

In the early recirculation period, the energy pool is restored more or less rapidly depending on the severity of the ischemic event (Kobayashi et al., 1977; Ljunggren et al., 1974; Mrsulja et al., 1976; Siesjö and Wieloch, 1985). This recovery period until 24 hours after ischemia was also characterized by hypermetabolic events including increased glucose concentration and increased availability of oxidizable substrates in TCAC, which are indeed used for energy formation.

Information on recovery of the energy pool for recirculation periods for 24 hours, or even longer, is, however, scarce (Arai et al., 1982; Pulsinelli and Duffy, 1983). Pulsinelli and Duffy (1983) found CrP to be increased in the paramedian neocortex 24 and 48 hours after a 30 min forebrain ischemia. 72 hours later, it was not different from that of the controls; this was also the case for ATP concentration except for a decrease at 72 h recirculation. Likewise, in this study a significant increase of creatine phosphate was observed at 24 h recirculation, but at 48 and 72 hours the values were the same as those of the controls.

The most remarkable abnormality in this study was found 48 and 72 hours after recirculation. At this recovery period, ATP and the energy charge potential diminished although the concentrations of oxidizable substrates such as glucose and C-skeletons of the TCA cycle intermediates increased. Of course, the delayed post-ischemic energy failure cannot be compromised by the increased availability of the substrates ready for energy production. Since the utilization of ATP was found to be elevated during the same period as was measured in the increased concentrations of ADP and AMP, it may be assumed that there was a metabolic abnormality in the ATP-producing pathway. It remains obscure as to which mechanism(s) cause(s) this transient abnormality. It may be speculated that the deficit in biologically available energy may produce further perturbation of cell homeostasis and therefore function. Normalization of the changes in substrate oxidation was observed after 96 hours of recovery from ischemia. It would be of further interest to study the repair mechanism underlying this improvement.

SUMMARY

In this study, the effect of a 15-minute complete cerebral ischemia (cci) on glucose metabolism and energy production in fronto-parieto-temporal brain cortex was investigated in 2-year-old rats during cci and in recovery periods of 60 min, 24 h, 48 h, 72 h and 96 h, respectively.

During ischemia, the concentrations of glucose, ATP, creatine phosphate, the sum of C-skeletons and of adenine nucleotides and energy charge potential dropped significantly whereas lactate ADP and AMP increased significantly. In the early recirculation period until 24 h, energy metabolism was rapidly restored. This recovery period was characterized by hypermetabolism including glycolysis, oxidation and energy production. The ATP and energy charge potential diminished after 48 h of recirculation and this change was more pronounced after 72 h, although the concentrations of oxidizable substrates such as glucose and the tricarboxylic acid cycle compounds as measured as C-skeletons increased. After a recirculation of 96 h, energy metabolism normalized again. A delayed postischemic damage in intermediate metabolism at 48 h and 72 h recirculation may cause the abnormality in energy metabolism, which is assumed to be responsible for further perturbation of cell homeostasis.

REFERENCES

Arai H, Lust WD, Passonneau JV (1982) Delayed metabolic changes induced by 5 min of ischemia in gerbil brain. Trans Am Soc Neurochem Abst 13: 177.

Borgström L, Johannsson H, Siesjö BK (1975) The influence of acute normovolemic anemia on cerebral blood flow and oxygen consumption of anaesthetized rats. Acta Physiol Scand 93: 505-514.

Fuller JH, Shipley MJ, Rose G, Jarrett RJ, Keen H (1983) Mortality from coronary heart disease and stroke in relation to degree of glycaemia: the Whitehall study. Br Med J 2: 867-870.

Hollander CF, van Zwieten MJ, Zurcher C (1983) The aged animal. In: Gispen WH, Traber J (eds): Aging of the brain. Elsevier, Amsterdam, pp 187-196.

Hoyer S, Krier C (1986) Ischemia and the aging brain. Studies on glucose and energy metabolism in rat cerebral cortex. Neurobiol Aging 7: 23-29.

Hubert HB, Feinleib M, Mc Namara PM, Castelli WP (1983) Obesity as an independent risk factor for cardiovascular disease: a 26-year follow-up of participants in the Framingham heart study. Circulation 67: 968-977.

Kobayashi M, Lust WD, Passonneau JV (1977) Concentrations of energy metabolites and cyclic

nucleotides during and after bilateral ischemia in the gerbil cerebral cortex. J Neurochem 29: 53-59.
Ljunggren B, Ratcheson RA, Siesjö BK (1974) Cerebral metabolic state following complete compression ischemia. Brain Res 73: 291-307.
Mrsulja BB, Lust WD, Mrsulja BJ, Passonneau JV, Klatzo I (1976) Post-ischemic changes in certain metabolites following prolonged ischemia in the gerbil cortex. J Neurochem 26: 1099-1103.
Price DL, Whitehouse PJ, Struble RG (1986) Cellular pathology in Alzheimer's and Parkinson's diseases. TINS 9: 29-33.
Pulsinelli WA, Duffy TE (1983) Regional energy balance in rat brain after transient forebrain ischemia. J Neurochem 40: 1500-1503.
Rosenwaike I, Yaffe N, Sagi PC (1980) The recent decline in mortality of the extreme aged: an analysis of statistical data. Am J Public Health 70: 1074-1080.
Siesjö BK (1984) Cerebral circulation and metabolism. J Neurosurg 60: 883-908.
Siesjö BK, Wieloch T (1985) Cerebral metabolism in ischaemia: neurochemical basis for therapy. Br J Anaesth 57: 47-62.
World Health Organization (1972) Psychogeriatrics. Report of a WHO scientific group. Technical Report, Series No 507. Geneva.

Section II

NEUROENDOCRINOLOGY AND BEHAVIOUR

New Trends in Aging Research
G. Pepeu, B. Tomlinson, C.M. Wischik (eds)
Fidia Research Series, vol. 15
Liviana Press, Padova © 1988

NEURAL CONTROL OF GROWTH HORMONE SECRETION IN AGED ANIMALS

E.E. Müller, S.G. Cella, L. Lima, M. Parenti, and D. Cocchi

Department of Pharmacology, Chemotherapy and Toxicology,
University of Milan, Via Vanvitelli 32, 20129 Milano, Italy

Several mechanisms have been proposed as causes of geriatric changes in structure and function: the irreversible effect of age, acting through cumulative unrepaired errors in DNA, loss of mitotic potential, loss of fidelity in protein synthesis, damage by free radicals, the cumulative effect of disease processes, the effects of physical inactivity or disease, and, in elderly women, the menopause. In 1985 Rudman proposed another mechanism for geriatric regression, a mechanism present in about half of the aged: the cessation of endogenous growth hormone (GH) secretion.

Rudman showed that there were some similarities between the alterations in structure and function occurring with advancing age and those occurring in GH-deficient patients. Both conditions are characterized by shrinkage of lean body mass, expansion of adipose mass, diminution in renal functions and decrease in the rate of cell division.

Moreover, both kinds of subjects exhibit a reduction in bone mass and density, dental deficits and a decrease in calcium absorption. Consistent with this proposition, one third of a large group of old subjects (55-80 yrs) evaluated by the same author (Rudman, 1985) presented very low levels of somatomedin C (Sm-C), the GH-related peptide that mediates most of the biological effects of GH (Van Wyk, 1984).

As defective GH secretion may be one of the pacemakers of aging, it is important to have an insight into the mechanisms underlying the reduced GH secretion in aged humans and animals (Rudman et al., 1981; Shibasaki et al., 1984; Meites, 1986), as this should allow us to pharmacologically counteract this age-related phenomenon.

Abbreviations: GH, growth hormone; GHRH, somatocrinin; GRF, growth hormone releasing factor; SmC, somatomedin C.

AGED RODENTS

As in humans, GH responses to different secretagogues are blunted in aged rats (Sonntag et al., 1980; 1981; Cocchi et al., 1986). In aged male and female rats, the GH pulsatile release is reduced (Sonntag et al., 1980; Takahashi et al., 1987), and the central nervous system or pituitary-operated stimuli evoke a significantly lower GH response than in young male and female rats (Sonntag et al., 1981; Cocchi et al., 1986). Parallel to the *in vivo* findings, an impaired responsiveness to somatocrinin (GHRH) is evident in pituitary somatotropes from aged (20-24 mos) and middle-aged (14 mos) male and female rats (Takahara et al., 1984; Cocchi et al., 1986). The reduced *in vitro* GH secretion after GHRH is linked with a diminished GHRH-induced stimulation of adenylate cyclase, the main intracellular transducing mechanism of the peptide signal in pituitary membranes from aged male and female rats. In addition, the basal adenylate cyclase in the pituitary membranes of aged rats is significantly higher than in young male, but not female, rats (Cocchi et al., 1986; Parenti et al., 1987).

A defective responsiveness of pituitary somatotrophs to GHRH may bring about a reduction in the intracellular content, a constant feature in aged rats (Cocchi et al., 1986; Meites, 1986; Takahashi et al., 1987). As GHRH can induce not only GH release but also synthesis (Gick et al., 1984) and prime the somatotrophs, at least in some circumstances (Borges et al., 1984; Janson et al., 1985), the diminished pituitary GH content and the reduced response to GHRH in aged rats may be due to a defective hypothalamic release of the neurohormone.

Studies using the GH bioassay as an end-point showed that GRF-activity was lower in the hypothalamus of aged than young rats (Pecile et al., 1965) and more recent studies have demonstrated that the hypothalami of aged rats release less GHRH *in vitro* than the hypothalami of younger counterparts (Ono et al., 1985).

We therefore thought it would be of interest to investigate the effect of a GHRH replacement regimen on the GHRH-induced adenylate cyclase activation in aged male and female rats (14 mos) and compare it to the pattern elicited by the same treatment in young rats (2 mos). In old male rats, short-term *ex vivo* treatment with a high GHRH dose (5 μg/rat/die for 3 days) reduced the high basal adenylate cyclase activity to values similar to those of young rats and caused a downward parallel shift of the GHRH dose-response curve (Parenti et al., 1987). Treatment of young male rats with the same GHRH schedule left basal adenylate cyclase activity unchanged in the anterior pituitaries, but it markedly reduced the effectiveness of acute exposure to GHRH to stimulate enzyme activity (Parenti et al., 1987).

These findings suggest that short-term GHRH treatment has a priming effect on pituitary GHRH receptors in old rats, whereas it induces desensitization of the same receptors in young rats.

The results obtained by measuring adenylate cyclase activity were supported by data on GH secretion from cultured pituitary cells. Pituitary cells from 14-month and 2-month-old female rats were enzymatically dissociated and cultured for 3-4 days in Ham's F-10 medium (Flow Laboratories) supplemented with 15% horse serum, 2.5% fetal calf serum and antibiotics. On the day of the experiments the attached cells were incubated in different concentrations of rGHRH (Peninsula, Belmont, Ca) in a randomized way for 2 hours. At the end of the incubation, the media were collected and the attached cells were extracted in 0.01N NaOH.

The growth hormone secretions from pituitary cells of aged and young female rats were similar, when expressed as ratio between the medium and the intracellular content. GHRH (10^{-8} and 10^{-9}M) induced a significantly lower release of GH into the medium of cells from old than from young rats (Fig. 1). *Ex vivo* pretreatment with GHRH (5 μg/rat daily for 3 days) reduced both the basal GH secretion and the acute responsiveness to GHRH of cells from young rats, but left both indices in cells from aged animals unchanged (Fig. 1).

These findings confirm the view that in aged animals a (primary?) deficiency of GHRH synthesis and/or release is the main event underlying a defective GH response to GHRH and CNS-acting stimuli. Therefore, the situation in old rats is reminiscent of the ability of a GHRH pretreatment to increase GH responsiveness to a bolus GHRH injection in GHRH/GH-deficiency states of animals, as shown in hypophysectomized rats with an ectopic pituitary (Janson et al., 1985), or GH-deficient humans (Borges et al., 1984).

If GHRH synthesis and/or release is deficient in humans, as it is in aged rats, it would be of paramount importance to establish whether somatotropes of elderly humans are also amenable to GHRH priming, and, if so, whether the enhanced GHRH-

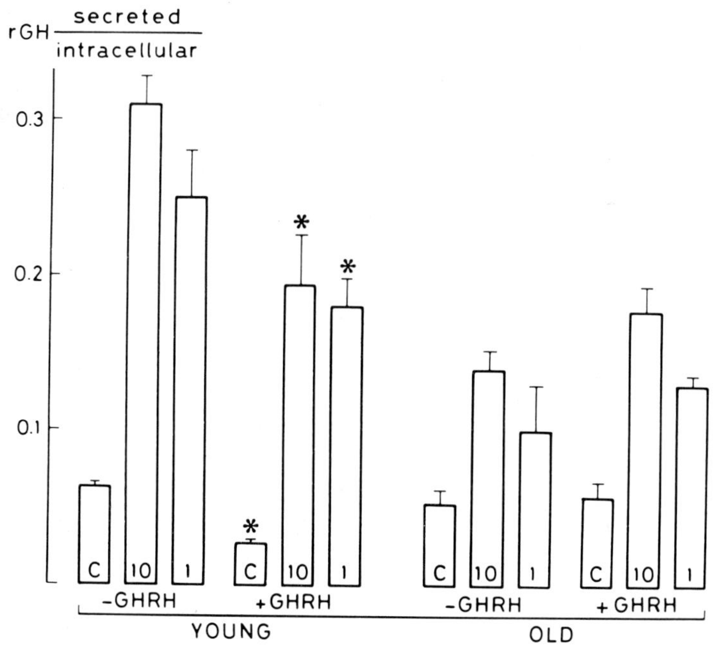

Figure 1. Effect of an *ex vivo* pretreatment with GHRH (+GHRH) on *in vitro* acute responsiveness to GHRH (10^{-8} and 10^{-9}M) of cultured cells from young (2 mos) and middle-aged (14 mos) female rats. Data are expressed as ratio between medium and intracellular GH content. Each column represents the mean ± SEM of 6-12 determinations. *p at least <0.05 vs young–GHRH.

induced GH release would be beneficial to counteract the catabolic processes of aging (Meites, 1986).

AGED DOGS

Before applying the above data to humans and starting a clinical investigation, we performed an analogous study on dogs. Data from our laboratory as well as from elsewhere have demonstrated that the dog is a particularly suitable animal for studies on the control of GH secretion since its GH regulation is similar to that of humans (Tsushima et al., 1971; Cocola et al., 1976). Four young (3 to 4 yrs, two males and 2 females) and four old (10 to 14 yrs, 2 males and 2 females) well trained beagle dogs were used in this study. Freely moving animals, after overnight fasting were taken into the surgery room. Blood samples were collected from the cephalic vein at time -60 and 0. Further blood samples were taken at 15, 30, 45 and 60 min after administration of GHRH or clonidine. Basal GH levels of the aged dogs were significantly lower than those of the young dogs (0.9 ± 0.05 ng/ml vs 1.48 ± 0.1 ng/ml $p < 0.05$). In old dogs, acute administration of GHRH (2 µg/kg iv) induced a plasma GH rise that was significantly lower than in young dogs, a response pattern which was also present after acute administration of clonidine (4 µg/kg iv), a selective agonist of α_2-adrenergic receptors (Fig. 2). Acute clonidine failed to elicit GH release in old dogs, and this finding is

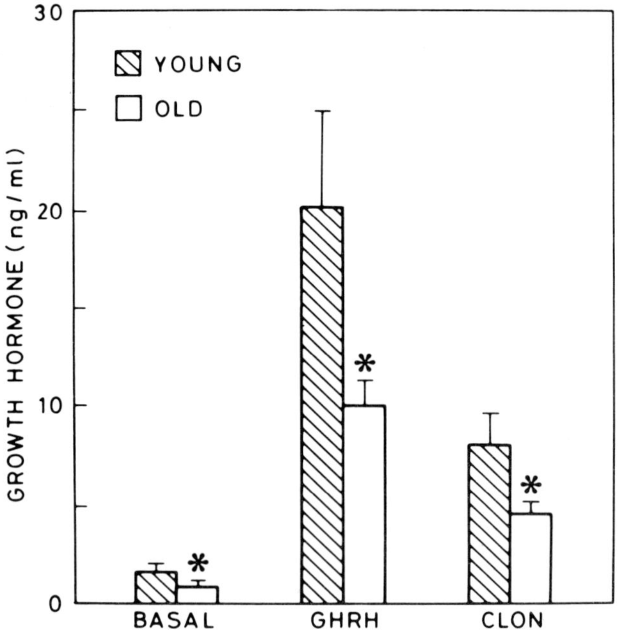

Figure 2. Effect of acute administration of GHRH (2 µg/kg iv) or clonidine (CLON, 4µg/kg, iv) on plasma GH levels in 8 young (3 to 4 yrs) and 4 aged (10 to 14 yrs) dogs of both sexes. Columns represent the mean ± SEM.

reminiscent of the finding that it fails to modify GH secretion in aged rats (Sonntag et al., 1981) and humans (author's unpublished results).

As mentioned previously, the spontaneous pulsatile release of GH is significantly reduced in aged with respect to young rats (Sonntag et al., 1980; Takahashi et al., 1987). No significant difference was found between the pulse frequency of the two age groups, but a 3-fold greater amplitude was found in the young rats. A lower pulsatile GH secretion also has been reported in elderly humans, particularly during sleep, when the amplitude of the pulses is significantly decreased or they may be completely absent (Vermeulen, 1987).

We then studied spontaneous GH secretion in aged dogs by repeatedly taking samples from the animals every 10 min through the cephalic vein for 6 hr (from 0900h to 1500 h) and comparing the pattern found to that found in young dogs. Data were analyzed using the "cluster analysis" (Veldhuis and Johnson, 1986). The peak of a GH pulse was defined as a statistically significant increase in a cluster of hormone values followed by a statistically significant decrease in a second cluster of values (cluster size, two peak values against two trough values; $t = 2.23$ for 10 degrees of freedom). The pulse interval was defined as the time interval in minutes between two successive peaks. Data were analyzed using Student's t test. Aged animals showed a release of GH that was less pulsatile than that of young animals (data not shown). The mean peak frequency was 3.6 ± 0.6/360 min vs 1.8 ± 0.3/360 min, $p < 0.05$ in young and old animals respectively; the mean peak amplitude was 2.8 ± 0.5 ng/ml vs 1.5 ± 0.1 ng/ml, $p < 0.05$ respectively; the mean peak area was 45.1 ± 13.1 ng/ml vs 20.2 ± 3.5 ng/ml, $p < 0.05$; the mean integrated area under the curve was 632.5 ± 68.6 vs 343.3 ± 67.3 ng/ml/360 min, $p < 0.01$.

Reduced output of hypothalamic GHRH, the GH regulatory peptide believed to be responsible for the occurrence of GH spikes (Thorner and Cronin, 1985), is the most likely cause of the diminished pulsatile release of GH in old rats. In view of the previous finding with rats that a GHRH priming could enhance sensitivity of pituitary receptors to the neurohormone, we decided to stimulate the function of the endogenous GHRH system also in aged dogs.

It has been clearly demonstrated that clonidine increases GH secretion through a GHRH-mediated mechanism. In the rat, pretreatment with anti GHRH-serum completely abolishes the GH-releasing effect of the drug (Miki et al., 1984; Cella et al., 1987). Moreover, like GHRH itself, a subacute treatment with the drug increases *de novo* synthesis of GH in pituitaries from ten-day-old rats (Cozzi et al., 1986). We therefore treated aged dogs with clonidine (150 μg/dog p.o. daily, for 14 days in two divided doses) in an attempt to activate the function of endogenous GHRH neurons. The dogs were sampled every 10 min for 6 hr before and 14 hr after a two week-treatment with clonidine.

Treatment with clonidine enhanced the pulsatile release of GH, although the effect was evident only in two out of four dogs (see Fig. 3). The mean GH peak frequency of all the dogs, irrespective of whether or not they responded to clonidine was significantly higher after clonidine treatment than before (3.0 ± 0.4/360 min vs 1.8 ± 0.3/360 min, $p < 0.05$); clonidine also markedly increased the mean peak amplitude (2.98 ± 0.7 ng/ml vs 1.5 ± 0.1 ng/ml, $p < 0.01$) and the mean peak area (54.3 ± 18.6 ng/ml/360 min vs 20.2 ± 3.5 ng/ml/360 min, $p < 0.01$).

In a second experiment, we tried to restore the defective GH secretion present in aged dogs by enhancing the endogenous GHRH secretion with fasting. In humans, fasting is associated with an increase in the GH pulse frequency and integrated GH secretion (Thorner et al., 1985). Four aged dogs were completely fasted for five days. Testing for pulsatile GH secretion was performed before and after the fifth day of fasting.

Two out of four dogs exhibited a more evident pattern of GH pulsatile release after fasting. An evaluation of the above described indices in all the dogs, gave the following: the mean peak frequency was strikingly increased (3.75 ± 0.5/360 min vs 1.8 ± 0.3/360 min, $p < 0.01$) as was the amplitude of peaks (2.54 ± 0.3 ng/ml vs 1.5 ± 0.1, $p < 0.05$) and the mean peak area (46.8 ± 8.6 ng/ml/360 min vs 20.2 ± 3.5 ng/ml/360 min, $p < 0.05$) (see Fig. 3).

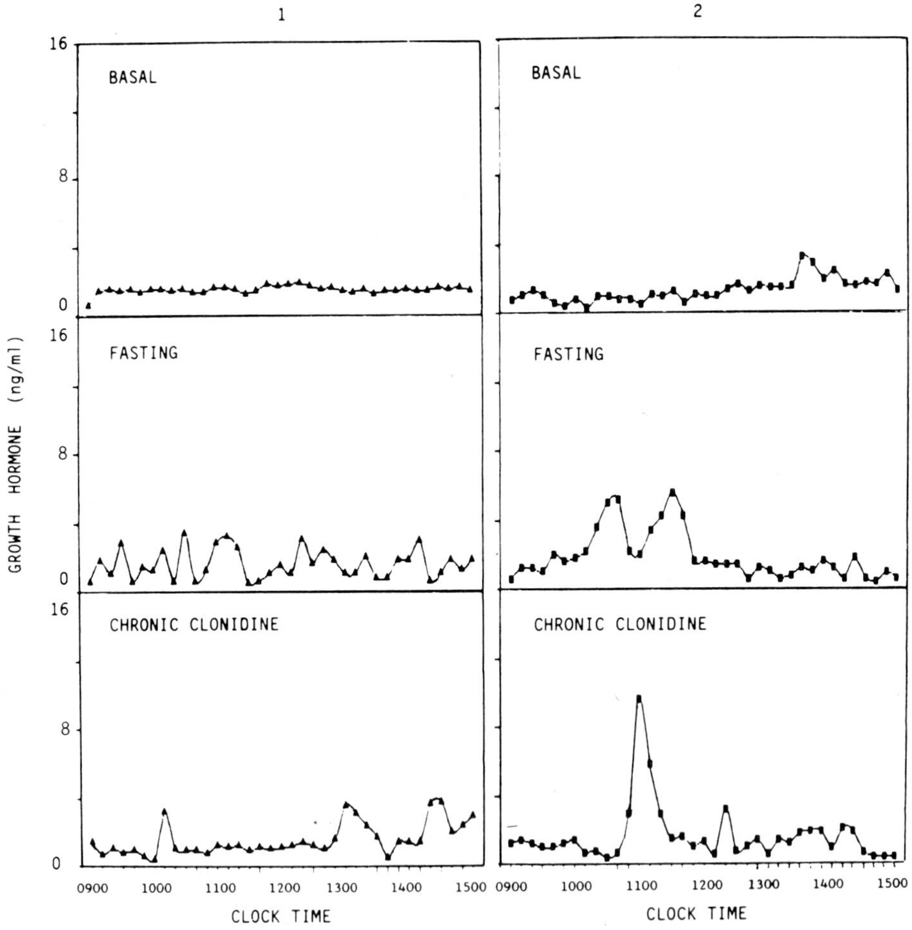

Figure 3. Effect of a 5-day fast (middle panel) or chronic clonidine (lower panel) on basal pulsatile GH secretion (upper panel) in two representative aged dogs. The dogs were sampled every 10 min for 6 hr before and 14 hr after a two week-treatment with clonidine (150 μg/dog/po daily for 14 days).

As yet the cause of the increased pulsatile GH secretion elicited by fasting in aged dogs is not known. Fasting in humans, however, is associated with a marked decrease in circulating Sm-C levels (Clemmons et al., 1981). Reportedly, Sm-C in the systemic circulation feeds back at the pituitary and/or hypothalamus to regulate the release of GH (Abe et al., 1983). Thus, the enhanced pulsatile secretion of GH during fasting may be considered a consequence of the lack of, or diminution in, this autoregulatory mechanism. In conditions of protein-calorie malnutrition, anorexia nervosa and starvation, the low Sm-C levels are associated with high GH levels (Van Wyk, 1984). However, a series of considerations might contradict this proposal; circulating levels of Sm-C are already considerably reduced in aged mammals (Florini et al., 1985) and probably dogs are no exception to this rule; prolonged fasting increases some blood constituents, such as non-esterified fatty acids, whose action on CNS-pituitary structures would counter that of Sm-C (Imaki et al., 1985); at present there is no proof that Sm-C feedbacks at the level of GHRH-secreting structures, as the increase in GH pulse frequency elicited by fasting in old dogs would imply.

The analogy observed between clonidine administration and fasting in restoring GH pulsatile secretion in old dogs would suggest that both stimuli depend upon a mechanism mediated via an increased catecholaminergic function. However, irrespective of the mechanism(s) of action of clonidine or fasting in triggering GH release, our present data demonstrate that in old dogs, as in old rats, the defective secretion of GH is not irreversible since it can ben restored by physiological or pharmacological means.

REFERENCES

Abe H, Molitch ME, Van Wyk JJ, Underwood LE (1983) Human growth hormone and somatomedin C suppress the spontaneous release of growth hormone in unanesthetized rats. Endocrinology 113:1319-1324.

Berelowitz M, Szabo M, Frohman LA, Firestone S, Chu L, Hintz RL (1981) Somatomedin-C mediates growth hormone negative feedback by effects on both the hypothalamus and the pituitary. Science 212:1279-1281.

Borges JCL, Blizzard RM, Evans WS, Furlanetto R, Rogol AD, Kaiser DI, Rivier J, Vale WW, Thorner MO (1984) Stimulation of growth hormone (GH) and somatomedin C in idiopathic GH-deficient subjects by intermittent pulsatile administration of synthetic human pancreatic tumor GH-releasing factor. J Clin Endocrinol Metab 59:1-6.

Cella SG, Locatelli V, De Gennaro V, Puggioni R, Pintor C, Müller EE (1985) Human pancreatic growth hormone (GH)-releasing hormone stimulates GH synthesis and release in infant rats. An in vivo study. Endocrinology 116:574-577.

Clemmons DR, Klibanski A, Underwood LE, McArthur JW, Ridgway EL, Beitins IZ, Van Wyk JJ (1981) Reduction of plasma immunoreactive somatomedin C during fasting in humans. J Clin Endocrinol Metab 53:1247-1250.

Cocchi D, Calderini G, Ganzetti I, Galbiati E, Parenti M, Müller EE (1986) Aspects of the control of prolactin and growth hormone secretion in aging. In: Müller EE, McLeod RM (eds): Neuroendocrine Perspectives, vol. 5, Elsevier, Amsterdam, pp. 191-204.

Cocola F, Udeschini G, Panerai AE, Neri F, Müller EE (1976) A rapid radioimmunoassay method for growth hormone in dog plasma. Proc Soc Exp Biol Med 151:140-144.

Cozzi MG, Zanini A, Locatelli V, Cella SG, Müller EE (1986) Growth hormone releasing hormone and clonidine stimulate biosynthesis of growth hormone in neonatal pituitaries. Biochem Biophys Res Comm 138:1223-1230.

Florini J, Prinz PN, Vitiello MV, Hintz RV (1985) Somatomedin-C levels in healthy young and old men. Relationship to peak and 24 hours integrated levels of growth hormone. J Gerontol 40:2-9.

Gick GG, Zeytin FN, Brazeau P, Ling NC, Esch FS, Bancroft C (1984) Growth hormone-releasing factor regulates growth hormone mRNA in primary cultures of rat pituitary cells. Proc Soc Acad Natl Sci USA 81:1553-1555.

Imaki T, Shibasaki T, Shizume K, Masuda A, Hotta M, Kiyosawa Y, Jibiki K, Demura H, Tsushima T, Ling N (1985) The effect of free fatty acids on growth hormone (GH)-releasing hormone mediated GH secretion in man. J Clin Endocrinol Metab 60:290-293.

Jansson JO, Carlsson L, Isaksson OGP (1985) Growth hormone (GH)-releasing factor (GRF) pretreatment enhances the GRF-induced GH secretion in rats with the pituitary auto-transplanted to the kidney capsule. Endocrinology 116:95-98.

Meites J (1986) The neuroendocrinology of hypothalamic aging. In: Müller EE, MacLeod RM (eds): Neuroendocrine Perspectives, vol. 5. Elsevier, Amsterdam, pp. 179-189.

Miki N, Ono M, Shizume K (1984) Evidence that opiatergic and α-adrenergic mechanisms stimulate rat growth hormone release via growth hormone-releasing factor. Endocrinology 114:1950-1956.

Ono M, Miki N, Shizume K (1986) Release of immunoreactive growth hormone-releasing factor (GRF) and somatostatin from incubated hypothalamus in young and old male rats. Abstract Book of lst International Congress of Neuroendocrinology, San Francisco, Ca, Abst. No. 342.

Parenti M, Dall'Ara A, Rusconi L, Cocchi D, Müller EE (1987) Different regulation of GHRH-sensitive adenylate cyclase in the anterior pituitary of young and old rats. Endocrinology 121:1649-1653.

Pecile A, Müller EE, Falconi G (1985) Growth hormone releasing activity of hypothalamic extracts at different ages. Endocrinology 77:241-246.

Rudman D, Kutner MH, Rogers CM, Lubin MF, Fleming GH, Bain RP (1981) Impaired growth hormone secretion in the adult population. J Clin Invest 67:1361-1369.

Rudman D (1985) Occasional hypothesis. J Am Geriatrics Soc 33:800-807.

Shibasaki T, Shizume K, Makahara M, Masuda A, Jibiki K, Demura H, Wakabayashi I, Ling V (1984) Age-related changes in plasma growth hormone response to growth hormone-releasing factor in man. J Clin Endocrinol Metab 58:212-214.

Sonntag WE, Steger RW, Forman LJ, Meites J (1980) Decreased pulsatile release of growth hormone in old male rats. Endocrinology 107:1875-1879.

Sonntag WE, Forman LJ, Miki N, Steger RW, Ramos T, Arimura A, Meites J (1981) Effects of CNS active drugs and somatostatin antiserum on growth hormone release in young and old male rats. Neuroendocrinology 33:73-78.

Takahara J, Niimi M, Kawanishi K, Irino S (1984) Effects of age on GH responsiveness to human pancreatic GHRH in rats. Abstract Book of 7th International Congress of Endocrinology, Excerpta Medica, Amsterdam, p. 1247.

Takahashi S, Gottschall PE, Quigley KL, Goya RG, Meites J (1987) Growth hormone secretory pattern in young, middle-aged and old female rats. Neuroendocrinology 46:137-142.

Thorner MO, Cronin MJ (1985) Growth hormone-releasing factor: clinical and basic studies. In: Müller EE, MacLeod RM, Frohman LA (eds): Neuroendocrine Perspectives, vol. 4. Elsevier, Amsterdam, pp. 95-133.

Thorner MO, Vance ML, Blizzard RM, Rogol AD, Evans WS, Ho K, Klingensmith G, Brook C, Smith P, Rivier J, Vale W (1986) Clinical studies with growth hormone releasing hormone.

In: Müller EE, MacLeod RM (eds): Neuroendocrine Perspectives, Vol. 5. Elsevier, Amsterdam, pp. 87-99.

Tsushima T, Irie M, Sakuma M (1971) Radioimmunoassay for canine growth hormone. Endocrinology 89:685-693.

Van Wyk JJ (1984) The somatomedins: biological actions and physiologic control mechanisms. In: Li CH (ed): "Growth Factors" Hormonal Proteins and Peptides, vol. 12. Academic Press, New York, pp. 81-125.

Veldhuis J, Johnson ML (1986) Cluster analysis: a simple, versatile, and robust algorithm for endocrine pulse detection. Am J Physiol 250:E486-E493.

Vermeulen A (1987) Nyctohemeral growth hormone profiles in young and aged men: correlation with somatomedin-C levels. J Clin Endocrinol Metab 64:884-888.

New Trends in Aging Research
G. Pepeu, B. Tomlinson, C.M. Wischik (eds)
Fidia Research Series, vol. 15
Liviana Press, Padova © 1988

AGE-RELATED CHANGES IN PLASTICITY OF VASOPRESSIN- AND OXYTOCIN-IMMUNOREACTIVE NEURONS IN RATS AND MICE

Seiichiro Kawashima and Keiichi Kawamoto

Zoological Institute, Faculty of Science, and
Department of Neurosurgery, School of Medicine,
Hiroshima University, Hiroshima 730, Japan

INTRODUCTION

A number of hypothalamic functions decline with age. The decline may be due either to the decrease in the neuron number or to impaired function of individual neurons, or both. Hsu and Peng (1978) reported a loss of neuron in the medial preoptic and anterior hypothalamic areas and the arcuate nucleus in female rats at 24-30 months of age. On the other hand, no significant neuronal loss was detected in the supraoptic (SON), paraventricular (PVN), ventromedial and dorsomedial nuclei. The stability of neuronal population of the SON and PVN was confirmed in our study in rats (Kawashima and Kobayashi, 1982) and mice (Kawamoto and Kawashima, 1985a). However, impaired function of the SON and PVN with age has been reported by several investigators (see, for review, Kawashima et al., 1986). By electron microscopic study, Wilkinson and Davies (1981) suggested that the rate of axonal transport from the SON and PVN to the neural lobe (NL) was decreased. Similarly, Sladek et al. (1980; 1983) found in rats a significant increase in the number of Herring bodies, a decrease in the number of axons immunoreactive to anti-AVP and -neurophysin sera, and a marked reduction in the number of immunoreactive magnocellular neurons. They suggested that in aged brain the availability of AVP is decreased.

Abbreviations: AVP, arginine vasopressin; hypox, hypophysectomy; ME, median eminence; NL, neural lobe; OXT, oxytocin; PVN, paraventricular nucleus; RNA, ribonucleic acid; SON, supraoptic nucleus.

The decrease in availability of AVP can be induced by total hypophysectomy (hypox) or neural-lobectomy, and polydiptic state appears in the operated animals. However, axonal growth and regeneration of a neural lobe (NL)-like tissue eventually take place at the cut of the hypophyseal stalk, and the operated animals show a recovery of the water metabolism (Moll and De Wied, 1962; Kawashima et al., 1966; Raisman, 1973; Ibata et al., 1983). We have reported the age-related difference of the infundibular stem and the neurosecretory neuronal perikarya during reorganization after hypox in rats and mice (Kawamoto and Kawashima, 1985a; 1985b; 1987). The capability of axonal rearrangement is regarded to represent the plasticity of neurons.

This paper aims to summarize our recent findings on the age-related changes in the neuronal population and the neuronal response to hypox in rats and mice.

THE NUMBER OF MAGNOCELLULAR NEURONS AND NEUROSECRETORY ACTIVITY

Although the total number of neurons of the principal regions of the SON and PVN was apparently stable in both mice and rats (Table 1), the neurosecretory activity showed a significant change as a function of age. In C57BL/Tw mice at 19 months of age, the perikarya of AVP-immunoreactive neurons (AVP neurons) in both the SON and PVN were stained less strongly than those in 3-month-old mice. At the same time, the density of AVP axons was decreased in the vicinity of the SON in aged mice. The immunoreactivity of OXT neurons and axons of the SON and PVN was somewhat weaker in aged mice than young mice, but the age-related decrease in stainability was less pronounced as compared with that in AVP neurons and axons (Kawamoto and Kawashima, 1985a).

In Wistar/Tw rats, the stainability of perikarya and axons of AVP and OXT

Table 1. *Total number of magnocellular neurons in the principal regions of the SON and PVN in young and aged mice and rats*

Animals	Age in months	No. of animals	SON	PVN
C57BL/Tw mice	3	5	5826 ± 224*	1860 ± 106
	19	5	5688 ± 196	1846 ± 100
Wistar/Tw rats	3	6	17600 ± 580	6800 ± 240
	17-18	7	16600 ± 570	6000 ± 220[a]

* Mean ± standard error. [a]$P < 0.02$ (young vs aged). (Data from Kawashima and Kobayashi, 1982, and Kawamoto and Kawashima, 1985a).

neurons was weaker at 16-18 months than at 3, 5 and 9 months. The decreased immunoreactivity is related with the increased release of AVP from the NL, because a significant increase in the AVP serum level and a decrease in the AVP concentration in the NL were noted in 16 to 18 month-old rats (serum, 4.42 ± 0.41 pg/ml; NL, 212 ± 29 ng/mg) as compared to 3-month-old rats (serum, 1.64 ± 0.13 pg/ml; NL, 852 ± 113 ng/mg) (Kobayashi et al., 1986). The enhanced release of AVP in Wistar/Tw rats is related to the development of polydipsia and polyuria at middle ages due to renal dysfunction and, therefore, they are in need of AVP. In fact, Sprague-Dawley/Tw rats, kept in the same laboratory conditions as Wistar/Tw rats, exhibited no significant age-related changes in the SON and PVN (Kawashima and Kobayashi, 1982). Zbuzek and Wu (1982) also reported that in Sprague-Dawley male rats AVP concentration was similar at 3, 12 and 30 months of age. These results may show that age-related changes are variable among strains of rats. However, the survey of literature indicates that excepting Wistar/Tw rats general trends during aging are toward a decrease in neurosecretory activity (Kawashima et al., 1986).

BASIC FEATURES OF AXONAL REARRANGEMENT AFTER HYPOPHYSECTOMY

The proximal end of the hypophyseal stalk is reorganized into a tissue resembling the NL. Animals operated on invariably exhibit polydipsia and polyuria as a result of lack in neurohypophyseal hormones, but concurrently with the reorganization of a NL-like tissue the animals show a resumption of normal water metabolism. Kawashima et al. (1966) found that the ratio of vasopressor to oxytocic activity was smaller in reorganized NL four weeks after hypox than in the NL of intact rats, suggesting the preferential release of AVP from the reorganized tissue.

The accumulation of immunoreactive AVP and OXT was observed not only at the proximal end of the hypophyseal stalk, but also in its anterior extension, in the external layer of the ME (Fig. 1). This indicates the enhanced loading of neurohypophyseal hormones in the pre-existing and newly sprouted axons after hypox. However, the projection of OXT axons to the external layer 10 days after hypox was less extensive than that observed for AVP axons. A marked increase in the number of AVP axons in the external layer of the ME was also reported in adrenalectomized rats by Stillman et al. (1977) and Silverman and Zimmerman (1982). They suggested that adrenalectomy could activate the loading of AVP in pre-existing and newly sprouted axons in the external layer. Furthermore, Stillman et al. (1977) found that such loading was suppressed by dexamethasone treatment. These results urged us to study whether the increase of AVP and OXT axons in the external layer after hypox is concerned with endogenous hormones. The increase of AVP and OXT immunoreactivity was not suppressed by dexamethasone injections (Kawamoto and Kawashima, 1986). Injections of vasopressin were also without effects on the enhanced loading of AVP and OXT. These results suggest that the sprouting of AVP axons and the loading of AVP after hypox are associated with intrinsic neuronal response to the extirpation of axonal terminals, and they are not directly related to the decline in circulating glucocorticoids and AVP.

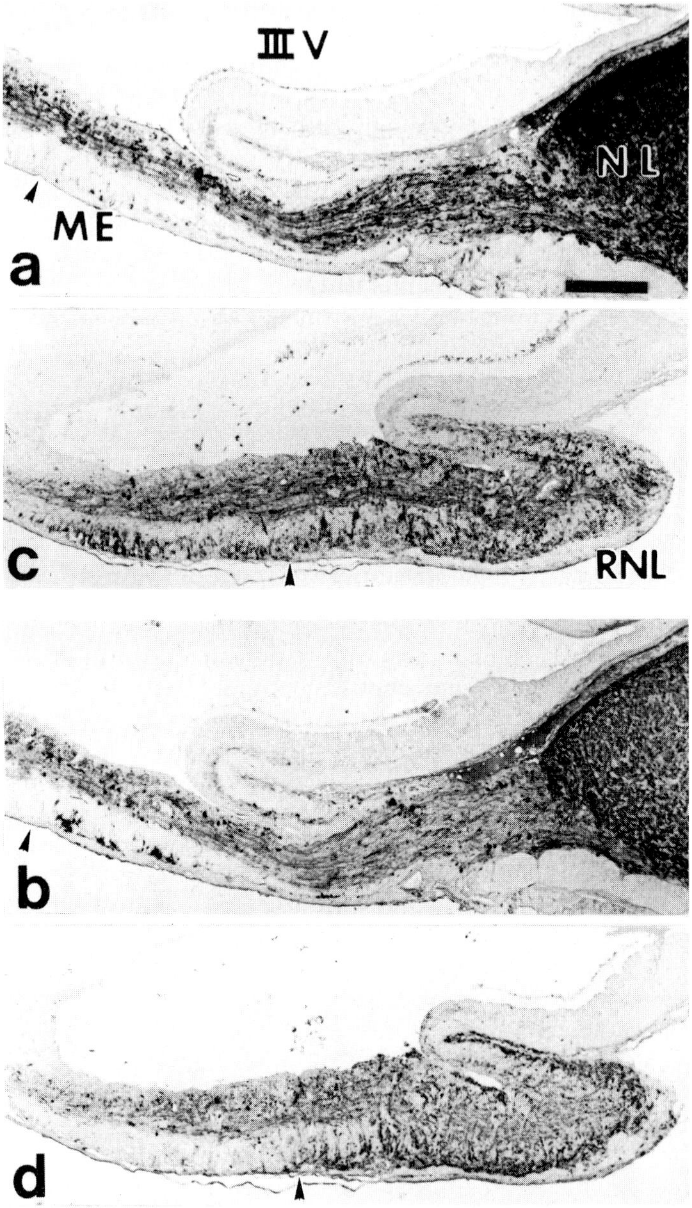

Figure 1. Sagittal sections of the neurohypophysis (NL) in a sham operated rat (a and b) and reorganized neural lobe (RNL)-like tissue in a hypophysectomized rat 10 days after the operation (c and d). a and c: Stained with anti-AVP serum, b and d: Stained with anti-OXT serum. Arrows indicate approximately the identical plane of the median eminence (ME). III V: third ventricle. Bar: 200 μm. (From Kawamoto and Kawashima, 1986; reprinted with permission).

COMPARISON OF NEURONAL RESPONSE BETWEEN YOUNG AND AGED MICE

In young hypophysectomized mice of the C57BL/Tw strain, AVP axons in the external layer of the ME showed a marked increase in number, while the amount of AVP immunoreactive material in the fiber layer of the ME significantly decreased as compared with the young unoperated mice. In contrast, in aged hypophysectomized mice, the increase in AVP immunoreactivity of the external layer was far less than in young mice. These results indicate that the plasticity of AVP neurons for the rearrangement and regrowth of axons was retarded at advanced ages. Changes in the number of AVP immunoreactive Herring bodies 10 days after hypox are presented in Table 2. Hypox significantly decreased the number of Herring bodies in young mice, but not in aged mice. In contrast, size distribution analysis revealed that smaller sizes of Herring bodies occupied a greater part of the population in hypophysectomized mice than unoperated mice of both age groups (Kawamoto and Kawashima, 1985b). Disintegration of Herring bodies may indicate the release of neurohypophyseal hormones into the general circulation. The stainability and the number of OXT axons in the external layer of the ME in aged hypophysectomized mice were similar to those in young hypophysectomized mice. The difference between AVP and OXT axons may be related to the greater need of the former in hypophysectomized animals.

After hypox, some neurons in the SON and PVN showed a remarkable deposition of AVP-immunoreactive material in their perikarya, whereas some other neurons were only weakly reactive to anti-AVP serum in both young and aged mice. The total numbers of AVP neurons in the SON and PVN were decidedly less in intact aged mice than in intact young mice. Ten days after hypox, the total number of AVP neurons of both nuclei was significantly decreased in both young and aged mice as compared to intact controls, and the difference between young and aged mice was no more statistically significant (Table 3). In intact aged mice, the total numbers of OXT neurons in the SON and PVN were significantly less than in intact young mice. Ten days after hypox the total number of OXT neurons in the PVN significantly decreased in young

Table 2. *Changes in the total number of AVP- and OXT-immunoreactive Herring bodies in the median eminence after hypophysectomy in young and aged mice*

Antigen	Group	Young (n = 5)	Aged (n = 5)
AVP	Control	39.0 ± 3.8*	128.4 ± 12.0^{a}
	Hypox	25.0 ± 2.3^{b}	116.3 ± 19.8^{c}
OXT	Control	24.2 ± 2.9	112.4 ± 24.5^{a}
	Hypox	24.8 ± 2.2	68.0 ± 8.2^{d}

* Mean ± standard error in 10 sections of the median eminence at 40 μm intervals. Herring bodies smaller than 30 μm^2 are omitted. Young, 3-month-old; Aged, 19-month-old; Hypox, 10 days after hypophysectomy. Difference from young control, $^{a}P < 0.01$; Difference from control, $^{b}P < 0.05$; Difference from young hypox, $^{c}P < 0.05$, $^{d}P < 0.01$. (Data from Kawamoto and Kawashima, 1985b).

Table 3. *Effects of hypophysectomy on the total number of AVP- and OXT-immunoreactive neurons in the SON and PVN of young and aged mice*

Antigen	Nucleus	Group	No. of mice	Young (3 months of age)	Aged (19 months of age)
AVP	SON	Control	5	4285±232*	2931±341[a]
		Hypox	4	1201± 53[d]	1130±204[d]
	PVN	Control	5	1627± 90	1000± 85[b]
		Hypox	4	661±100[d]	604±146[c]
OXT	SON	Control	5	964± 91	740± 49[b]
		Hypox	4	791±149	648± 92
	PVN	Control	5	2103± 77	1319±103[b]
		Hypox	4	1371±143[d]	1238±198

* Mean ± standard error. Hypox, 10 days after hypophysectomy. Difference from young, $^{a}P<0.05$, $^{b}P<0.01$. Difference from matched control, $^{c}P<0.05$, $^{d}P<0.01$. (Data from Kawamoto and Kawashima, 1985a).

mice, but not in aged mice. In the SON the total number of OXT neurons was not affected by hypox in either young or aged animals.

The present morphometric analyses showed a decrease in the number of AVP neurons in the SON decidedly and, to a lesser extent, in the PVN. This difference between the two nuclei may relate to their difference in the axonal length from the cut end to the perikarya, if the rate of retrograde axonal degeneration is assumed to be the same for neurons of the SON and PVN. The present findings also suggest that neurosecretory neurons, in particular AVP neurons of young mice, are composed of the population of neurons that are more readily affected by hypox than those of aged mice. Thus, approximately the same number of AVP neurons was observed in both young and aged mice 10 days after hypox. These neurons may be responsible for the reorganization of the NL after hypox. However, as mentioned before, the increase in the number of AVP axons in the external layer of the ME 10 days after hypox was greater in 3-month-old mice than that observed in 19-month-old ones, suggesting a decrease in plasticity in aged animals.

REGENERATION OF NEUROHYPOPHYSEAL HORMONE-CONTAINING AXONS IN IMMATURE RATS

Age-related changes in the plasticity of AVP and OXT neurons after hypox were also studied during immature life in rats of the Wistar/Tw strain (Kawamoto and Kawashima, 1987). Rats were hypophysectomized at 9, 16, 23, 30 and 90 days of age by transaural approach, and sacrificed 10 days after the operation. AVP or OXT immunoreactivity in the external layer of the ME was generally stronger in hypophysectomized immature rats than hypophysectomized adult rats, and the age-related difference in immunoreactivity was more conspicuous for AVP axons than OXT ones. Immunohistochemical studies during postnatal development have been reported by Choy and Watkins (1979) and Watkins and Choy (1979). They found that OXT immunoreactivity of the NL, hypothalamus and fiber layer of the ME was weaker than AVP immunoreactivity during early postnatal period. Therefore, the difference between AVP and OXT immunoreactivity of the ME after hypox in the present study may be related with the delayed sprouting of OXT axons to the external layer after hypox in immature rats.

Recently, van Tol et al. (1986) showed that the increase in AVP content in the hypothalamus and NL coincided well with the increase in mRNA coding AVP precursor molecule in the SON and PVN. In the present study, the acridine orange staining was performed according to the method of Rigler (1966) for the detection of RNA. The fluorescence in neuronal perikarya was more intense in immature rats than in adult rats. With the assumption that detected RNA relates with the synthesis of neurohypophyseal hormones, the age-related changes in immunoreactivity in the external layer of the ME after hypox may be concerned with the difference in the rate of synthesis of neurohypophyseal hormones.

The cell body size of AVP and OXT neurons in hypophysectomized adult rats was not significantly different from the value of unoperated or initial control rats. However, the neurons in immature rats became significantly larger after hypox compared with those of initial controls. This size growth in immature rats during the 10 postoperative days may be a normal maturational change.

In conclusion, the present results indicate that AVP- and OXT-producing neurons in immature rats, as early as at 9 days of age, are endowed with the capacity of axonal rearrangement to the external layer of the ME after hypox, and that the stronger immunoreactivity in the external layer of the ME in immature rats than the adult may be due to the differences in the rate of synthesis of neurohypophyseal hormones and the regenerative potency of neurons.

ACKNOWLEDGEMENT

This work was supported by a Grant-in-Aid for Scientific Research from the Ministry of Education, Science and Culture, Japan (No. 62480023).

REFERENCES

Choy VJ, Watkins WB (1979) Maturation of the hypothalamo-neurohypophyseal system. I. Localization of neurophysin, oxytocin and vasopressin in the hypothalamus and neural lobe of the developing rat brain. Cell Tissue Res 197:325-336.

Hsu HK, Peng MT (1978) Hypothalamic neuron number of old female rats. Gerontology 24:434-440.

Ibata Y, Fukui K, Obata-Tsuto HL, Murabe Y, Kawata M (1983) Changes in the hypothalamo-hypophyseal neuron system following hypophysectomy. In: Sano Y, Ibata Y, Zimmerman

EA (eds): Structure and function of peptidergic and aminergic neurons. Japan Sci Soc Press, Tokyo, pp. 129-147.

Kawamoto K, Kawashima S (1985a) Changes of vasopressin- and oxytocin-immunoreactive neurons after hypophysectomy in young and old mice. Exp Gerontol 20:295-304.

Kawamoto K, Kawashima S (1985b) Plasticity of vasopressin- and oxytocin-containing fibers in the median eminence in hypophysectomized young and old mice. Brain Res 330:189-193.

Kawamoto K, Kawashima S (1986) Effects of glucocorticoids and vasopressin on the regeneration of neurohypophyseal hormone-containing axons after hypophysectomy. Zool Sci 3:723-726.

Kawamoto K, Kawashima S (1987) Regeneration of neurohypophyseal hormone-producing neurons in hypophysectomized immature rats. Brain Res 422:106-117.

Kawashima S, Kobayashi Y (1982) Morphometric study of the hypothalamo-neurohypophyseal system in aged rats. J Sci Hiroshima Univ, Ser B Div 1, 30:229-242.

Kawashima S, Hirano T, Matsui T, Takewaki K (1966) Neurosecretion and neurohypophyseal hormones in the rat median eminence after total hypophysectomy, with reference to histological and fine structure of the region. J Fac Sci Univ Tokyo IV 11:11-28.

Kawashima S, Kawamoto K, Kobayashi Y (1986) Aging of the hypothalamo-neurohypophyseal system and water metabolism in rats. Zool Sci 3:227-244.

Kobayashi Y, Lederis K, Kawashima S (1986) Neural lobe function in aged Wistar/Tw strain rats showing polydipsia and polyuria. Endocrinol Japon 33:617-627.

Moll J, De Wied D (1962) Observations on the hypothalamo-posthypophyseal system of the posterior lobectomized rat. Gen Comp Endocrinol 2:215-228.

Raisman G (1973) Electron microscopic studies of the development of new neurohaemal contacts in the median eminence of the rat after hypophysectomy. Brain Res 55:245-261.

Rigler R Jr (1966) Microfluorometric characterization of nucleic acids and nucleoproteins by acridine orange. Acta Physiol Scand 67 (Suppl 267): 1-122.

Silverman AJ, Zimmerman EA (1982) Adrenalectomy increases sprouting in a peptidergic neurosecretory system. Neurosci 7:2705-2714.

Sladek JR Jr, McNeill TH, Khachaturian H, Zimmerman EA (1980) Chemical neuroanatomy of monoamine-neuropeptide interactions in the hypothalamic magnocellular system. In: Yoshida S, Share L, Yagi K (eds): Antidiuretic hormone. Japan Sci Soc Press, Tokyo, pp. 3-17.

Sladek JR Jr, Schöler J, Armstrong WE (1983) Norepinephrine-vasopressin interactions during aging. In: Sano Y, Ibata Y, Zimmerman EA (eds): Structure and function of peptidergic and aminergic neurons. Japan Sci Soc Press, Tokyo, pp. 289-298.

Stillman MA, Recht LD, Rosario SL, Seif SM, Robinson AG, Zimmerman EA (1977) The effects of adrenalectomy and glucocorticoid replacement on vasopressin-neurophysin in the zona externa of the median eminence of the rat. Endocrinology 101:42-49.

van Tol HHM, Snijdewint FGM, Boer GJ, Burbach JPH (1986) Postnatal development of vasopressin mRNA content in supraoptic and paraventricular nuclei of the Wistar rat. Neurosci Lett 65:1-6.

Watkins WB, Choy VJ (1979) Maturation of the hypothalamo-neurohypophyseal system. II. Neurophysin, vasopressin and oxytocin in the median eminence of the developing rat brain. Cell Tissue Res 197:337-346.

Wilkinson A, Davies I (1981) The influence of age on the hypothalamo-neurohypophyseal system of the mouse: a quantitative ultrastructural analysis of the posterior pituitary. Mech Ageing Devel 15:129-139.

Zbuzek VK, Wu W-H (1982) Age-related vasopressin changes in rat plasma and the hypothalamo-hypophyseal system. Exp Gerontol 17:133-138.

New Trends in Aging Research
G. Pepeu, B. Tomlinson, C.M. Wischik (eds)
Fidia Research Series, vol. 15
Liviana Press, Padova © 1988

DESTRUCTIVE HORMONAL INFLUENCES ON BRAIN AGING: THE RESULT OF INTERACTING MODULATORS?

Bruce S. McEwen

Laboratory of Neuroendocrinology, Rockefeller University
1230 York Avenue, New York, N.Y. 10021, USA

INTRODUCTION

The endocrine system, which is under the control of the brain, has a profound influence on the structure and function of the nervous system throughout the lifespan of each individual. The interplay of experiences, experimentally-altered hormone secretion and the feedback actions of hormones on the brain and the rest of the body constitutes a powerful force which shapes each individual both in adult life and during development. Not only is the behavior and personality of each individual subject to modification through this pathway, but also the disease susceptibility is maleable through the interplay between the brain, hormones and the immune system (Cotman et al., 1987).

A central component of the endocrine portion of this tri-partite system is the hypothalamo-pituitary-adrenal (HPA) axis. Hypothalamic neurons, under the influence of other parts of the nervous system, release chemical signals (releasing hormones such as corticotrophin releasing factor, CRF, and vasopressin) which trigger release of ACTH from the pituitary. ACTH, in its turn, promotes secretion of glucocorticoid steroids by the adrenal cortex. The widespread actions of glucocorticoids throughout the body, together with actions of ACTH and its partner, beta endorphin, and the more local effects of the releasing hormone, CRF, are responsible for a myriad of effects. Much of this endocrine mechanism is deemed of benefit for the organism in its adaptation to stressful and other disequilibrating events, and these hormone effects are ones which protect the organism from its own tendency to overreact to stressful stimuli through other defense mechanisms (Munck et al., 1984).

There is a negative aspect which is dramatized by the fate of the migrating salmon, whose efforts to climb up a series of waterfalls in order to reach breeding grounds culminate in a crisis of hypersecretion of adrenal steroids that terminates the lifespan of most individuals after spawning has occurred (Robertson and Wexler, 1960). In at least one other vertebrate species (Bradley et al., 1980) there is a similar form of glucocorticoid-induced self destruction, but these are the exceptional cases. Nevertheless, some elements of endocrine involvement in degenerative aspects of senescence can be seen in the loss of neurons in the hippocampal formation of two-year-old rats which can be attenuated by adrenalectomy in mid-life (Landfield et al., 1978; 1981). Glucocorticoid administration to guinea pigs induces some loss of neurons in hippocampus and several hypothalamic and thalamic nuclei (Muhlen and Ockenfels, 1969), and repeated glucocorticoid treatment of young rats induces neuronal loss in hippocampus which mimics that seen in aging (Sapolsky et al., 1986). Moreover, the hippocampus is a structure in which ischaemia induces neuronal loss to a greater extent than in other brain regions, and this damage is also exacerbated by elevated glucocorticoids (Sapolsky and Pulsinelli, 1985), although excitatory amino acids and calcium ions are believed to play an important role as well (Nayler, 1981; Choi, 1985; Garthwaite and Garthwaite, 1986; Sakamoto et al., 1986).

The hippocampus is also a brain structure endowed with high levels of glucocorticoid receptors (McEwen et al., 1968). Over the past 19 years, we and other laboratories have attempted to unravel the mystery of what glucocorticoids do in the hippocampus. This article is a progress report of these attempts. It also discusses other factors which are involved in regulating neuronal loss, with which the glucocorticoids may be interacting in producing both their adaptive and deleterious effects.

THE GLUCOCORTICOID RECEPTOR SYSTEM OF THE BRAIN AND ITS ROLE IN THE DIURNAL RHYTHM AND IN ADAPTATION TO STRESS

The glucocorticoid receptor system of the brain is made up of two principal components with different regional distributions. Uptake studies in adrenalectomized rats and rhesus monkeys revealed that one of these components is located principally in the hippocampus, with lesser concentrations in septum and amygdala (McEwen, 1982).

Subsequent measurements of cytosolic receptor sites by in vitro binding assays uncovered the second site, although it was not identified as such until recently (McEwen et al., 1986). The introduction of synthetic steroids such as Ru26988 (glucocorticoid agonist) and Ru38486 (glucocorticoid antagonist) by Roussel-Uclaf provided the tools necessary to dissociate the two components (Veldhuis and DeKloet, 1982; Reul and DeKloet, 1985). The major component, called the Type 2 receptor, is found throughout the brain in both neurons and glial cells, and it appears to be identical with the major glucocorticoid receptor species of the liver (McEwen et al., 1986). Its presence accounts for the brain-wide cytosol binding of 3H dexamethasone. The minor component, called the Type 1 receptor, is very similar to the mineralocorticoid receptor of the kidney, but in the hippocampus, where its concentration is highest, it binds corticosterone preferentially in vivo. This is because of at least two factors:

1. the Type 1 receptor has a slightly higher affinity for corticosterone over the mineralocorticoid, aldosterone; and

2. concentrations of corticosterone are 100 times higher than aldosterone.

It is therefore surprising and puzzling why the kidney Type 1 receptor apparently preferentially binds aldosterone over corticosterone (Sheppard and Funder, 1987).

What is the function of these two receptor types in the brain? Because the Type 1 receptors have a ten-fold higher affinity for corticosterone than the Type 2 receptor, they may function as sensors for low and high levels of corticosterone, respectively (Reul and DeKloet, 1985; McEwen and Brinton, 1987). Low to moderate levels of corticosterone are achieved during the diurnal cycle of pituitary adrenal activity, whereas stress brings about high levels of corticosterone. It therefore appears that Type 1 receptors in hippocampus, septum and amygdala may function as sensors for diurnally-varying levels of corticosterone, whereas Type 2 receptors in these brain regions and elsewhere in the brain may function as sensors for stress-induced corticosterone elevations, which are much higher than the diurnal peak.

What are the functions mediated by these two receptor systems? Diurnally-varying corticosterone levels are responsible for coordinating daily activity and sleep behavior with the time of the light-dark cycle. The daily glucocorticoid peak prior to waking helps to arouse animals from sleep and promotes food seeking behavior, increases appetite and also delays sleep (McEwen and Brinton, 1987). Jet lag is a phenomenon associated with the displacement of this rhythm by rapidly moving across time zones. We do not yet know of the neurochemical correlates of glucocorticoid actions during the diurnal cycle, but there are reports indicating adrenally-modulated diurnal cycles of synaptic efficacy, measured electrophysiologically, in hippocampus associated with long-term potentiation, which is a simplified model system relevant to learning (Dana and Martinez, 1984).

As for stress-induced glucocorticoid secretion, we are becoming increasingly aware of long-term effects of glucocorticoids which modify neurochemistry throughout the brain. These may be classified into three categories of potential relevance:

1. synaptic plasticity;
2. stress-induced analgesia; and
3. post-synaptic responsivity to endogenous neurotransmitters.

With regard to synaptic plasticity, we have found that 3-5d treatment with corticosterone elevates levels of the synaptic phosphoprotein, Synapsin 1, in hippocampus and apparently nowhere else in the brain (Nestler et al., 1981). We are currently investigating the effects of stress-induced corticosterone secretion on Synapsin 1 levels. Most likely, increases in Synapsin 1 reflect either increased synaptic size or increased numbers of synaptic endings. With regard to opiate analgesia, part of which is centrally mediated through the septo-hippocampal system (Kelsey and Baker, 1983), we are currently investigating effects of corticosterone and stress on levels of mRNA for proenkephalin in CNS regions. Thus far it appears that proenkephalin mRNA in at least one brain region, the corpus striatum, decreases after adrenalectomy and increases after corticosterone treatment (Chao et al., 1987). This is consistent with studies on cultured cells showing glucocorticoid modulation of proenkephalin mRNA (Yoshikawa and Sabol, 1986; Comb et al., 1986). Finally, with regard to CNS sensitivity to neurotransmitters, chronic glucocorticoid treatment modifies the response to a number of neurotransmitters and neuromodulators, including serotonin, noradrenaline, VIP, histamine and glutamic acid (Table 1). Prominent among the affected brain structures are the hippocampus and cerebral cortex, and prominent among the affected neurotransmitters is noradrenaline. Cortical and hippocampal sensitivity to noradrenaline is dampened, in terms of the cAMP response, by repeated glucocorticoid treatment or by repeated stress (Stone et al., 1985; 1986; Roberts et al., 1984; Mobley et al., 1983; Harrelson et al., 1987). This may have some relevance for the consequences after severe stress, which are often attributed to hyper-reactivity of the CNS noradrenergic system (Gold et al., 1987; Weiss et al., 1986). Taken together, the changes induced in brain by glucocorticoids are consistent with the notion of a role for the adrenal cortex in the adaptation of the brain to stressful events.

Table 1. *Glucocorticoid effects on sensitivity of neuroactive substances*

Neuroactive substance	Brain region	Direction of effect
Noradrenaline[1]	Cortex	down
Noradrenaline[1]	Hippocampus	down
VIP[1]	Hippocampus	down
Histamine[1]	Hippocampus	up
Serotonin[2]	Hippocampus	down
Glutamate[3]	Hippocampus	biphasic

[1] Cyclic AMP measured (Harrelson et al., 1987; Mobley et al., 1983; Stone et al., 1985; 1986).
[2] 5HT-1 receptor binding measured (Biegon et al., 1985; DeKloet et al., 1986).
[3] Glutamate receptor binding measured (Halpain et al., 1985).

GLUCOCORTICOIDS AS A FACTOR IN NEURAL DAMAGE AND CHANGES OCCURRING DURING THE AGING PROCESS

Whereas the organism cannot easily survive without the adrenal cortex, there are instances in which adrenocortical secretions have damaging effects upon the brain as well as suppressing immunity and resistance to disease and tumors (Cotman et al., 1987). In the brain, glucocorticoid actions exacerbate damage after hypoxia (Sapolsky and Pulsinelli, 1985) and promote neuronal loss with age (Sapolsky et al., 1986; Landfield et al., 1978; 1981). Adrenalectomy reduces the magnitude of such damage. In this section and the next section, we address the mechanism by which this damage occurs and how it may be prevented.

A first line of defense against damaging effects of glucocorticoids may well be the down-regulation of glucocorticoid receptors induced by stress or by repeated glucocorticoid administration (Sapolsky et al., 1986). However, the magnitude of this down-regulation is not profound, even in hippocampus, and moreover it is associated with hypersecretion of adrenal steroids in the aftermath of stress (Sapolsky et al., 1986). Such hypersecretion may, in fact, worsen or potentiate damage if it is allowed to continue. Therefore, the principal line of defense is the cessation of adrenocortical secretion — that is to say, prolonged secretion of, or exposure to, adrenal steroids is believed to be the key to facilitation of damage (Sapolsky et al., 1986).

As far as the mechanism of the damaging effects of glucocorticoids are concerned, there are indications that glucocorticoids interact with at least 5 different processes which are linked to neuronal damage (Table 2). Most of the relevant evidence has come from studies of excitotoxin-induced neuronal death and also from the study of hypoxia-induced damage, which is thought to occur through elevated excitatory amino acids (Pulsinelli, 1985). Hypoxic-damage may have relevance to age-related neuronal loss because of the similarity in structures affected (notably hippocampus) and because of the parallel facilitation by glucocorticoids. As indicated in Table 2, glucocorticoids retard glucose entry into brain as well as into other tissues; were this retardation to occur at times of maximal excitation, some neurons might be unable to get enough energy to maintain ion balance and death would ensue (Sapolsky, 1986). Arguing for this mechanism is the fact that supplementation with brain fuels reduces damage produced by exogenous excitotoxins (Sapolsky, 1986).

Excitotoxins induce the entry of Ca^{++} ions into neurons (Choi, 1985, and Ca^{++} entry which overwhelms the neuron's ability to pump it out or sequester it in mitochondria can initiate neuronal self-destruction through proteolysis (Garthwaite and Garthwaite, 1986). There are two sites of entry of Ca^{++}, the nerve endings and the neuron cell body. At the nerve endings, Ca^{++} entry is linked to exocytosis and neurotransmitter release, and studies on aging indicate that nerve ending Ca^{++} entry may actually decline with aging (Peterson et al., 1985). Other studies point to the possibility of an age-related increase in internal Ca^{++} levels in neurons which would be consistent with a greater vulnerability for cell loss (Martinez et al., 1987). Glucocorticoids have been reported to increase Ca^{++} entry at nerve endings (Sze, 1985) and have diverse effects in other tissues which include inhibition of mitochondrial uptake of Ca^{++} in liver (Kimura and Rasmussen, 1977), induction of Ca^{++} uptake by hepatic microsomes (Friedman and Johnson, 1980) and inhibition of active transport of Ca^{++} in

Table 2. *Systems involved in neuronal loss*

System	Influence	Nature of glucocorticoid effect
Excitatory amino acids	Hyperexcitation believed to be responsible for ischaemic damage possibly through Ca^{++} entry	Biphasic effects on glutamate receptors
Calcium	Elevated cytosolic Ca^{++} may trigger neuronal self-destruction	Increase Ca^{++} entry?
Glucose	Entry important as source of energy	Retards glucose entry
Noradrenaline	6-OHDA lesions increase ischaemic damage	Retards Na cAMP response
Serotonin	Tryptophan loading reduces ischaemic damage	Reduces CNS sensitivity to 5HT

the intestine (Harrison and Harrison, 1960). It remains to be seen whether glucocorticoids would also increase Ca^{++} entry into neuron cell bodies, or at least alter the balance of internal Ca^{++} buffering mechanisms so as to increase internal Ca^{++} levels in neuronal cytoplasm. In contrast to glucocorticoids, Ca^{++} channel blockers like verapamil interfere with Ca^{++} entry and retard ischaemia-induced damage in the heart (Nayler, 1981). However, neuronal cell body uptake of Ca^{++} may be dependent on other types of Ca^{++} channels, and other channel blockers may be required to interfere with this process in the CNS (Reynolds et al., 1986).

Two principal neurotransmitter systems, noradrenaline (NA) and serotonin (5HT), are implicated in the ability of the brain to withstand ischaemic damage (Table 2). Denervation of NA input by 6 hydroxydopamine lesions leads to increased damage from hypoxia (Blomqvist et al., 1985). Involvement of indoleamines are inferred from studies which show that supplementation of tryptophan reduces ischaemic damage (Carney, 1986). Potentially, glucocorticoids may modulate both systems, since they potentiate acutely catecholamine and 5HT turnover and yet, given chronically, they dampen CNS sensitivity to NA and to 5HT (McEwen, 1987) (Table 1). Thus glucocorticoids may have biphasic effects on the ability of monoamines to modulate neuronal susceptibility to ischaemic damage. The fact that both noradrenaline and 5HT innervation may decline in Alzheimer's disease (Palmer et al., 1987) and that declines in NA and dopamine occur in normal aging must be borne in mind as factors which are likely to increase the vulnerability of the brain to damage.

In contrast to NA and 5HT, excitatory amino acids appear to play a causal role in neural damage (see above) and glucocorticoids modulate the level of excitatory amino acid binding sites in hippocampus (Halpain and McEwen, 1988). Curiously, glucocorticoid treatment causes changes in putative excitatory amino acid receptor sites which are confined to hippocampus and which show a triphasic time course: facilitation of binding at one day, inhibition after 5 d of treatment and no effect after 15 d (Halpain and McEwen, 1988). These results imply that glucocorticoids may modulate sensitivity to excitatory amino acids and that duration of exposure to hormone determines the degree of the effect.

Another aspect of neural damage concerns the potential role of free radicals, which can induce cellular destruction. According to one hypothesis (Yoshida et al., 1983), the conversion of prostaglandin G2 to prostaglandin H2 release active oxygen species; in turn, these active oxygen may propagate free radical chain reactions among free polyunsaturated fatty acids. Free fatty acid levels are known to increase following ischaemia, a condition which may catalyze the increased vulnerability to damage through a free radical cascade (Yoshida et al., 1983). Several substances are known which may reduce free radical formation and interrupt the cascade. These include anaesthetics like thiopental (Yoshida et al., 1983; Bendo et al., 1987) and possibly the naturally occurring substance, acetylcarnitine (Fariello et al., 1985). Acetylcarnitine has found some success in use as an anti-aging agent (Angelucci et al., this volume) and it remains to be seen whether its effects occur through interruption of free radical mechanisms, improvements of cerebral energy metabolism, interference with Ca^{++} entry, reduction of circulating glucocorticoid levels or antagonism of endogenous excitotoxin actions, or a combination of several mechanisms.

A final consideration in relation to neuronal death is the relationship between turnover of cytoskeletal and membrane components and the influence of endogenous factors like excitatory amino acids and Ca ions and exogenous factors like glucose and glucocorticoids. Failure of normal degradative mechanisms, or over-production, may be responsible for accumulation of cytoskeletal elements in plaques and tangles and membrane elements in the amyloid bodies of the Alzheimer brain (Maragos et al., 1987; Selkoe, 1986; Mori et al., 1987; Kang et al., 1987). It remains to be established whether the various extrinsic and intrinsic factors noted above may promote cytoskeletal and beta amyloid protein accumulation. Moreover, because the gene for the beta amyloid protein on chromosome 21 may be present in multiple copies in Down's syndrome and familial Alzheimer's brains (Delabar et al., 1987), it is important to find out whether the same exogenous and endogenous factors which promote neuronal damage may exacerbate expression of beta amyloid gene products and thus accelerate the accumulation of these substances in Down's and Alzheimer's victims.

CONCLUSIONS

This article has summarized a complex series of interactions by which substances that are endogenous and exogenous to the brain may lead to neuronal damage. Glucocorticoids are in the ambivalent position of both protecting the brain from itself during acute periods of adjustment to stress and exacerbating damage brought about by ischaemia and by the wear and tear of the aging process. Growing evidence indicates that glucocorticoids interact with many different cellular processes, and that the balance between protection and destruction is the product of how much glucocorticoid is present, the time course and duration of exposure, and the intrinsic state of the neurons at the time of exposure. The intrinsic state of the neurons is related to factors such as the level of glucose and oxygen as well as the genetic constitution which determines the nature and number of genes that contribute essential factors for neuronal structure and function. Given this complexity, what can be said about possible treatment strategies which might benefit victims of premature aging and progressive dementia?

From the standpoint of the glucocorticoids which are the central focus of this article, it is unlikely that stress or adrenal steroids *per se* are the cause of any premature aging or progressive dementia. However, stress may be an accelerator of degeneration in individuals whose genetic composition and nutrition or state of cerebrovascular function may predispose towards progressive dementia. Therefore, one step might be to control adrenocortical secretion by means of steroid synthesis inhibitors in individuals who appear to be vulnerable. Likewise, supplementation of tryptophan and tyrosine might help to improve monoaminergic function which appears to protect the brain from ischaemic damage due to cerebrovascular malfunction. Moreover, adjusting blood glucose levels and administering low levels of Ca channel blockers may also assist in maintaining normal energy metabolism and reducing abnormal Ca^{++} accumulation, respectively. Finally, anti-aging agents such as acetylcarnitine, which may act via free radical scavanging, show promise as a long-term means of reducing the impact of endogenous aging factors. Whereas none of these treatments alone may have significant value in prophylaxis and prevention, the combined use of several treatments might be of some benefit in slowing down the progression of the disease process.

ACKNOWLEDGMENTS

Grant support for research described herein was obtained from NIMH (MH41256) and from Sigma Tau. Ms. Inna Perlin provided editorial assistance.

REFERENCES

Bendo A, Kass I, Cottrell J (1987) Anesthetic protection against anoxic damage in the rat hippocampal slice. Brain Res 403:136-141.

Biegon A, Rainbow T, McEwen BS (1985) Corticosterone modulation of neurotransmitter receptors in rat hippocampus: a quantitative autoradiographic study. Brain Res 332:309-314.

Blomqvist P, Lindvall O, Wieloch T (1985) Lesions of the locus coeruleus system aggravate ischemic damage in the rat brain. Neurosci Letts 58: 353-358.

Bradley A, McDonald I, Lee A (1980) Stress and mortality in a small marsupial (antechinus stuartii, Macley). Gen Comp Endo 40:188-200.

Carney J (1986) Acute tryptophan pretreatment protects against behavioral changes caused by cerebral ischemia. Neurosci Letts 66:127-130.

Chao H, Blum M, Roberts J, McEwen BS (1987) Glucocorticoid regulation of preproenkephalin and mRNA level in rat striatum. Abstr Soc Neurosci 13:1086.

Choi D (1985) Glutamate neurotoxicity in cortical cell culture is calcium dependent. Neurosci Letts 58:293-297.

Comb M, Birnberg N, Seasholtz A, Herbert E, Goodman H (1986) A cyclic AMP- and phorbol ester-inducible DNA element. Nature 323:353-356.

Cotman C, Brinton R, Galaburda A, McEwen B, Schneider D (1987) The Neuro-Immune-Endocrine Connection. Raven Press, New York.

Dana RC, Martinez J (1984) Effect of adrenalectomy on the circadian rhythm of LTP. Brain Res 308:392-395.

DeKloet ER, Sybersma H, Reul H (1986) Selective control by corticosterone of $serotonin_1$ receptor capacity in raphe-hippocampal system. Neuroendocrinology 42:513-521.

Delabar J-M, Goldgaber D, Lamour Y, Nicole A, Huret J-L, Grouchy J, Brown P, Gajdusek D, Sinet P-M (1987) Beta-amyloid gene duplication in Alzheimer's disease and karyotypically normal Down's syndrome. Science 1390-1392.

Fariello RG, Ferraro TN, Golden GT, DeMattei M, Phillips T, Shug AL (1985) Hypotheses on the role of the carnitine system in normal and aging brain. IVth World Congress of Biological Psychiatry. Philadelphia, PA.

Friedmann N, Johnson F (1980) Induction of hepatic microsomal calcium uptake by glucocorticoids. Life Sci 27:837-842.

Garthwaite G, Garthwaite J (1986) Amino acid neurotoxicity: intracellular sites of calcium accumulation associated with the onset of irreversible damage to rat cerebellar neurons in vitro. Neurosci Letts 71:53-58.

Gold PW, Goodwin FK, Chrousos GP (1987) Clinical and biomedical manifestation of depression: relationship to the neurobiology of stress. New Engl J Med 319:413-420.

Halpain S, McEwen BS (1988) Corticosterone decreases ^{3}H-glutamate binding in rat hippocampal formation. Neuroendocrinology, in press.

Harrelson A, Rostene W, McEwen BS (1987) Adrenocortical steroids modify neurotransmitter-stimulated cAMP accumulation in the hippocampus and limbic brain of the rat. J Neurochem 48:1648-1655.

Harrison H, Harrison H (1960) Transfer of Ca across intestinal wall in vitro in relation to action of vitamin D and cortisol. Am J Physiol 199:265-271.

Kang J, Lemaire H-G, Unterbeck A, Salbaum JM, Masters C, Grzeschik K-H, Multhaup G, Beyreuther K, Muller-Hill B (1987) The precursor of Alzheimer's disease amylid A4 protein resembles a cell-surface receptor. Nature 325:733-736.

Kelsey J, Baker M (1983) Ventromedial septal lesions in rats reduce the effects of inescapable shock on escape performance and analgesia. Behav Neurosci 97: 945-961.

Kimura S, Rasmussen H (1977) Adrenal glucocorticoids, adenine nucleotide translocation, and mitochondrial calcium accumulation. J Biol Chem 252:1217-1225.

Landfield P, Baskin R, Pitter TA (1981) Brain-aging correlates: retardation by hormonal-pharmacological treatments. Science 214:581-584.

Landfield P, Waymire J, Lynch G (1978) Hippocampal aging and adrenocorticoids quantitative correlation. Science 202: 1098-1101.

Maragos W, Greenamyre T, Penney J, Young A (1987) Glutamate dysfunction in Alzheimer's disease: an hypothesis. TINS 10:65-68.

Martinez A, Vitorica J, Bogonez E, Satrustegui J (1987) Intrasynaptosomal free calcium levels and aging. Abstracts New Trends in Aging Research, Italian Study Group on Brain Aging, Sirmione, Italy.

McEwen BS (1987) Glucocorticoid-biogenic amine interactions in relation to mood and behavior. Biochem Pharm 36:1755-1763.

McEwen BS (1982) Glucocorticoids and hippocampus: receptor in search of a function. In: Ganten D and Pfaff D (eds): Current Topics in Neuroendocrinology. Springer, New York, pp. 1-22.

McEwen BS, Brinton RE (1987) Neuroendocrine aspects of adaptation. In: DeKloet ER, Wiegandt V, DeWied D (eds): Prog Brain Res, Elsevier, Amsterdam, vol. 72, pp. 11-26.

McEwen BS, DeKloet ER, Rostene W (1986) Adrenal steroid receptors and actions in the nervous system. Physiol Rev 66:1121-1188.

McEwen BS, Weiss J, Schwartz L (1968) Selective retention of corticosterone by limbic structures in rat brain. Nature 220:911-912.

Mobley P, Manier D, Sulser F (1983) Norepinephrine-sensitive adenylate cyclase system in rat brain: role of adrenal corticosteroids. J Pharm Therap 226:71-77.

Mori H, Kondo J, Ihara Y (1987) Ubiquitin is a component of paired helical filaments in Alzheimer's disease. Science 1641-1644.

Muhlen K, Ockenfels H (1969) Morphologische Veranderungen im Diencephalon und Telencephalon nach Storungen des Regelkreises Adenohypophyse-Nebennierenrinde. III. Ergebnisse bein Meerschweinchen nach Verabreichung von Cortison und Hydrocortison. Zeitschift für Zellforschung 93:126-141.

Munck A, Guyre P, Holbrook N (1984) Physiological functions of glucocorticoids in stress and their relation to pharmacological actions. Endocr Rev 5:25-44.

Nayler W (1981) The role of calcium in the ischemic myocardium. Am J Pathol 102:262-270.

Nestler E, Rainbow T, McEwen BS, Greengard P (1981) Corticosterone increases the level of protein I, a neuron-specific protein in rat hippocampus. Science 212:1162-1164.

Palmer A, Wilcock G, Esiri M, Francis P, Bowen D (1987) Monoaminergic innervation of the frontal and temporal lobes in Alzheimer's disease. Brain Res 401:231-238.

Peterson C, Nicholls D, Gibson C (1985) Subsynaptosomal distribution of calcium during aging and 3,4-diaminopyridine treatment. Neurobiol Aging 6:297-304.

Pulsinelli WA (1985) Selective neuronal vulnerability: morphological and molecular characteristics. In Kogure K, Hossmann K-A, Siesjo BK, Welsh FA (eds): Prog Brain Res 63:29-38.

Reul J, DeKloet ER (1985) Two receptor systems for corticosterone in rat brain: microdistribution and differential occupation. Endocrinology 117:2505-2511.

Reynolds I, Wagner J, Snyder S, Thayer S, Olivera B, Miller R (1986) Brain voltage-sensitive calcium channel subtypes differentiated by w-conotoxin fraction GVIA. Proc Natl Acad Sci 83:8804-8807.

Roberts V, Singhal R, Roberts D (1984) Corticosterone prevents the increase in noradrenaline-stimulated adenyl cyclase activity in rat hippocampus following adrenalectomy or metopirone. Eur J Pharm 103:235-240.

Robertson O, Wexler B (1960) Histological changes in the organs and tissues of migrating and spawning pacific salmon (genus oncorhynchus). Endocrinology 66:222-239.

Sakamoto N, Kogure K, Kato H, Ohtomo H (1986) Disturbed Ca^{++} homeostasis in the gerbil hippocampus following brief transient ischemia. Brain Res 364:372-376.

Sapolsky RM, Krey LC, McEwen BS (1986) The neuroendocrinology of stress and aging: the glucocorticoid cascade hypothesis. Endocr Rev 7:284-301.

Sapolsky RM, Pulsinelli W (1985) Glucocorticoids potentiate ischemic injury to neurons: therapeutic implications. Science 229:1397-1399.

Sapolsky RM (1986) Glucocorticoid toxicity in the hippocampus: reversal by supplementation with brain fuels. J Neurosci 2240-2244.

Selkoe D (1986) Altered structural proteins in plaques and tangles: What do they tell us about the biology of Alzheimer's disease? Neurobiol Aging 7:425-432.

Sheppard K, Funder J (1987) Mineralocorticoid specificity of renal type I receptors: in vivo binding studies. Am J Physiol 252:E224-E229.

Stone E, Slucky A, Platt J, Trullas R (1985) Reduction of the cyclic adenosine 3'5'-monophosphate response to catecholamines in rat brain slices after repeated restraint stress. J Pharm Exp Therap 233:382-388.

Stone E, Herrera A, Carr K, McEwen BS (1986) Selective regulation of brain beta adrenergic receptors by the noradrenergic system and brain alpha adrenergic receptors by the pituitary adrenal system. Abst Soc Neurosci 12:394.1.

Sze P (1985) Effects of corticosterone on calcium uptake by rat brain synaptosomes. Trans Amer Soc Neurochem Abstr 264:16.

Veldhuis HD, Van Koppen C, Van Ittersum M, DeKloet ER (1982) Specificity of the adrenal steroid receptor system in rat hippocampus. Endocrinology 110:2044-2051.

Weiss J, Simpson P (1986) Depression in an animal model: focus on the locus coeruleus in antidepressants and receptor function. In: Murphy D (ed): Ciba Foundation Symposium 123. Chichester, John Wiley and Sons, pp. 191-209.

Yoshida S, Inoh S, Asano T, Sano K, Shimasaki H, Ueta N (1983) Brain free fatty acids, edema, and mortality in gerbils subjected to transient, bilateral ischemia, and effect of barbiturate anesthesia. J Neurochem 40:1278-1286.

Yoshikawa K, Sabol S (1986) Glucocorticoids and cyclic AMP synergistically regulate the abundance of preproenkephalin messenger RNA in neuroblastoma-glioma hybrid cells. Biochem Biophys Res Commun 139:1-10.

New Trends in Aging Research
G. Pepeu, B. Tomlinson, C.M. Wischik (eds)
Fidia Research Series, vol. 15
Liviana Press, Padova © 1988

ALTERATION OF NOVELTY-INDUCED EXCESSIVE GROOMING BEHAVIOR IN AGED MALE RATS AND THE POSSIBLE NEUROCHEMICAL SUBSTRATE

Filippo Drago, Giuseppe Continella, Pier Luigi Canonico and Umberto Scapagnini

Institute of Pharmacology, University of Catania Medical School,
Viale A. Doria 6, 95125 Catania, Italy

INTRODUCTION

A decrease in adaptability to various physiological and pharmacological manipulations is known to occur during aging (Basen, 1979). Aged rats exhibit a reduction in thermoregulative adaptation (Mc Dougal et al., 1980) and an impaired learning ability (Drago et al., 1981), which may be considered as an aspect of adaptation to environmental changes. These alterations in adaptability may depend on the regression of brain functions occurring during aging (for a review, see Pradham, 1980).

Grooming behavior in rodents has been shown to undergo influences by environmental changes and stressors (Sprujt and Gispen, 1983). It has been suggested that this behavior plays a deactivating role in restoring behavioral homeostasis, thus facilitating adaptation to stressor stimuli (Gispen and Isaacson, 1981; Sprujt and Gispen, 1983). In fact, grooming occurs under extremely arousing conditions, as well as during the exposure to mild stressors, such as novelty, or to conflict and frustration (for a review, see Sprujt and Gispen, 1983). For this reason, quantitation of novelty-induced grooming allows an evaluation of adaptive capacity of animals to mild stressors, such as a novel environmental situation.

NOVELTY-INDUCED GROOMING IN AGED RATS

We have studied the novelty-induced grooming in 24-month-old male rats compared to young animals (3 months old). When put in a novel environmental situation, aged rats exhibited a grooming activity markedly greater than that shown by young rats (Table 1). Such behavior did not disappear over a 30 min observation. Furthermore, no significant change in ambulation, rearing and defecation was observed in aged rats subjected to an open field test as compared to young animals (Continella et al., 1985). These findings agree with a previous study carried out on female rats (Kametani et al., 1984).

Table 1. *Novelty-induced grooming in young and aged rats over a 30-min observation test*

	Blocks of minutes		
	0-10	11-20	21-30
Young rats (15)	8.5±0.5	3.2±0.2	0.8±0.2
Aged rats (15)	23.7±1.2	12.7±1.0	7.4±0.9

Values are mean ± SEM. In parentheses the number of animals per each group.
Significant interaction age/behavior, $F(5,168)=2.39$, $p<0.05$.

Physiological "excessive" grooming behavior observed in aged rats may represent a sign of impaired ability of aged rats to adapt to novel environmental situations.

During aging, a number of alterations in brain functions have been found. Among others, an impairment of central neurotransmission, namely dopaminergic neurotransmission, has been demonstrated (Finch, 1973; Pradham, 1980). Brain mechanisms underlying grooming activity seem to involve deeply central dopaminergic neurotransmission (Wiegant et al., 1977; Drago et al., 1984). Thus, a disruption of dopamine mechanisms in the aging brain may be involved in the excessive grooming induced by novelty in the rat.

PROTEIN KINASE C AND GROOMING IN THE AGED RAT

Although the central mechanisms underlying novelty-induced grooming are not completely known, it has been demonstrated that pituitary hormones can markedly affect grooming behavior of the rat (reviewed in Drago and Scapagnini, 1984). One possibility is that the behavioral activity elicited by ACTH involves the phospholipid-dependent protein kinase (protein kinase C, PKC) (Gispen and Isaacson, 1981), an enzymatic system involved in the processes of transduction of biological signals. Gispen and Isaacson (1981) demonstrated a close correlation between the behavioral effects of ACTH fragments on grooming behavior and the activity that they exert on PKC activity *in vitro*. Gispen et al. (1985) reported also that the injection of PKC activator 1,2-dioctanoylglycerol (DOG) produces a reduction of ACTH-induced excessive grooming.

In a pilot study, we have investigated the effects of intracerebroventricular and intraperitoneal injection of the protein kinase C activators, phorbol esters, on novelty-induced grooming behavior in young rats and on adrenocorticotropin (ACTH) secretion. Phorbol esters had a dose-dependent inhibitory effect on grooming behavior after either central or peripheral injection, whereas they produced different secretory ACTH responses, depending upon the route of administration (Continella et al., 1987). These findings suggest that modulation of protein kinase C activity may be involved in the neurochemical mechanisms controlling grooming behavior in the rat.

Recently, marked modifications in PKC activity and distribution in aging brain have been reported (Calderini et al., 1986). We therefore investigated the effects of PKC activator phorbol 12-myristate 13-acetate (TPA) on novelty-induced grooming behavior of aged rats in comparison to young rats. In some of these experiments, another PKC activator, phosphatidylserine, was used. In fact, among phospholipids this drug is the most potent in supporting either TPA-mediated enzyme activation or enzyme activity itself (Couturier et al., 1984).

Table 2 shows that the total amount of grooming behavior was reduced in both young and aged rats by 50, 100, 150 and 200 µg/kg of TPA, and most completely abolished by the two greatest doses. A statistical analysis of the dose-response pattern showed that the behavioral responsiveness of old rats to TPA injection was significantly greater than that of young rats (ANOVA, $F=6.37$ 1/64, $p<0.05$), and a significant interaction dose level-effect was found ($F=4.55$ 4/64, $p<0.01$). The ED50 inhibiting grooming activity of aged rats resulted lower than that calculated for young rats (48 and 80 µg/kg, respectively).

Phosphatidylserine (20 and 30 mg/kg, i.p. for 20 days) did not affect the grooming activity of young rats. However, both doses of the drug significantly reduced grooming behavior of aged rats (Table 3).

Table 2. *Effects of TPA administration on novelty-induced grooming of young and aged rats*

	Grooming score
Young rats	
Vehicle (10)	18.5±0.7
TPA 50 µg/kg (8)	15.6±0.6
100 µg/kg (8)	12.4±0.7
150 µg/kg (8)	8.7±0.5
200 µg/kg (8)	6.8±0.5
Aged rats	
Vehicle (8)	38.6±2.1
TPA 50 µg/kg (6)	18.6±1.1
100 µg/kg (6)	6.4±0.6
150 µg/kg (6)	5.8±0.6
200 µg/kg (6)	4.2±0.5

Values are mean ± SEM. In parentheses the number of animals per each group.
Significant interaction treatment/behavior, $F(2,35)=3.54$, $p<0.05$.

Table 3. *Effects of phosphatidylserine administration on novelty-induced grooming of young and aged rats*

	Grooming score
Young rats	
Vehicle (6)	12.0 ± 3.3
PS 25 mg/kg/die (6)	16.7 ± 3.1
35 mg/kg/die (6)	13.3 ± 4.0
Aged rats	
Vehicle (6)	38.0 ± 5.4
PS 25 mg/kg/die (6)	22.5 ± 3.3*
35 mg/kg/die (6)	18.7 ± 2.7*

Values are mean $\pm$ SEM. In parentheses the number of animals per each group.
* Significant difference as compared to vehicle-treated animals ($p < 0.05$, Dunnett's test for multiple comparisons).

These findings suggest that PKC activity plays a crucial role in the central mechanisms controlling grooming behavior. Since deep modifications have been detected in PKC distribution in the brain of aged rats (Calderini et al., 1986), this may account for the excessive grooming of aged rats exposed to a novel environment. This is indirectly supported by the finding that ACTH-induced PKC inhibition is associated to an increase in grooming behavior (Gispen and Isaacson, 1981).

That aged animals were more responsive than young animals to the TPA-induced grooming inhibition may be caused by different pharmacokinetics of the phorbol ester or, more likely, by a greater sensitivity to TPA of the neurons responsible for grooming behavior under conditions of chronic impairment of PKC activity. It remains to be elucidated whether, in contrast to TPA, PS failed to reduce grooming activity in young rats. The different potency of the drugs in stimulating PKC may at least partly explain this discrepancy.

These findings suggest that PKC activity may play a role in the behavioral modifications of aged rats. The fact that the excessive novelty-induced grooming behavior in these animals was counteracted by the activation of PKC allows us to suggest that modulation of PKC activity may provide a valuable experimental tool to further investigate the behavioral modifications associated to the aging of the brain.

REFERENCES

Basen MM (1979) The aging processes and psychoactive drug use. US Dept of HEW 79-813, Washington.

Calderini G, Bellini F, Bonetti AC, Galbiati E, Rubini R, Zanotti A, Toffano G (1986) Pharmacological properties of phosphatidylserine in the aging brain: biochemical aspects and therapeutical potential. In: Horrocks LA, Freysz L (eds): Phospholipid Research and the Nervous System. Liviana Press, Padova, pp. 123-132.

Continella G, Drago F, Auditore S, Scapagnini U (1985) Quantitative alteration of grooming behavior in aged male rats. Physiol Behav 35:839-842.

Continella G, Drago F, Rapisarda E, Scapagnini U, Canonico PL (1988) Protein kinase C activators decrease grooming behavior in the rat. Brain Res Bull, in press.

Couturier A, Baygar S, Castagna M (1984) Further characterization of tumor-promoter-mediated activation of protein kinase C. Biochem Biophys Res Comm 121:448-455.

Drago F, Scapagnini U (1984) Prolactin-ACTH interactions in the neuroendocrine responses to stress. In: Usdin E (ed): Stress: The role of catecholamines and other neurotransmitters. Gordon and Breach, New York, pp. 311-324.

Drago F, Canonico PL, Scapagnini U (1981) Behavioral effects of phosphatidylserine in aged rats. Neurobiol Aging 2:209-213.

Drago F, Kovacs GL, Continella G, Scapagnini U (1984) Dopamine in the nucleus accumbens: its role in prolactin-enhanced grooming behavior of the rat. Biogen Amines 1:75-81.

Finch CE (1973) Catecholamine metabolism in the brains of ageing mice. Brain Res 52:261-276.

Gispen WH, Isaacson RL (1981) ACTH-induced excessive grooming in the rat. Pharmacol Ther 12:209-222.

Gispen WH, Schrama LH, Eichberg J (1985) Stimulation of protein kinase C reduces excessive grooming. Eur J Pharmacol 114: 339-400.

Kametani H, Osada H, Inoue K (1984) Increased novelty-induced grooming in aged rats: a preliminary observation. Behav Neur Biol 42:73-80.

Mc Dougal JN, Marques PR, Burks TF (1980) Age-related changes in body temperature responses to morphine in rats. Life Sci 27: 2679-2685.

Pradham SN (1980) Central neurotransmitters and aging. Life Sci 26:1643-1656.

Sprujt B, Gispen WH (1983) ACTH and grooming behavior in the rat. In: Baltazart J, Prove E, Gilles R (eds): Hormones and Behavior in Higher Vertebrates. Springer-Verlag, Berlin, pp. 118-136.

Wiegant VM, Cools AR, Gispen WH (1977) ACTH-induced excessive grooming involves brain dopamine. Eur J Pharmacol 41:343-345.

New Trends in Aging Research
G. Pepeu, B. Tomlinson, C.M. Wischik (eds)
Fidia Research Series, vol. 15
Liviana Press, Padova © 1988

BEHAVIORAL EFFECTS OF AGE-RELATED DEGENERATION IN THE ACETYLCHOLINERGIC AND SEROTONERGIC NEURAL SYSTEMS IN MONKEYS AND RATS

Gary L. Wenk, Linda C. Cork and David S. Olton

Departments of Psychology and Neuropathology
Johns Hopkins University, Baltimore, MD 21218, USA

INTRODUCTION

An investigation of the age-related changes in behavior and the acetylcholinergic and serotonergic neural systems will be presented in three parts:

1. The data on age-related changes in selected neurochemical measures in both the rhesus monkey and the rat;
2. The behavioral changes that occur following the destruction of these two systems; and
3. The behavioral effects of the simultaneous destruction of both acetylcholinergic and serotonergic systems in rats. The purpose of these studies is to determine whether the age-related degeneration of these two neurotransmitter systems is related to the behavioral changes that accompany aging, and whether they interact to influence behavior.

Aging is associated with a decline in many cognitive processes (Folstein and Whitehouse, 1983). Our studies emphasized the age-related changes characterized by an impairment in learning and recent memory. In addition, aging is associated with a variety of biochemical changes, including the loss of acetylcholinergic and serotonergic

---

Abbreviations: ChAT, choline acetyltransferase; S2, serotonergic type 2 receptors; AD, Alzheimer's Disease; QNB, quinuclidinyl benzylate.

systems that project to the hippocampus and neocortex (Gottfries, 1981; McGeer, 1981). We have examined the brains of aging rodents and monkeys for similar age-related biochemical changes.

STUDIES IN MONKEYS

Rhesus monkeys (2 to 37 yrs old) were sacrificed and various cortical and subcortical areas were sampled and prepared for the analysis of selected cholinergic and serotonergic neurotransmitter markers.

The level of ChAT activity in the superior frontal gyrus of the monkeys declined with age (Fig. 1). Each vertical bar represents the value of ChAT activity for an individual monkey. We noted a wide variation between individuals in the level of this cholinergic marker throughout the neocortex. Depending upon the particular monkeys that are sampled, it is possible to demonstrate a statistically significant decline with age in this particular cholinergic marker. However, an overall analysis (by ANOVA) across all age groups found only a decreasing trend that was not statistically significant.

The density of ^{3}H-pirenzepine binding sites (putatively the postsynaptic muscarinic M-1 receptor) in the frontal pole of the monkeys decreased significantly with age

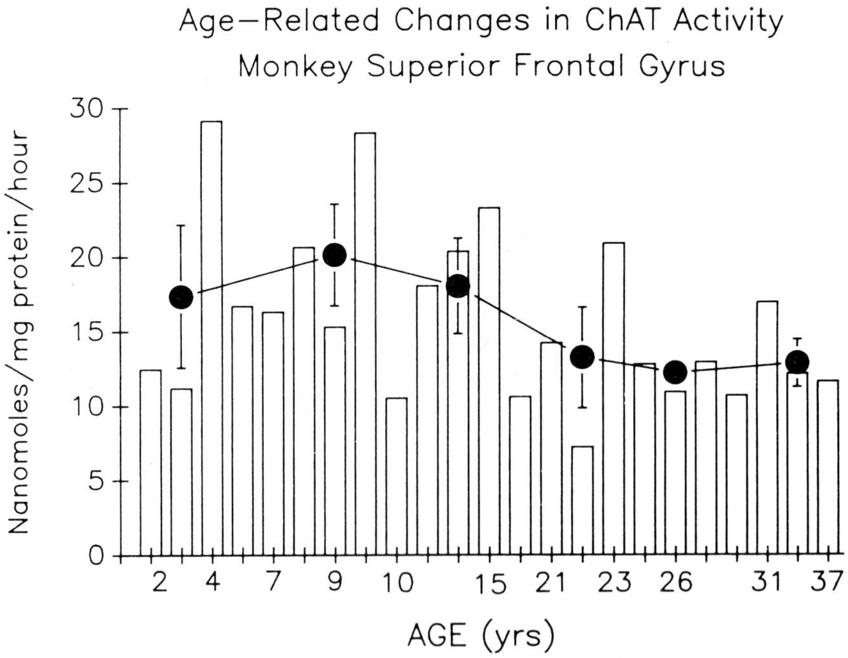

Figure 1. Age-related changes in choline acetyltransferase activity in the superior frontal gyrus of rhesus monkeys.

(Fig. 2). In contrast, the density of ³H-nicotine binding sites was not significantly decreased with age (Fig. 3).

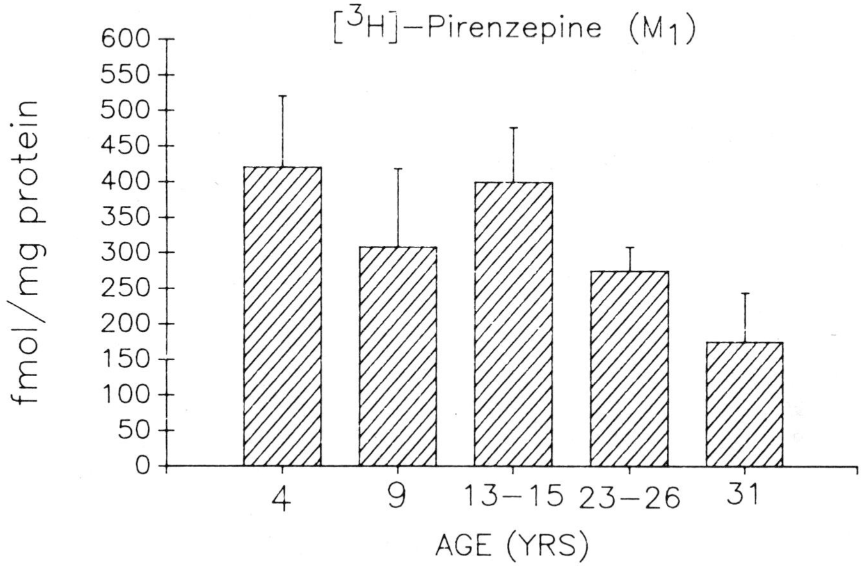

Figure 2. Age-related changes in [³H]-pirenzepine binding in frontal pole of rhesus monkeys.

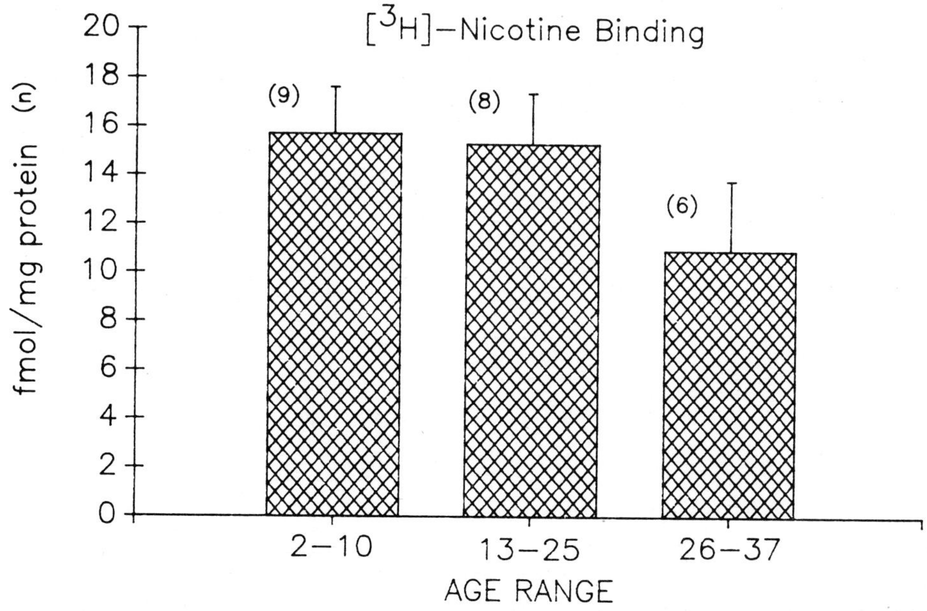

Figure 3. Age-related changes in [³H]-nicotine binding in the frontal pole of rhesus monkeys.

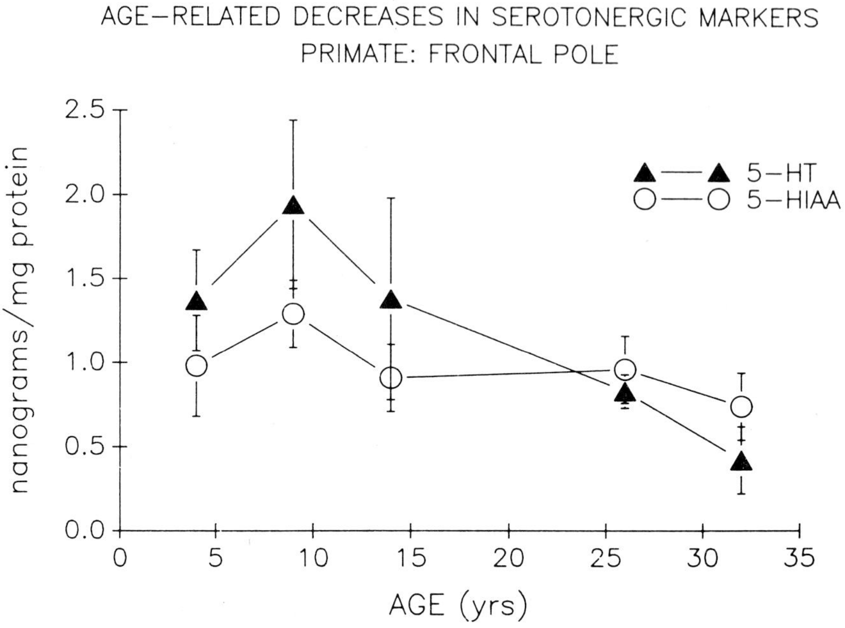

Figure 4. Age-related changes in endogenous levels of serotonin and 5-hydroxyindoleacetic acid in the frontal pole of rhesus monkeys.

Similar age-related changes in the serotonergic system were found in monkeys. Endogenous levels of serotonin and its primary metabolite, 5-hydroxyindoleacetic acid, were decreased in the frontal pole, but the changes were not statistically significant due to the small number of animals and the large variation among individuals (Fig. 4). In contrast, the density of serotonergic type-2 (S2) receptors decreased significantly throughout the primate brain with age (Fig. 5). S2 receptors decreased most dramatically between the ages of 10 and 31 years. In particular, the density of S2 receptors in the parahippocampal gyrus decreased to nearly undetectable levels with aging. These data demonstrate a significant age-related decrease in the levels of cholinergic and serotonergic neurotransmitter markers in the brains of aging monkeys that parallels that reported for aging humans.

STUDIES IN RODENTS

Three cholinergic markers were examined in aging rodents (4-30 months). The level of ChAT activity and the density of muscarinic receptors, as determined by ^{3}H-quinuclidinyl benzylate (^{3}H-QNB) binding, decreased with age (Fig. 6). The age-related increase and the level of sodium-dependent high affinity choline uptake may be related to increased activity of the cholinergic cells that survive the aging process. As cholinergic cells degenerate with aging, the remaining cholinergic cells may become more active to compensate for the cell loss. This increased activity may in turn accelerate their degeneration (Horwitz, 1987).

The effects on behavior of the loss of cholinergic markers that is associated with aging can be examined by selectively destroying the basal forebrain neurons that provide cholinergic input to the cortex and hippocampus. The loss of these cells is associated with an impairment in learning and memory (For reviews of this literature, see Wenk

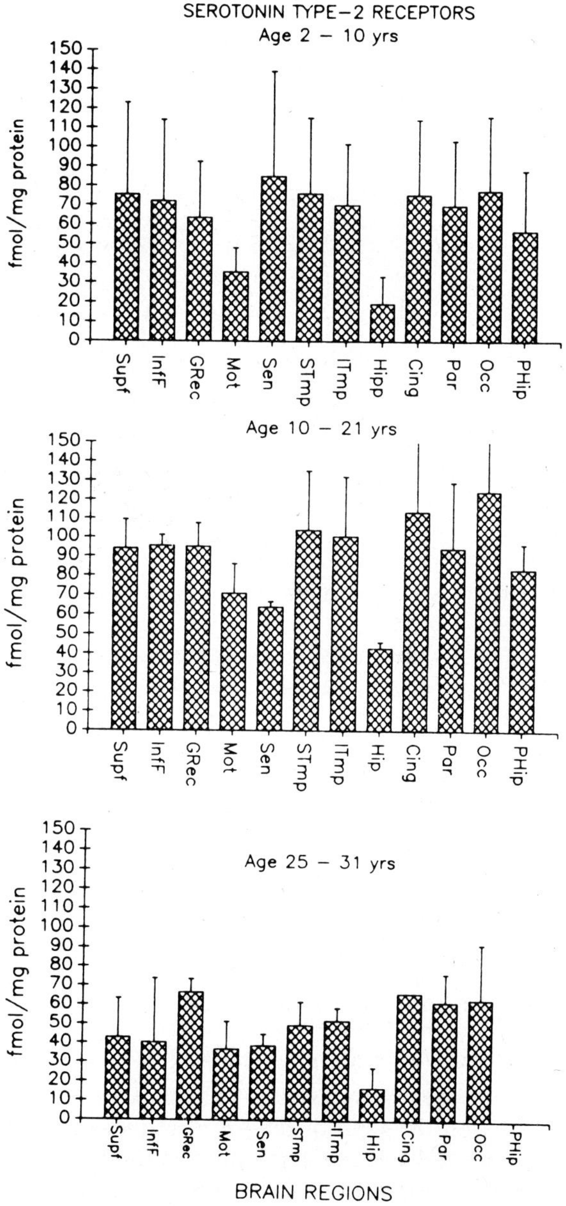

Figure 5. Age-related changes in the density of serotonergic type-2 receptors in the brain of rhesus monkeys.

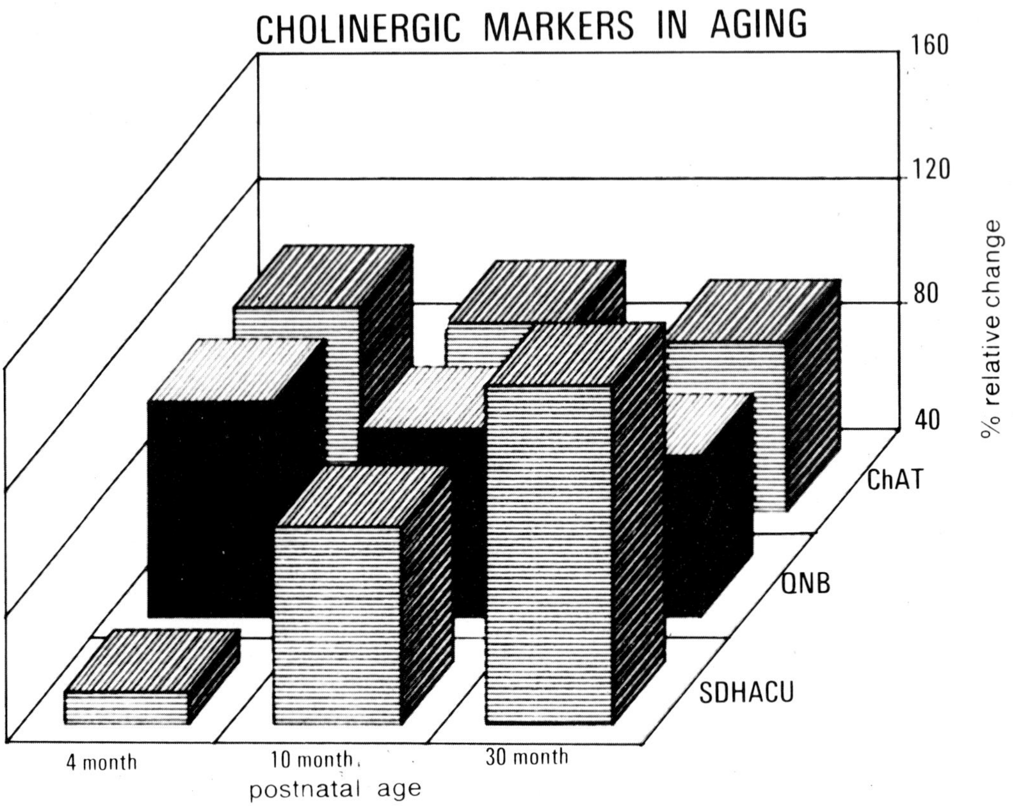

Figure 6. Age-related changes in choline acetyltransferase activity, muscarinic receptors (QNB) and sodium-dependent high affinity choline uptake in rodents.

and Olton, 1987; Olton and Wenk, 1987). Recent studies using this animal model support the hypothesis that cholinergic hypofunction is directly related to the amnesia observed in aging humans (Bartus et al., 1982).

We also investigated whether the loss of cholinergic and serotonergic neural systems can produce amnesia and whether these two neural systems interact to influence learning and memory. In order to reproduce the age-related loss of cholinergic and serotonergic markers, selective lesions were made using two neurotoxins. Ibotenic acid was injected into the basal forebrain to destroy cholinergic cells that project to the cortex and hippocampus (Wenk et al., 1984). Serotonergic cells in the midbrain raphe were destroyed by injecting 5,7-dihydroxytryptamine. After the rats recovered from the surgery, they were tested in a T maze alternation task (Wenk et al., 1987). Each rat was placed on the stem of the maze and was allowed to walk down the stem to the choice point of the T maze. Each rat was forced to one arm determined randomly on the first trial of 10 consecutive trials each day. After the rat ate the food at the end of the arm, it was returned to the stem for a variable interval (5, 3 or 60 seconds). For each subsequent trial, the food was placed in the arm not entered by the rat during the previous trial, and the rat was allowed to enter either arm. The optimal strategy for the rat was to remember the arm entered on the previous trial and enter the opposite arm on the present trial. Rats with basal forebrain cholinergic lesions were impaired at all intertrial delay intervals. Rats with raphe lesions were impaired only when the intertrial delay was 60 seconds. We concluded that the basal forebrain cholinergic system was involved in the performance of this task, and the raphe serotonergic system was only involved when task difficulty was high (Wenk et al., 1987).

When the rats with basal forebrain lesions were sacrificed four months after surgery, the following cholinergic and serotonergic changes were found (Wenk and Engisch, 1986; Wenk et al., 1986). ChAT activity was decreased significantly in the cortex and hippocampus and the density of S2 receptors in the cortex was increased significantly. The density of muscarinic receptors, as determined by ^{3}H-QNB, did not change. High affinity uptake of ^{3}H-serotonin into synaptosomes was decreased significantly (by 16%) in the frontal cortex but not in the hippocampus. These data suggest that long term changes in the serotonergic system can occur following the selective loss of basal forebrain cholinergic neurons. When similar basal forebrain cholinergic lesions were made in young rhesus monkeys, S2 receptor density increased throughout the cortex but not within the hippocampus (Wenk et al., 1986). The decrease in ChAT activity throughout various neocortical regions was correlated with the increase in S2 receptor density (Fig. 7).

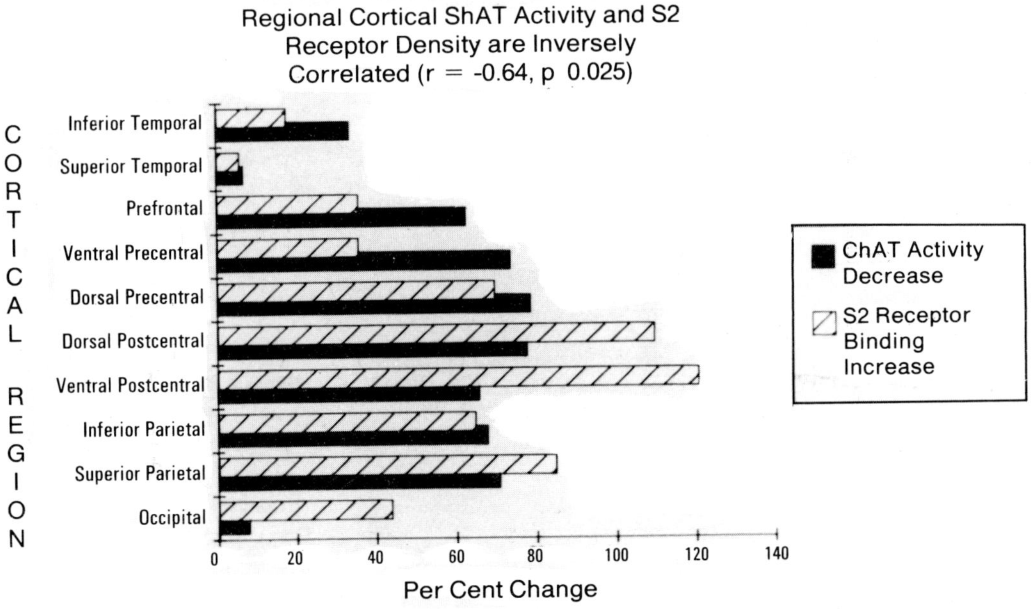

Figure 7. Correlation between the regional decrease in ChAT activity and increase in S2 receptors in the cortex of the rhesus monkey 11 months after basal forebrain lesions using ibotenic acid.

These biochemical and behavioral studies suggested that the serotonergic and cholinergic systems might interact to influence behavior. To test this hypothesis, lesions were produced in the basal forebrain cholinergic system and midbrain raphe. After the rats recovered from surgery, they were tested in the T-maze alternation task. The loss of basal forebrain cholinergic cells, but not raphe serotonergic cells, impaired performance in this task (Fig. 8). When both lesions were produced simultaneously, performance was similar to that in rats with the basal forebrain lesion alone. The data indicate that these two neural systems do not interact in any synergistic or antagonistic way to influence performance in this task.

These studies may have some clinical relevance to the age-related amnesia associated with Alzheimer's disease (AD). The loss of cholinergic and serotonergic markers was significant in patients who died with AD (Gottfries, 1981). Within the first year following the initial onset of the symptoms of dementia, cortical biopsy studies found a specific decrease in cholinergic presynaptic markers, including ChAT activity and high affinity choline uptake. The second detectable biochemical change was a loss of presynaptic serotonergic markers (Bowen and Davison, 1986; Francis et al., 1985; Palmer et al., 1987). The studies presented here suggest that the loss of cholinergic markers may not only precede the loss of serotonergic markers but may actually induce the loss of this neural system in AD and aging. Further, the behavioral studies suggest that the presence of amnesia during the early stages of AD may be due to the loss of cholinergic markers. As the changes in the serotonergic system proceed, following the

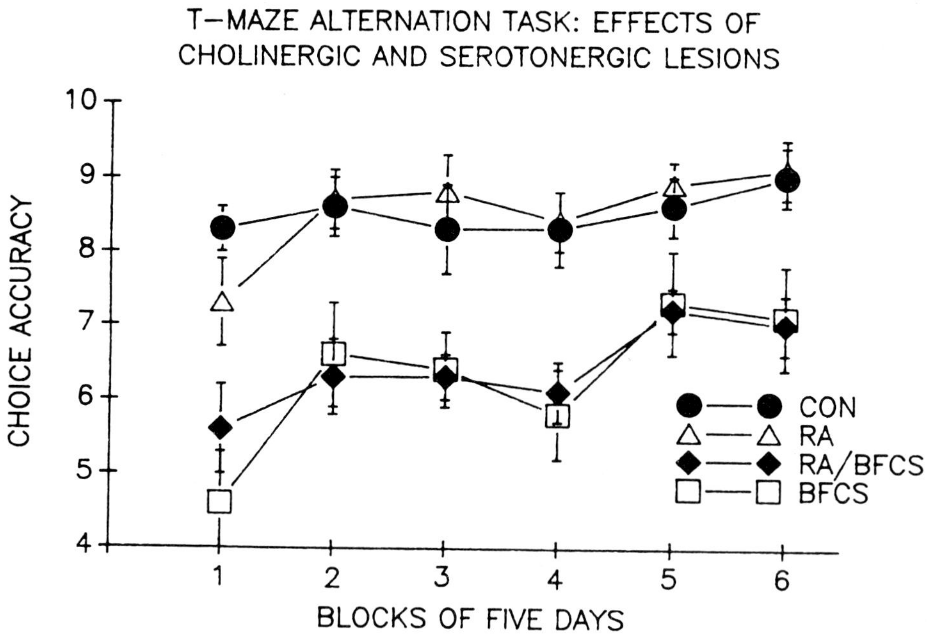

Figure 8. Performance of rats given lesions in the basal forebrain cholinergic system (BFCS), raphe (RA), or both, in the T-maze alternation task.

loss of cholinergic cells in the basal forebrain, there may be an exacerbation of the learning and memory impairment, as well as other changes, such as the hallucinations that can occur during the final stages of AD.

In summary, our studies confirm that the basal forebrain cholinergic system and midbrain serotonergic raphe degenerate with aging in primates and rodents. The loss of these systems may underlie some of the behavioral symptoms that are associated with aging. Although the cholinergic and serotonergic systems may not interact to influcence performance directly in the T-maze alternation task, they may interact in the control of other more complex behaviors. The two systems probably interact at a structural or biochemical level as indicated by the changes in the serotonergic system following the loss of basal forebrain cholinergic cells in the lesioned rodents or monkeys. The progression of these changes and the behavioral changes associated with them may provide a model of the progression of the dementia associated with Alzheimer's disease.

These data may also have therapeutic significance. Recent attempts to reverse the cognitive impairments associated with AD have augmented the cholinergic system by providing precursors for the production of acetylcholine, or by inhibiting the destruction of released acetylcholine. These therapies have been unsuccessful (Bartus et al., 1982). Patients with AD may benefit, however, from a therapeutic approach that manipulates cholinergic and serotonergic systems simultaneously.

ACKNOWLEDGMENTS

This research was supported in part by a grant from the U.S. Public Health Service (NIH AG 05146 and NS 20471). The authors thank D. Pierce and B. Cribbs for excellent technical assistance and R. Struble and L. Walker for dissection of the monkey brains.

REFERENCES

Bartus RT, Dean RL, Beer B, Lippa AS (1982) The cholinergic hypothesis of geriatric memory dysfunction. Science 217:408-417.

Bowen DM, Davison AN (1986) Biochemical studies of nerve cells and energy metabolism in Alzheimer's disease. Br Med Bull 42:1-7.

Folstein MF, Whitehouse PJ (1983) Cognitive impairment of Alzheimer disease. Neurobehav Toxicol Teratol 5:631-634.

Francis PT, Palmer AM, Sims NR, Bowen DM, Davison AN, Esiri MM, Neary D, Snowden JS, Wilcock GK (1985) Neurochemical studies of early-onset Alzheimer's disease. New Engl J Med 313:7-11.

Gottfries CG (1981) Levels of monoamines, monoamine metabolites, and activity of related enzyme systems correlated to normal aging and in patients with dementia of Alzheimer type. In: Corsini GU, Gessa GL (eds): Apomorphine and other dopaminomimetics, Vol. 2. Raven Press, New York, pp. 243-249.

Horwitz B (1987) Neuroplasticity and the progression of Alzheimer's disease. Brain Res, in press.

McGeer EG (1981) Neurotransmitter systems in aging and senile dementia. Prog Neuro-Psychopharmacol 5:435-445.

Olton DS, Wenk GL (1987) Dementia: Animal models of the cognitive impairments produced by degeneration of the basal forebrain cholinergic system. In: Meltzer HY (ed): Psychopharmacology: the third generation of progress. Raven Press, New York, pp. 941-953.

Palmer AM, Francis PT, Benton JS, Sims NR, Mann DMA, Neary D, Snowden JS, Bowen DM (1987) Presynaptic serotonergic dysfunction in patients with Alzheimer's disease. J Neurochem 48:8-15.

Wenk GL, Cribbs B, McCall L (1984) Nucleus basalis magnocellularis: Optimal coordinates for selective reductions of choline acetyltransferase in frontal neocortex by ibotenic acid injections. Exp Brain Res 56:335-340.

Wenk GL, Engisch KL, McCall LD, Mitchell SJ, Aigner TG, Struble RL, Price DL, Olton DS (1986) [^{3}H]Ketanserin binding increases in monkey cortex following basal forebrain lesions with ibotenic acid. Neurochem Int 9:557-562.

Wenk GL, Engisch KL (1986) [^{3}H]Ketanserin (serotonin type 2) binding increases in rat cortex following basal forebrain lesions with ibotenic acid. J Neurochem 47:845-850.

Wenk GL, Hughey D, Boundy V, Kim A, Walker L, Olton D (1987) Neurotransmitters and memory: The role of cholinergic, serotonergic and noradrenergic systems. Behav Neurosci 101:325-332.

Wenk GL, Olton DS (1987) Basal forebrain cholinergic neurons and Alzheimer's disease. In: Coyle JT (ed): Experimental models of dementing disorders: A synaptic neurochemical perspective. Alan Liss, New York, vol. 33, pp. 81-101.

Section III

NEUROIMMUNOLOGY

New Trends in Aging Research
G. Pepeu, B. Tomlinson, C.M. Wischik (eds)
Fidia Research Series, vol. 15
Liviana Press, Padova © 1988

NEUROENDOCRINE INFLUENCES ON THE IMMUNE SYSTEM IN AGING

Nicola Fabris

Chair of Immunology, Faculty of Medicine, University of Pavia, Pavia, Italy, and Immunol. Ctr., Gerontol. Res. Dept., Italian National Research Centres on Aging, I.N.R.C.A., Ancona, Italy

NEUROENDOCRINE INFLUENCE ON THE IMMUNE SYSTEM

It is generally accepted that although the immune system is regulated to a large extent by intrinsic cellular and humoral events, it is sensitive to signals from the immune network, namely those in the nervous and endocrine systems (Fabris, 1987; Fabris et al., 1987). This assumption is supported by two lines of experimental observation: first, that spontaneous or induced alterations in the neuroendocrine system may cause functional modifications in immune reactivity and, second, that receptor sites for many low molecular weight and protein hormones are present on the membrane of lymphoid cells.

As shown in Table 1, quite a high number of hormones, neurotransmitters and neuropeptides secreted by one neuroendocrine tissue or more, which may have a modulatory effect on the immune system, is likely to further increase in the future (Fabris, 1987).

The homeostatic circuits maintained through these factors are interdependent, and it is therefore hard to differentiate between the modulatory action of one of them free from that of the others. For the sake of clarity, we illustrate the regulatory action of the neuroendocrine system in relation to the network primarily involved: the central nervous system (CNS), the autonomous nervous system (ANS) and the endocrine system. The influence of psychosocial factors is also taken into consideration, because alterations in neuroendocrine balance can certainly be induced by macroenvironmental factors (Ader, 1981; 1984).

Table 1. *Neuroendocrines that may be involved immune functions*

Pituitary	Autonomic nervous system	Sensory ganglia	Brain Secretion
FSH LH - Gonadal steroids	Acetylcholine	Substance P	Pineal (Melatonin, others)
TSH - Thyroid hormones	Norepinephrine	Somatostatin	Somatostatin
ACTH	Serotonin	VIP	Fibroblast growth factor
Adrenocortical hormones	Somatostatin		Neurotensin
Vasopressin oxytocin	VIP		Bombesin
Neurophysin	Enkephalins		CCK
Beta-lipotropin	Substance P		Enkephalins
Beta-endorphin	Cholecystokinin		
Fibroblast growth factor			
Thymocyte growth factor			

Each of the four categories is controlled by the brain and may directly or indirectly provide feedback information to the brain.

Psychosocial Factors

The idea that extrinsic noxae may influence immune efficiency was first suggested on the basis of clinical and experimental observations which showed that psychological stress, such as that related to avoidance learning procedures, overcrowding and exposure to complex stimulations, might modify susceptibility to both viral and parasitic infections, to the development and course of experimentally induced tumors, and the serum levels of antibodies directed towards various antigens. Experimental research has also demonstrated that different immunological parameters such as primary and secondary immune responses, mitogen responsiveness, cytotoxic reactions, NK activity and interferon production may be increased and/or decreased in different stressful situations (Spector, 1983; Ader, 1984).

Similar phenomena have also been observed in humans; emotional situations, such as bereavement, are associated with immunodepression, even in the absence of dietary alterations or modifications in cortisone turnover. Hypnosis has also been found to influence the immune system: skin-positive patients may, under hypnosis, behave as if negative (Ader, 1983).

Since the central nervous system (CNS) is the primary organ that, through its peripheral sensory apparatus, filters most psychosocial information and coordinates (through the involvement of the hypothalamic regions), the most appropriate response, it is likely that it also mediates the psychosocially induced immunological modifications.

Central Nervous System (CNS)

The induction of electrolytic focal lesions in selected areas of the brain allows us to define the functional role of different brain formations, such as the hypothalamus, reticular formation, thalamus, superior colliculus, caudate nucleus and amigdaloid complex (Stein et al., 1976; Jsakovic, 1977; Jankovic, 1973); it has shown that only lesions in the hypothalamus and reticular formation induce depressed Arthus and delayed skin reactions to bovine serum albumin, together with a reduction in circulating antibody titers. Hypothalamic lesions also cause a reduction in spleen cellularity with the disappearance of germinal centers. A marked involution of the thymus is observed in brain lesioned rats irrespective of the area affected, although more pronounced changes have been documented in rats with lesions in the hypothalamic, reticular formation, and superior colliculus areas. Electric or mechanical stimulation, on the other hand, may also modify the immune efficiency, but only in few cases was it possible to demonstrate that its effect was the inverse of that obtained by the lesions to the same area (Korneva and Klimenko, 1976).

It is quite difficult to interpret these findings since interconnections between brain areas, the autonomic nervous system (ANS), and the endocrine system, which are known to influence the immune system, are complex and not well understood. Two main possibilities should be taken into account:

1) in the hypothalamic areas there are cells involved in programming the releasing factors that control the secretion of hypophyseal hormones; and

2) the same areas, in particular the anterior hypothalamus and reticular formation, are also involved in the central control of the ANS.

Endocrine System

The assumption that the endocrine system may have a consistent modulatory effect on immune functioning is now supported by a considerable amount of experimental evidence. All the endocrine glands appear to be involved, although a definite role has not yet been established for each hormone produced by them. This assumption is based on findings both from endocrine gland deprivation experiments (hypofunctional states) and successive reconstitution therapy, and from the exogenous administration of a given hormone in otherwise normal animals (hyperfunctional states) (Fabris, 1981). Further support comes from the identification of receptors for different hormones on the membrane of lymphoid cells. Specific binding has been documented for the somatotropic hormone, insulin, calcitonin, T3 and T4 and steroid hormones (Archer et al., 1973; Lesniak, 1974; Gavin III, 1977; Lemarchand-Beraud, 1977).

The effect of a single hormone, measured by the alterations induced in different immune parameters, may be positive or negative: it may enhance the efficiency of the immune system or reduce it. The developmental hormones, such as somatotropic hormone, thyroxine, and insulin have a positive effect. Depression of immune functions has been observed with gonadotropins, progesteroids and testosterone as well as with corticosteroids.

Due to the concomitant presence of both stimulator and antagonist hormones, the efficiency of the immune system at a given moment should be interpreted, therefore, as one permitted by the actual hormonal balance.

The hormonal action may vary in intensity, depending on the age of the animal: during development a higher hormonal supply or a more critical hormone concentration seems to be required than that needed in old age (Fabris, 1981a; 1981b). This is probably linked to the importance that some hormones have in the proliferation of lymphoid cells. The organism is more sensitive to modification of its hormonal balance during those periods of its life that are characterized by a high turnover of cells than during periods in which the proliferation is relatively low. Even in adulthood, however, a hormone-dependent modification of the immune efficiency may be demonstrable. Thus, dysendocrinopathies, such as hypo- and hyperthyroidism and diabetes, are associated both in animals and in man with substantial variations in the immune efficiency (Fabris, 1981b; Irvine, 1980). Of even greater interest is the fact that the distribution of the lymphocytes subset as well as the mitotic index of the thymus follows a circadian rhythmicity (Abo et al., 1980). Less well-known are the immune modifications associated with seasonal variations in the neuroendocrinal balance (Fabris, 1981b).

Hormones do not affect all kinds of lymphoid cells to an equal extent. On a functional basis, insulin and gonadotropins seem to act differently on humoral or cell-mediated immune responses. Many hormones are quite active in thymocyte differentiation while they are only required to an extremely limited extent by mature lymphocytes (Arrembrecht, 1974). This differential action may in certain instances be due to a different concentration of hormone receptor being on the surface of different lymphocyte subpopulations. Thus, insulin receptors are found in greater concentrations in B- than in T-cells (Gavin III, 1977). A grater somatotropic hormone binding occurs on thymocytes than on mature lymphocytes.

Moreover, even within different steps of the same immune response, the sensitivity to hormones may vary: thus, corticosteroids may play a positive role during the sensitization phase of the immune response, whereas in subsequent periods they are not required or may even be harmful (Stavy, 1974). Insulin receptors, which are not usually found on the membrane of lymphocytes capable of responding to Con A, appear during the early phase following mitogen stimulation (Krug et al., 1972).

Autonomic Nervous System (ANS)

The assumption that the lymphoid system is sensitive to the action of ANS is supported by two types of observation:

1) all lymphoid organs are innervated by ANS fibers (Spector, 1983); and

2) receptors for vasoactive amines have been found in the membranes of lymphoid cells both in humans and in laboratory animals (Hadden, 1977; 1983).

Regarding point 1), an innervation by the ANS has been demonstrated both in central lymphoid organs such as the thymus (Ghali et al., 1980) and bone marrow (Calvo, 1968) and in peripheral lymphoid tissues (Reilly et al., 1976; Kudoh et al., 1979). Similar nervous fibers have been found in the remaining lymphoid tissues and it has also been proven that any interruption of these fibers causes functional alterations both in cell-mediated and in humoral immune responses. Regarding point 2), receptors have been found on lymphoid cells; they can respond to stimuli from the parasympathetic system (acetylcholine-muscarinic), from the sympathetic system (norepinephrine-beta-adrenergics), from the neuro-adrenalinic system (epinephrine-beta-adrenergics) (Melmon, 1977), and from humoral mediators which are secreted in the course of inflammatory phenomena, such as E and F series prostaglandins, serotonin and histamine (H1 and H2). The receptors for these low-molecular-weight hormones are not present in all lymphocyte subpopulations. Beta-mimetic amines, histamine and prostaglandin E, as well as affecting the inflammatory process, act on both B- and

T-derived cells; in particular they inhibit both the cytolytic functions and the production of lymphokines by T-effector cells (antibody-dependent lymphocyte-mediated cytotoxicity also appears to be inhibited) and T-cell suppressor activity. They can also, with the exception of histamine, inhibit the B-cell production and release of specific antibodies.

On the other hand, cholinomimetic drugs, particularly of the muscarinic type, increase T-cell proliferation under mitogen stimulation and T-cell mediated cytolysis (Hadden, 1977; 1983).

These findings have been interpreted in the light of the role played by the cyclic nucleotides, cAMP and cGMP, in the physiological control of proliferation and differentiation of lymphocytes.

Neuro-hormonal action does not only affect peripheral cells (T, B, NK cells), it also may have an important effect on the thymus as a producer of hormonal factors. To investigate this possibility the circulating level of the "facteur thymique serique" (FTS), (Bach et al., 1972) more recently called thymulin in its zinc-bound form, was measured in different experimental and human disendocrinopathies (Fabris et al., 1983; 1985).

Figure 1 summarizes the data obtained in animals deprived of different endocrine glands, either because of a congenital absence, or because they had been excised or subjected to chemical blockade. Congenital hypopituitarism, experimental diabetes and thyroidectomy all cause a reduction in the thymulin plasma level, whereas removal of the gonads or of the adrenals induces no significant modification. Reconstitution experiments by means of substitutive hormonal therapy have demonstrated that the

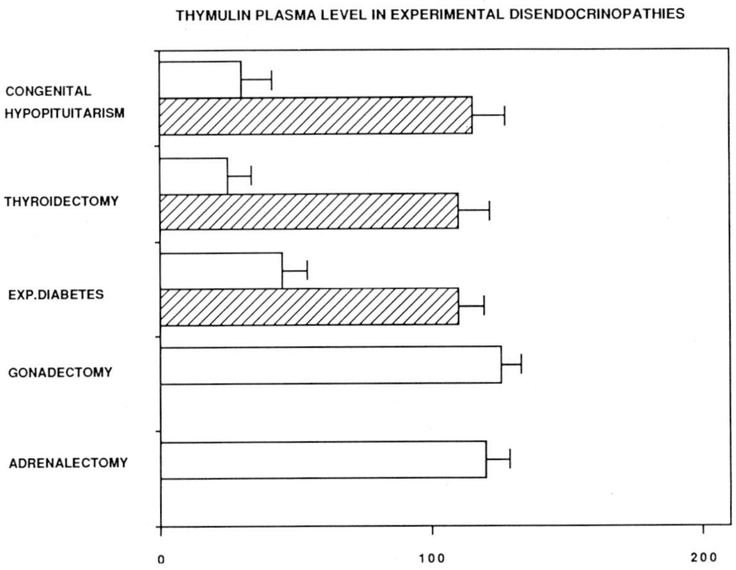

Figure 1. Reduced plasma thymulin concentration in different experimental endocrine imbalances (open columns) when compared to normal values (age-matched control = 100) and recovery of physiological levels (dashed columns) by means of appropriate therapy.

circulating level of thymulin returns to normal only a few days after initiation of the hormonal treatment (Fabris et al., 1985).

Also in humans, many dysendocrinopathies are associated with an alteration in circulating thymulin (Fig. 2). Thus congenital hypopituitarism and hypothyroidism following surgical thyroidectomy, are associated with a consistent reduction in the thymulin level, whereas hyperthyroidism, due to diffuse nodular goitre, is associated with high levels of thymulin; this is particularly evident in the aged, because in later life the physiological level of thymulin is usually quite low (Fabris et al., 1986). These data clearly confirm the finding made in mice that any modification in the turnover of different hormones may influence the synthesis and/or the secretion of thymulin.

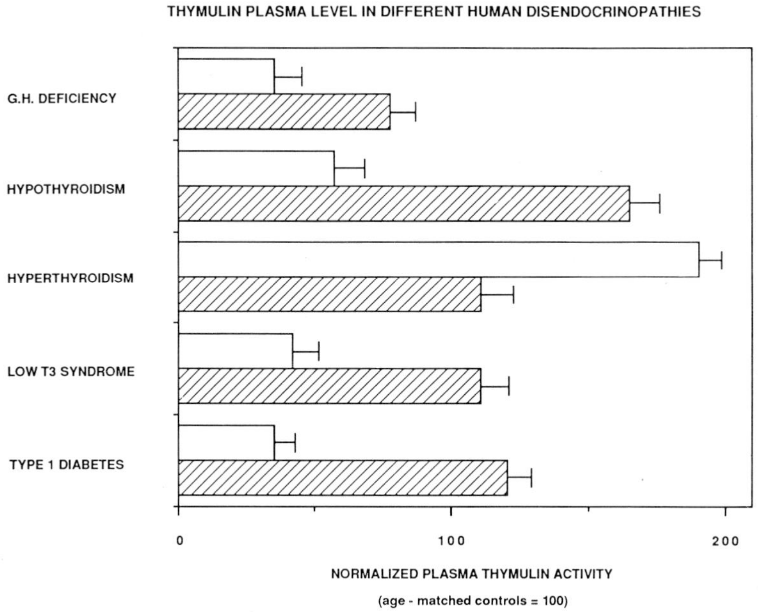

Figure 2. Modifications in plasma thymulin concentrations in different human dysendocrinopathies (open columns) when compared to normal values (age-matched controls = 100) and recovery of physiological levels (dashed columns) by means of appropriate therapy.

NEUROENDOCRINE-IMMUNE INTERACTION IN AGING

Our knowledge of neuroendocrine-immune systems interactions or the aging of neuroendocrine homeostasis is incomplete and any statement concerning the role that the latter might play in the aging of the immune system itself would appear to be almost totally speculative. It is likely, however, that a role in immunological aging should be ascribed to the complex regulatory mechanisms which, at least during development and maturity, have been shown to modulate some immune reactions. This assumption is supported by the following observations.

Some hormones and neurotransmitters seem to play a role in the aging of lymphoid cells (Dilman, 1978). It is generally accepted that with advancing age a decrease in thyroid-dependent body functions does occur although it is not necessarily revealed by modified serum levels of thyroid hormones. The assumption that modification of thyroid hormonc blood levels or their peripheral utilization may be responsible for some age-related immunodeficiencies is supported by other observations; in aged animals the exogenous administration of thyroxine can increase both the plaque-forming-cell capacity and the PHA response of the spleen cells (Fabris et al., 1982). These findings are in agreement with the observation that a progressive decline in peripheral conversion rate of T4 to T3 occurs with advancing age and that the exogenous injection of T4 may activate this conversion.

With advacing age a progressive decline in the concentration of membrane receptor for glucocorticoids has been documented in the spleen cell population (Roth, 1975). This alteration may depend either on an age-related modification of the ratio among various subsets of lymphoid cells carrying different receptor densities, or rather on an intrinsic failure of aged cells, which might be unable to maintain an adequate receptor molecules turnover. The age-related defect in cell receptors may be responsible for the altered functional responsiveness of old cells to the glucocorticoid action: the ability of these hormones to inhibit the metabolism of lymphoid cells is greatly reduced in old age (Roth, 1979).

Also with advancing age the concentration of membrane receptors for low-molecular-weight hormones on lymphoid cells shows alterations quite similar to those recorded for the glucocorticoid receptor (Schoken et al., 1977). It has been shown that the number of receptor molecules decreases with advancing age whereas the affinity does not seem to change. These findings, together with those obtained for glucocorticoid receptors in lymphoid cells and thosc documented in other systems of hormone-target cell receptor interaction, suggest that receptor loss is a generally age-related phenomenon, although the causes may vary depending upon the system under investigation. In the case of catecholamines, the reduced receptor density may represent, in fact, a compensatory phenomenon directed to adjusting cell responsiveness to the increased plasma hormone level (Ziegler et al., 1976).

It is here worthwhile to note that the intracellular level of both cAMP and cGMP increases with a consequent decline in the cAMP/cGMP ratio (Tan et al., 1978). Whether this imbalance is due to the alteration in the catecholamine receptor or to modifications in other hormonal balances, which may also affect the cyclic nucleotide pattern, has yet to be established.

Age-associated neuroendocrine alterations seem to also play a role in the progressive decline in thymulin production. The thymus, in fact, attains its maximum size at puberty, after which it starts to progressively involute, being replaced by fat. This process is nearly complete in man by the 5th to 6th decade: in the cortical areas there is lymphoid cell depletion and the epithelial cells show cystic changes and a reduction in intracellular granules.

The measurement of circulating levels of thymic factors has demonstrated that both in animals and in man the serum level of thymulin declines relatively early in life. It has been shown in rodents that thymulin is virtually undetectable in animals of over 15 months of age, and in man in individuals of over 50 years of age. Recent data from our laboratory, confirm these observations and, moreover, demonstrate that the thymus is not as involuted in the aged as might be deduced from the thymulin level. This assumption is based on the finding that in old age subjects the thymus can still produce FTS molecules, though to a lesser extent than in young subjects but a large proportion of these molecules are not biologically active because of the marginal zinc deficiency usually present in the elderly (Fabris et al., 1984).

The progressive decline in thymic endocrine activity with advancing age may be due either to alterations in epithelial cells which become unable to synthesize and/or release thymic factors or to alterations in the extrinsic mechanisms that seem to control the function of the endocrine epithelium. Experiments in mice have demonstrated that both intrinsic and extrinsic factors can play a role: in fact, thymuses from old mice, when grafted into adult thymectomized recipients, can partially restore the circulating thymulin level of the recipients, whereas newborn thymuses are less efficient in restoring the thymulin level in old recipients than in young adult thymectomized mice (Bach et al., 1979).

Direct experimental evidence that neuroendocrine factors are of primary relevance in this context comes from the recent observation that the circulating levels of thymulin can be restored in old mice by treating them with thyroxine, a hormone which, at least in mice, shows a progressive reduction in its turnover with advancing age. The recovery or thymulin secretion in old mice induces an increased functionality of the peripheral immune system as assessed by the reconstitution of the number of T-lymphocytes and of their responsiveness to mitogen stimulation; these are extremely low in aged mice (Fabris et al., 1982; 1985).

These data show that the microenvironmental effect on immunological aging has quite complex attributes, which may in the future be clarified by a coordinated interdisciplinary investigation.

ACKNOWLEDGMENTS

This study was supported in part by the "Consiglio Nazionale delle Ricerche", through grants Nos. 85.0555.56 and 86.01765.56 and by the Italian Ministry of Health through the "Progetto Finalizzato - Farmacologia Geriatrica" to I.N.R.C.A.

REFERENCES

Albo T, Kawate T, Hinuma S, Itoh K, Abo W, Sato J, Kumagai K (1980) The circardian periodicities of lymphocyte sub-populations and the role of corticosteroid in human beings and mice. In: Smolensky (ed): Recent advances in chronobiology of allergy and immunobiology. Pergamon Press, pp. 301-316.

Ader R (ed) (1981) Psychoneuroimmunology. Academic Press, New York.

Ader R (1984) Psychoneuroimmunology. In: Ballieux RE (ed): Breakdown in human adaptation to "stress", Vol. 2(3). Martinus Nijoff, Hingham, USA, pp. 653-670.

Archer JA, Gorden P, Gavin JR III, Lensniak MA, Roth J (1973) Insulin receptors in human circulating lymphocytes: application to the study of insulin resistance in man. J Clin Endocrinol Met 36:627-635.

Arrembrecht S (1974) Specific binding of growth hormone to the thymocytes. Nature 252:255-257.

Bach JF, Dardenne M, Papiernik M, Barvis A, Lavasseur P, Lebrand H (1972) Evidence for a serum-factor secreted by the human thymus. Lancet ii:1056-1058.

Calvo W (1968) The innervation of the bone marrow in laboratory animals. Am J Anat 123(2):315-322.

Dardenne M, Pleau JM, Nabama B, Lefancier P, Denien M, Choay J, Bach JF (1982) Contribution of zinc and other metals to the biological activity of the serum thymic factor. Proc Natl Acad Sci Usa 79:5370-5373.

Dilman VM (1978) Ageing, metabolic immunodepression and carcinogenesis. Mech Ageing Develop 8:153-164.

Fabris N (1981a) Body homeostatic mechanisms and aging of the immune system. In: Kay MMB, Makinodan T (eds): Immunology in Aging. CRC Press, Boca Raton, Florida, pp. 61-78.

Fabris N (1981b) Ontogenic and phylogenetic aspects of neuroendocrine-immune network. Develop and Comparat Immunol 5(Suppl 1):46-53.

Fabris N, Muzzioli M, Mocchegiani E (1982) Recovery of age-dependent immunological deterioration in Balb-c mice by short-term treatment with L-thyroxine. Mech Ageing Develop 18:327-338.

Fabris N, Garaci E, Hadden J, Mitchison NA (eds) (1983) Immunoregulation. Plenum Press, pp. 1-477.

Fabris N, Mocchegiani E (1985) Endocrine control of thymic serum factor in young-adult and old mice. Cell Immunol 91:325-335.

Fabris N, Mocchegiani E, Mariotti S, Pacini F, Pinchera A (1986) Thyroid function modulates thymus endocrine activity. J Clin Metab 62:474-478.

Fabris N, Mocchegiani E, Amadio L, Zanotti M, Licastro F, Franceschi C (1984) Thymic hormone deficiency in normal ageing and Down's syndrome; is there a primary failure of the thymus. Lancet i:983-986.

Fabris N, Mocchegiani E, Muzzioli M, Provinciali M (1988) Neuroendocrine-thymus interactions: perspectives for intervention in aging. In: Pierpaoli W, Spector NH (eds): Neuro-immunomodulation: interventions in aging and cancer. Annals NY Acad Sci, pp. 145-157.

Fabris N (1988) In: Nelson D (ed): Hormones and natural immunity. Academic Press, New York, in press.

Gavin JR III (1977) Polypeptide hormone receptor on lymphoid cells. In: Hadden JW, Coffey RG, Spreafico F (eds): Immunopharmacology, Comprehensive Immunology, No. 3. Plenum Press, New York, pp. 357-373.

Ghali WM, Abdel-Rahman S, Hagib M, Mahran ZY (1980) Intrinsic innervation and vasculature of pre- and post-natal human thymus. Acta Anat 108:115-125.

Hadden JW (1977) Cyclic Nucleotides in Lymphocyte proliferation and differentiation. In: Hadden JW, Coffey RF, Spreafico F (eds): Immunopharmacology, Comprehensive Immunology No. 3. Plenum Press, New York, pp. 1-30.

Hadden JW (1983) Cyclic nucleotides and related mechanisms in immune regulation: a mini review. In: Fabris N, Garaci E, Hadden J, Mitchison NA (eds): Immunoregulation. Plenum Press, New York, pp. 201-230.

Irvine J (ed) (1980) Immunology of diabetes. Teviot Scientific Publications, Edinburgh.

Isakovic K, Jankovic BD (1973) Neuroendocrine correlates of immune response. II. Changes in the lymphatic organs of brain lesioned rats. Int Arch Allergy 45:373-380.

Jankovic BD, Isakovic K (1973) Neuroendocrine correlates of immune response. I. Effects of brain lesions on antibody production, Arthus reactivity and delayed hypersensitivity in the rat. Int Arch Allergy 45:360-70.

Korneva EA, Klimenko VM (1976) Neuronale hypotalamusaktivitat und homostatische reactionen. Ergeb Exp Med 23:373-78.

Krug U, Krug F, Cuatrecacas P (1972) Emergence of insulin receptors on human lymphocytes during in vitro transformation. Proc Nat Acad Sci USA 9:2604-08.

Kudoh G, Hoshi K, Murakami T (1979) Fluorescence of microscopic and enzyme histochemical studies of the innervation of the human spleen. Arch Hitol Jap 42(2):169-76.

Lemarchand-Beraud T, Hom AC, Scazziga BR (1977) Triidothyronine and thyroxine nuclear receptors in lymphocytes from normal, hyper and hypothyroid patients. Acta Endocrinol 85:44-49.

Lesniak MA (1974) Binding of I-125 human growth hormone to specific receptors in human cultures lymphocytes: characterization of the interaction and sensitivity of radioreceptor assay. J Biol Chem 249:1661-68.

Melmon KL, Weinstain J, Poon TC, Bourne MR, Shearer GM, Coffino P, Insel PA (1977) Receptors for low-molecular-weight hormones on lymphocytes. In: Hadden JW, Coffey RG, Spreafico F (eds): Immunopharmacology, Comprehensive Immunology, Vol. 3. Plenum Press, New York, pp. 331-50.

Reilly FD, Mc Cuskey RS, Meineke HA (1986) Studies of the hemopoietic microenvironment. VIII. Adrenergic and cholinergic innervation of the murine spleen. Anat Rec 185:109-115.

Roth GS (1975) Age related changes in glucocorticoid binding by rat splenic leukocytes: possible cause of altered adaptive responsiveness. Fed Am Soc Biol 34:183-187.

Roth GS (1979) Hormone action during aging: alterations and mechanisms. Mech Ageing Develop 9:479-487.

Shocken DD, Roth GS (1987) Reduced beta adrenergic receptor concentrations in aging man. Nature (London) 267:856-858.

Spector NH (1983) Anatomical and physiological connections between central nervous and the immune systems. In: Fabris N, Garaci E, Hadden J, Mitchison Na (eds): Immunoregulation. Plenum Press, London, pp. 231-258.

Stavy L (1974) Stimulation of rat lymphocyte proliferation by hydrocortisone during the induction of cell-mediated immunity in vitro. Transplantation 17:173-178.

Stein M, Schiavi RC, Camerino M (1976) Influence of brain and behaviour on the immune system. Science 191:435-38.

Tam CF, Walford RL (1978) Cyclic nucleotide levels in resting and mitogen-stimulated spleen cell suspensions from young and old mice. Mech Aging Develop 7:309-318.

Ziegler Mg, Lake Cr, Koping IJ (1976) Plasma noradrenaline increases with age. Nature (London) 261:333-335.

New Trends in Aging Research
G. Pepeu, B. Tomlinson, C.M. Wischik (eds)
Fidia Research Series, vol. 15
Liviana Press, Padova © 1988

IMMUNOPATHOLOGICAL ASPECTS OF SENILE BRAIN AMYLOIDOSIS

Frans C. Stam, Johanna M Rozemuller and Piet Eikelenboom

Department of Neuropathology, Pathology Institute, Academic Hospital, Free University, Postbus 7057, 1007 MB Amsterdam, the Netherlands

In 1927 Divry demonstrated that the centre of many senile plaques has the histochemical properties of amyloid. In his opinion the deposition of amyloid in the neuropil should be the start of the plaque formation. In later stages astrocytes proliferate around the periphery of the central amyloid core. Furthermore, in this periphery degenerating and regenerating neurites are found (Simchowicz, 1911).

Divry characterized the neuropathological changes in senile dementia and Alzheimer's disease as a disseminated miliary-amyloidosis. Later on, congophilic angiopathy was included in this concept (Scholz, 1938; Pantelakis, 1954). According to Wisniewski and Terry (1973) it should be unlikely that deposition of amyloid forms the initiating factor in the formation of senile plaques. According to these authors amyloid deposition is secondary to neuritic degeneration.

Wigboldus (1959), Stam (1965) Schwartz (1970) and Eikelenboom (1982), on the contrary, supported the vision of Divry. The opinion of Wisniewski and Terry was briefly formulated in the concept of the neuritic plaque. This term has been widely accepted and is still beloved by investigators studying specific transmittor systems. In 1981, however, Wisniewski et al. concluded from their studies of experimental scrapie disease in mice that whatever causes the local amyloid production is simultaneously responsible for neuritic degeneration.

Senile plaques progress through a series of stages (Wigboldus, 1959; Stam, 1965; Terry and Wisniewski, 1970). The central amyloid core can finally be resolved (Wigboldus, 1959; Stam, 1965; Shelanski, 1970; Brun and Englund, 1981) leaving empty glial nests ore disciform densifications of the neuropil.

Senile brain amyloidosis is not restricted to human pathology, it is also found in old dogs and monkeys (Schwartz, 1965; Selkoe, 1987). In order to get some basic information about the prevalence and incidence of senile brain amyloidosis in man, Stam et al. (1986) examined 1400 successive autopsies in general and mental hospitals. The authors did not find senile plaques in 184 autopsies of patients under the age of 50 years. In 41% of 1216 autopsies of people aged over 50 years of life senile plaques were found, whereas congophilic angiopathy was found in 13.5% of cases. Linear regression analysis strongly suggested that senile brain amyloidosis increases linearly with age.

There was a statistically significant difference between females and males. Congophilic angiopathy did not show this difference. In the last decade of life the prevalence of congophilic angiopathy was even higher in males. Study of the clinical records of the patients with senile plaques revealed the number of clinical manifestations of senile dementia in this population (Fig. 2). In total, 59% of males and 55% of females with senile plaques had a clinical manifestation of dementia. Linear regression analysis, again, revealed that senile dementia linearly increases with age. The difference between males and females was also statistically significant.

The etiology of senile brain amyloidosis is still elusive. We even do not know if this type of amyloidosis is an expression of normal aging or an age related manifestation of a distinct pathological process. Glenner et al. (1972; 1973) supposed that senile amyloid is the result of degradation of immunoglobulins in lysosomes. Mumenthal (1976) attributed senile brain amyloidosis to a failure of the adaptive immune response for the removal of deviant neurons. Behan and Behan (1979) concluded that different indexes in literature suggest that the immune system may be involved in the pathogenesis of Alzheimer's disease. The possibility that senile brain amyloid is derived from immunoglobulins seemed to be supported by the demonstration of immunoglobulins in senile plaques (Stam, 1965; Ishii, 1975; Powers et al., 1981).

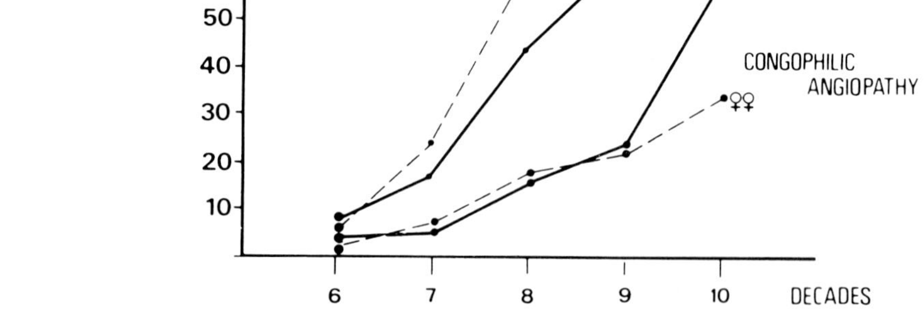

Figure 1. Senile brain amyloidosis linear increase with age.

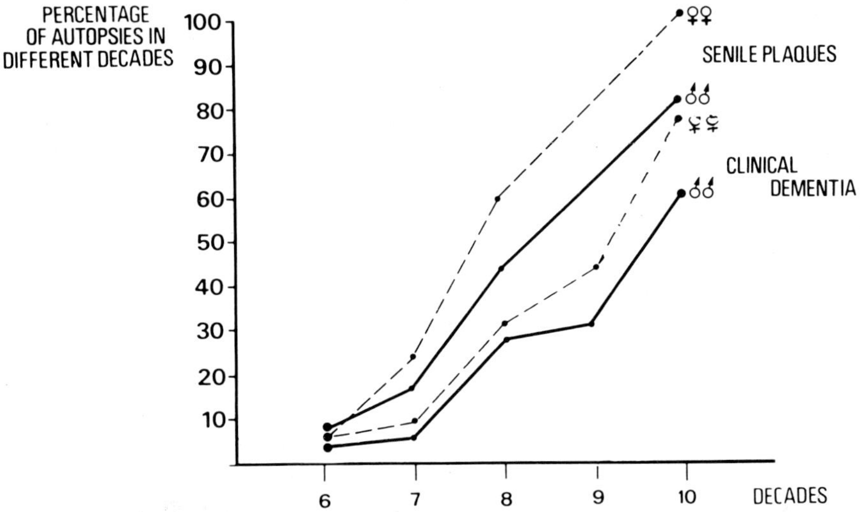

Figure 2. Clinical manifestation of dementia in patients with senile brain amyloidosis.

Continuing studies in our laboratory revealed that positive reactions with antisera against immunoglobulins could only be obtained in formol fixed paraffin sections. In unfixed brains tissue no immunoglobulins or light chains could be detected (Stam and Eikelenboom, 1985; Table 1). These findings were in accordance with the results of the chemical analysis of isolated plaque cores (Kidd et al., 1985). Goust et al. (1984)

Table 1. *Immunohistochemical differences between unfixed frozen sections and formol fixed paraffin sections*

	Unifixed frozen sections		Formol-fixed paraffin material	
	amyloid angiopathy	amyloid core of senile plaques	amyloid angiopathy	amyloid core of senile plaques
IgG (Y-specific)	—	—	—	+
Kappa	—	—	—	+
Lambda	—	—	—	++
Fibrinogen	—	—	—	++
P component	+ or ±	—	—	—
Prealbumin	—	—	—	—
AA amyloid	—	—	—	—
C_1q	—	+	—	— or ±
C_3c	—	+	—	— or ±

+ = Positive; ± = weakly positive.

demonstrated that immunoglobulins, which can be eluted from brain tissue at neutral pH are probably not bound to tissue antigens by their Fab fragment, while the immunoglobulins eluted at acid pH may reflect immunologic binding. In cases of senile brain amyloidosis only the neutral eluates contained significant amounts of IgG, which were usually polyclonal.

A very remarkable finding in our study was the presence of complement factors in the amyloid core of senile plaques. These factors could also be found in congophilic vessels if the sections were stained without delay. The absence of immune complexes and properdin in senile plaques made it clear that the activation of complement factors in senile brain amyloid is due to an unusual cause. Around the amyloid core of senile plaques non neuronal cells can be found. According to Wisniewski et al. (1981) these non neuronal cells belong to the microglial system. The authors were of the opinion that the amyloid in the plaques is made by these cells. The concept of the microglia, however, is still under discussion. For a long time the predominant view was that microglial cells form a phagocytic system specific to the brain. In the last decade many authors have shown that the so called reactive microglial cells belong to the monocyte-macrophage system. Fujita and Kitamura (1976) concluded from their study that all phagocytes in the brain are derived from the blood and suggested that monocytes invading the brain may transform into microglial cells. Oehmichem and Huber (1976) have pointed out that the so called reactive microglia is characterized by the activity of non specific esterase and by membrane markers identical with those of monocytes. Do the glial cells around amyloid cores in senile plaques show these membrane markers? Immunohistochemical studies of cases of senile brain amyloidosis in our laboratory revealed that the glial cells around the amyloid cores in senile plaques did not show the membrane markers of blood derived phagocytes (Table 2). The cells around the amyloid cores had often hyperchromatic nuclei and sometimes showed lipofuscin in their

Table 2. *Immunohistochemical properties of glial cells around amyloid cores of senile plaques*

Embedding	Antibody	Predominant specifity	Results
f	OKIa	HLA-DR	+/—*
f	DAKO LC	leucocytic lineage	—
f	a-C-3brec	C3b-receptor	—
f	a-Leu M3	monocytes, phagocytes	—
f	MO1	idem	—
f	FK24	idem	—
f	5D2	part of macrophages	—
p	1-anti chymotrypsin	histiocytes	—
p	a-lysozyme	monocytes and reactive histiocytes	—
p	lectin WGA	macrophages	—

p= paraffin sections; f= frozen sections; *the same pattern of reaction was found in neuroglial cells.

perikaryon. This light microscopical aspect is in accordance with the "regressive glial cells" described by Spielmeyer (1922).

Up to this time the histochemistry of senile amyloid brings little support for the hypothesis that senile amyloidosis is the result of an autoimmune response. A possible support was found in the demonstration of circulating brain reactive antibodies. Daar and Fabre (1981) demonstrated an almost universal incidence of multiple autoantibodies in normal individuals. In every normal serum they found organ-specific IgM antibodies to brain, liver and heart. Robinson et al. (1984) have demonstrated that Epstein-Barr virus-transformed lymphocytes from normal individuals produce multiple auto-antibodies that react with diverse antigens. This viral effect demonstrates that damage of the target organ is not required for the production of organ-specific autoantibodies. B-lymphocytes from Alzheimer patients in the nature of the case show an identical reaction (Simpson et al., 1986). Another general aspect of autoantibodies is their increase with age (Hallgren et al., 1973; Goodwin et al., 1982).

Nandy (1972) found an increase of brain reactive antibodies with age in sera of mice. In 1978 he demonstrated brain reactive antibodies in human sera and found higher levels of antibodies in Alzheimer patients than in age-matched controls. Watts et al. (1981) also found antibodies against specific neural cell types in sera and cerebrospinal fluid of Alzheimer patients, patients suffering from other neurological disorders and normal controls. The authors found varying degrees of surface staining of neurons with both sera and cerebrospinal fluid within all groups.

Fillit et al. (1985) reported that sera from a subpopulation of Alzheimer patients react with cholinergic areas of normal rat and human brain. These antibodies were not found in age matched controls. Antibodies against neurofibrillary tangles were found by Felicia Gaskin et al. in 1987. These antibodies were also found in normal controls. The highest frequency of the antibodies, however, was found in Alzheimer patients. The significance of the above mentioned autoantibodies with regard to the pathogenesis of Alzheimer's disease in still elusive. In any case cerebral immune responses are only possible when there is a dysfunction of the blood-brain barrier.

In normal conditions the blood-brain barrier effectively impedes the access of antibodies to the brain (Aarli, 1983). Consequently, an auto-immune response can only be initiated by a dysfunction of this barrier. Wisniewski and Koslowski (1982), using immunohistochemical techniques, found albumin and globulin in senile plaques, neuroglial cells and neuronal perikarya in the cortex of Alzheimer patients. The authors suggested that these findings illustrate a dysfunction of the blood-brain barrier. In our laboratory we could not confirm these findings. We have examined 28 cases of Alzheimer's disease and 31 age matched controls. In 13 cases of the Alzheimer group no, or only a few, neurons showed a positive reaction with antialbumin, antiglobulin and antifibrinogen sera. Of the 31 control cases, 20 showed the same pattern of reaction. In 15 cases of the Alzheimer group and 11 control cases positively stained clusters of neurons were found. The senile plaques within these clusters were usually also stained, whereas outside of these clusters no stained cells or plaques were found. In frozen unfixed sections the results were very variable. The amyloid cores of senile plaques, however, were always negative. From these results we concluded that serumproteins are absent in the amyloid cores and may be present in clusters of cortical neurons in Alzheimer patients and in age matched controls. We had the impression, however, that the clusters of staining neurons were somewhat greater in Alzheimer patients. These results do not support the hypothesis of an Alzheimer-specific dysfunction of the blood-brain barrier. The results are much too inconsistent.

On the basis of their positron emission tomographic studies, Frieland et al. (1983) came to the conclusion that in Alzheimer's disease there is a normally impermeable blood-brain barrier for rubidium, a small ion. Altogether, it is very unlikely that a dysfunction of the blood-brain barrier allows circulating antibodies or immunoglobulins to enter the brain and to initiate immune responses and deposition of senile amyloid. The amyloid cores of senile plaques have been isolated and sequenced in several laboratories (Anderton, 1987). It appeared that the protein component of senile amyloid is an aggregated polypeptide with a subunit mass of 4 kd, the so called A4 monomer (Colin Masters et al., 1985).

Recently, it became evident that the A4 is of neuronal origin and is the cleavage product of a larger precursor protein. This precursor contains features of glycosylated cell surface receptors (Kang et al., 1987). The A4 amino acid sequence is encoded by a gene located on human chromosome 21. This scientific breakthrough has revealed that senile amyloid is of neuronal origin. It can no longer be held that immunologic factors play a major role in the pathogenesis of senile amyloidosis with or without clinical manifestations of dementia.

REFERENCES

Aarli JA (1983) The immune system and the nervous system. J Neurol 229: 137-154.

Anderton BH (1987) Alzheimer's disease, progress in molecular pathology. Nature 325: 658-659.

Behan PO, Behan WMH (1979) Possible immunological factors in Alzheimer's disease. In: Glen AIM, Whalle LJ (eds): Alzheimer's disease early recognition of potentially reversible deficits. Churchill Livingstone, Edinburgh, London, New York, p. 35.

Brun A, Englund E (1981) Regional pattern of degeneration in Alzheimer's disease. Histopathology 5: 549-564.

Daar AS, Fabre JW (1981) Organ specific IgM autoantibodies to liver heart and brain. Clin Exp Immunol 45: 37-47.

Divry G (1927) Étude histo-chémique des plaques séniles. Journal Belge de Neurologie et de Psychiatrie 27: 643-657.

Eikelenboom P, Stam FC (1982) Immunoglobulins and complement factors in senile plaques. Acta Neuropathol (Berl) 57: 239-242.

Fillit H, Luine VN, Reisberg B, Amador R, Mc Ewen B, Zebriskie JB (1985) Studies on the specifity of antibrain antibodies in Alzheimer's disease. In: Senile dementia of the Alzheimer type. Alan Riss Inc, pp. 307-318.

Frieland RP, Yukio Yano, Budinger ThF, Ganz E, Huesman RH, Derenzo SE, Knittel E (1983) Quantitative evaluation of blood-brain barrier integrity in Alzheimer-type dementia. Emission tomographic studies with Rubidium-82. Europ Neurol 22 (suppl): 19-20.

Fujita S, Kitamura T (1976) Origin of brain macrophages and the nature of microglia. In: Zimmerman HM (ed): Progress in Neuropathology, Vol III. Grune and Stratton, New York, pp 1-50.

Gaskin F, Kingsley BS, Shu Man Fu (1987) Autoantibodies to neurofibrillary tangles and brain tissue in Alzheimer's disease. J Exp Med 165: 245-250.

Glenner GG, Terry WD, Isersky (1973) Amyloidosis, its nature and pathogenesis. Semin Hematol 10: 65-82.

Goodwin JS, Searks RP, Tung KSK (1982) Immunological responses of a healthy elderly population. Clin Exp Immunol 48: 403-410.

Goust JM, Mangren M, Powers JM (1984) An immunologic assessment of brain associated IgG in senile brain amyloidosis. J Neuropathol and Exp Neurol 43: 481-488.

Hallgren HM, Buckley CE, Gilbersten VA, Yunis EJ (1973) Lymphocyte phytohemagglutinin responsiveness, immunoglobulins and autoantibodies in aging humans. J Immunol 111: 1101-1107.

Ishii T, Haga S, Shimuzu F (1975) Identification of components of immunoglobulins in senile plaques by means of fluorescent antibody technique. Acta Neuropathol (Berl) 32: 157-162.

Kang J, Lemaire HG, Unterbeck A, Salbaum M, Masters CL, Grzeschik KH, Multhaup G, Beyreuther C, Müller-Hill B (1987) The precursor of Alzheimer's disease amyloid A4 protein resembles a cell-surface receptor. Nature 325: 733-736.

Kidd M, Allsop D, Landon M (1985) Senile plaque amyloid. Modern approaches to the dementias. F. Clifford Rose des Karger, London, pp. 114-126.

Masters CL, Multhaup G, Simms G, Pottgiesser J, Martins RN, Beyreuther K (1985) Neuronal origin of a cerebral amyloid: neurofibrillary tangles of Alzheimer's disease contain the same protein as the amyloid of plaque cores and blood vessels. The EMBO Journal (4) 11: 2757-2763.

Mumenthal HT (1976) Immunological aspects of the aging brain. In: Terry RD, Gershan S (eds): Neurobiology of Aging. Raven Press, pp. 313-334.

Nandy K (1972) Brain-reactive antibodies in mouse serum as a function of age. J Gerontol 27: 173-177.

Nandy K (1978) Brain-reactive antibodies in aging and senile dementia. In: Katzman R, Terry RD, Bick KL (eds): Aging, vol 7. Raven Press, New York, pp. 503-512.

Oehmichen M, Huber H (1976) Reactive microglia with membrane features of mononuclear phagocytes. J Neuropath Exp Neurol 35: 30-39.

Pantelakis S (1954) Un type particulier d'angiopathie sénile du système nerveux centrale. Mschr Psych Neurol 128:219-256.

Powers JM, Schlaepfer WW, Willingham MC, Hall BJ (1981) An immunoperoxidase study of senile brain amyloidosis with pathogenetic considerations. J Neuropath Exp Neurol 6:592-612.

Robinson JE, Stevens KC (1984) Production of autoantibodies. Clin Immunol Immunopathol 33:339-350.

Schattner A (1987) The origin of autoantibodies. Immunology Letters 14:143-153.

Scholz W (1938) Die drusige Entartung der Hirnarterien und Kapillaren. Zschr ges Neurol Psych 140:333-397.

Schorlemmer HU, Davies P, Allison AC (1976) Ability of activated complement components to induce lysosomal enzyme release from macrophages. Nature (5555) 261:48-49.

Selkoe DJ, Bell DS, Podlinsny MB, Price DL, Cork CL (1987) Conservation of brain amyloid proteins in aged mammals and humans with Alzheimer's disease. Science 235:873-876.

Schwartz P (1970) Amyloidosis: cause and manifestation of senile deterioration. Thomas Springfield 1L.

Shelanski ML (1970) In: Wolstenholme G and O'Connor M (eds): Alzheimer's disease and related conditions. Churchill Livingstone, Edinburgh, pp. 249-261.

Simchowicz T (1911) Histologische Studien über die Senile Demenz. Hist und Histopath Arbeiten Fr Nissl (ed) IV: 267-444.

Simpson J, Boyd JE, Janice E, Yates CM, Christie JE, Fink G, James K, Gordon A (1986)

Autoantibodies to Alzheimer and normal brain structures from virus-transformed lymphocytes. J of Neuroimmunol 13:1-8.

Spielmeyer W (1922) Histopathologie des Nervensystems I. Julius Springer Berlin, pp. 149-156.

Stam FC (1965) Histochemistry of senile involution of the brain. Proc 5th Intern Foundation, Amsterdam, New York, London, Milan, Tokyo, Buenos Aires, pp. 513-517.

Stam FC, Wigboldus JM, Smeulders AWM (1986) Age incidence of senile brain amyloidosis. Path Res Pract 181:558-562.

Stam FC, Eikelenboom P (1985) Senile amyloid. In: F Clifford Rose (ed): Modern Approaches to the Dementias S. Karger, London, pp. 127-130.

Watts H, Kennedy PGE, Thomas M (1981) The significance of anti-neuronal antibodies in Alzheimer's disease. J Neuroimmunol 1:107-116.

Wigboldus JM (1959) Over de aard en genese van seniele plaques. Dissertatie Amsterdam VU. Dijkstra's Drukkerij Groningen.

Wisniewski HM, Koslowski PJ (1982) Evidence for blood-brain barrier changes in senile dementia of the Alzheimer type. Ann Acad Science 396:119-129.

Wisniewski HM, Terry RD (1973) Re-examination of the pathogenesis of the senile plaque. Progress in Neuropathology 2:1-26. Ed HM Zimmerman.

Wisniewski HM (1981) Evidence for induction of localized amyloid deposits and neuritic plaques by an infectious agent. Annal Neurol 10:517-522.

Wood JG, Mirra SS, Pollock NJ, Binder LJ (1986) Neurofibrillary tangles of Alzheimer's disease share antigenic determinants with the axonal microtubule-associated protein tau. Proc Natl Acad Sci USA 83:4040-4043.

New Trends in Aging Research
G. Pepeu, B. Tomlinson, C.M. Wischik (eds)
Fidia Research Series, vol. 15
Liviana Press, Padova © 1988

THYMOSIN α_1: A SYNTHETIC IMMUNOTRANSMITTER THAT INDUCES RECOVERY OF T CELL FUNCTIONS IN AGING

Gino Doria and Daniela Frasca

Laboratory of Pathology, ENEA C.R.E., Casaccia, C.P. 2400,
00100 Roma A.D., Italy

There is increasing evidence that the nervous and the immune systems are functionally interconnected. Both systems are critically involved in the ability of the organism to respond to environmental changes so that homeostasis can be maintained. The high level of versatility of both the immune system and the central nervous system (CNS) suggests the existence of a complex network involving different cell types, structures and molecules able to transmit and to receive bidirectional signals. Activated immune cells are able to emit messages addressed to the brain or to other brain-related systems, so that the CNS may receive signals from immune responses under way. On the other hand, through innervation of some lymphoid tissues (thymus) the CNS may respond by emitting chemical signals with regulatory function, such as acetylcholine, dopamine, norepinephrine, epinephrine, serotonin, γ-aminobutyric acid, glutamate, glycine, and neuropeptides (met-enkephalin, leu-enkephalin, substance P, neurotensin, angiotensin II, somatostatin, etc.). All these molecules act as neurotransmitters at the synapses, where they are released and destroyed, and as neuroregulators which are also released from nerve terminals but then diffuse locally to influence a large number of receptor-bearing cells. Besides, the immune system is able to autoregulate its response by several mechanisms such as antibody feedback, idiotype-anti-idiotype network, and regulatory cells and molecules. Cells of the immune system, in particular lymphocytes, express receptors for an unusually large number of different hormones and other cell-to-cell mediators. Results from several laboratories show that peripheral lymphoid cells are responsive to signals released by the CNS, thymus, adrenals and other endocrine

---

Abbreviations: CNS, central nervous system; IL-1, interleukin 1; IL-2, interleukin 2; NK, natural killer.

glands. Many effects of these signals are mediated by intracellular second messengers, such as Ca^{++} ions and cyclic nucleotides.

The endocrine system and the CNS are physically and functionally interconnected by the hypothalamus, which in turn is directly connected to the pituitary gland by the pituitary stalk. The bridging function of the hypothalamus is exerted by cells that have properties of both nerve cells and endocrine cells and for this reason are called neurosecretory cells. These hypothalamic cells can be stimulated by other nerve cells located in higher regions of the brain to secrete specific peptide hormones into the blood vessels of the pituitary stalk. Such hormones then specifically stimulate or suppress the secretion of other hormones from the pituitary. Many of the pituitary hormones regulated by the hypothalamus in this way stimulate other endocrine glands to secrete their hormones.

Several examples document that the neuroendocrine system influences immune responses. Enkephalin and endorphins increase a variety of immune functions, including human NK (natural killer) activity and lymphocyte proliferation to suboptimal mitogen stimulation (Wybran, 1985). The expression of MHC cass II molecules and the production of interleukin 1 (IL-1) by macrophages (Snyder and Unanue, 1982), as well as lymphokine release by T cell clones (Kelso and Munck, 1984), are inhibited by glucocorticoids. The neurohypophyseal hormones arginine vasopressin and oxytocin are able to satisfy the interleukin 2 (IL-2) requirement for immune interferon production by mitogen-activated murine spleen cells (Johnson and Torres, 1985). Insulin and the growth hormone potentiate T lymphocyte activation (Snow, 1985).

The immunopeptides acting on the CNS are defined as immunotransmitters (Hall et al., 1985) and their biological activities are listed in Table 1. Many investigations have

Table 1. *Immunotransmitters are molecules produced by the immune system which are also biologically active in the central nervous system*

Immunotransmitter	Biological activity
Thymosins	Stimulate the production of: — ACTH — Prolactin — LH — GH — β-endorphin
Interleukin 1	Stimulates thermoregulatory centers Stimulates slow-wave sleep
Interleukin 2	Stimulates the production of ACTH Decreases brain levels of norepinephrine Stimulates glial cells
α-interferon	Induces lethargy and depression
C 3a	Modulates feeding behaviour
ACTH	Stimulates the production of corticosteroids
TSH	Stimulates thyroid function
β-endorphin	Induces insensitivity to pain

been addressed to understanding the biological role of thymosins. One of the most studied is thymosin α_1, a 28 amino acid residues peptide with thymic hormone-like activity. Thymosin α_1 was the first peptide to be purified, sequenced (Goldstein et al., 1977) and synthesized (Goldstein, 1978) by solution or solid phase methods (Wang et al., 1979) and by recombinant DNA technology (Wetzel et al., 1980), among the several peptides present in the calf thymus extract denominated Fraction 5. Several tests performed both *in vivo* and *in vitro* have shown that thymosin α_1 is 10-1000 times more active than Fraction 5 in promoting T cell differentiation.

Several studies were carried out in our laboratory to investigate immunological effects of synthetic thymosin α_1. Results showed that injection of immunodeficient old mice with thymosin α_1 recovers to a significant extent helper T cell activity, IL-2 production and IL-2 receptor expression by spleen cells (Frasca et al., 1986). These biological activities are restricted to the first 14 amino acids of the thymosin α_1 molecule. Table 2 shows the results of four independent experiments in which spleen cells from aging (3-18 month old) mice, primed with Horse Red Blood Cells (HRBC) 4 days before culture, were assayed for helper T cell activity, IL-2 production and IL-2 receptor expression. Mice were left uninjected or injected with 10 μg thymosin α_1, 5 μg N_{14}

Table 2. *Enhanced helper T cell activity, IL-2 production and IL-2 receptor expression by spleen cells from aging mice injected with thymosin peptides*

Exp. No.	Age (months)	Treatment	Helper T cell activity	IL-2 production	IL-2 receptor expression
1	3	none	100	100	100
	3	α_1 (10 μg)	107	78	93
	3	N_{14} (5 μg)	106	82	77
	3	C_{14} (5 μg)	116	84	95
2	3	none	100	100	100
	6	none	57	47	25
	6	α_1 (10 μg)	74	87	99
	6	N_{14} (5 μg)	104	85	66
	6	C_{14} (5 μg)	59	23	18
3	3	none	100	100	100
	12	none	53	52	0
	12	α_1 (10 μg)	81	71	89
	12	N_{14} (5 μg)	114	78	134
	12	C_{14} (5 μg)	43	28	9
4	3	none	100	100	100
	18	none	43	0	23
	18	α_1 (10 μg)	74	47	82
	18	N_{14} (5 μg)	86	99	81
	18	C_{14} (5 μg)	46	0	0

Results are expressed as percent of 3-month-old untreated controls.

(N-terminal amino acid residues 1-14) or 5 μg C_{14} (C-terminal amino acid residues 15-28) synthetic fragment of the thymosin α_1 molecule, 3 days before HRBC priming. Results indicate that helper T cell activity, IL-2 production and IL-2 receptor expression are impaired by aging but are restored to a large extent by a single injection of 10 μg thymosin α_1. Injection of an equimolar amount of the N_{14} fragment is at least as effective as the entire molecule in restoring these T cell activities, whereas injection of the C_{14} fragment has no demonstrable effect. It is noteworthy that thymosin and its N_{14} fragment are effective when injected in 6, 12 and 18 month old mice, but not in 3 month old mice. Our data support the possibility that the thymosin α_1-induced enhancement of helper T cell activity in old mice results from an increase in the T cell precursor frequency.

Results from limiting dilution analysis of T cell precursors (Table 3) indicate that injection of thymosin α_1 or its N_{14} fragment 3 days before the assay increases the frequency of mitogen responsive T lymphocytes in old, but not in young mice, whereas injection of the C_{14} fragment is devoid of any effect in both young and old mice. Thus, thymosin α_1 amplifies the pool of T cell precursors in immunodeficient old mice.

Our studies on the T cell precursor frequency were performed on spleen cells which comprise an extrathymic T cell pool of mature T cells and immature T cells undergoing the final maturation steps (Weissman et al., 1975; Stutman, 1978; Scollay et al., 1984). The effects observed after the short time interval between the injection of thymosin peptides and the assay are likely due to induced proliferation of mature T cells rather than to enhanced T cell maturation (Frasca et al., 1987). This rapid amplification of the

Table 3. *Precursor frequency of proliferating T cells from mice of different ages uninjected or injected with thymosin peptides*

Exp. No.	Age (months)	Treatment	Precursors per 10^4 cells
1	3	none	27 (1.35)
	3	α_1 (10 μg)	41 (1.28)
	19	none	9 (1.65)
	19	α_1 (10 μg)	23 (1.38)
2	3	none	79 (1.21)
	3	N_{14} (5 μg)	91 (1.20)
	19	none	24 (1.37)
	19	N_{14} (5 μg)	95 (1.19)
3	3	none	42 (1.28)
	3	C_{14} (5 μg)	51 (1.25)
	20	none	11 (1.57)
	20	C_{14} (5 μg)	13 (1.51)

Numbers in parentheses are error factors by which precursor frequencies should be multiplied or divided to obtain the variations due to one standard error.

mature T cell compartment is a biological effect of practical value for the therapy of age-related T cell immunodeficiency.

In conclusion, our results altogether demonstrate the possibility of repairing T cell functions in aging mice by injection of thymosin peptides. These findings are very promising as they suggest possible applications of these immunotransmitters to prevent or treat immune disorders in the elderly.

ACKNOWLEDGMENTS

Work supported by ENEA-Euratom Contract and Pasteur Institute - Cenci Bolognetti Foundation. It is publication No. 2405 of the Euratom Biology Division.

REFERENCES

Frasca D, Adorini L, Doria G (1987) Enhanced frequency of mitogen-responsive T cell precursors in old mice injected with thymosin α_1. Eur J Immunol 17:727-730.

Frasca D, Adorini L, Mancini C, Doria G (1986) Reconstitution of T cell functions in aging mice by thymosin α_1. Immunopharmacology 11:155-163.

Goldstein AL (1978) Thymosin: basic properties and clinical potential in the treatment of patients with immunodeficiency diseases and cancer. Antibiotics Chemother 24:47-59.

Goldstein AL, Low TLK, Mc Adoo M, Mc Clure J, Thurman GB, Rossio J, Lai CY, Chang D, Wang SS, Harvey C, Ramel AH, Meienhofer J (1977) Thymosin α_1: isolation and sequence analysis of an immunologically active thymic polypeptide. Proc Natl Acad Sci USA 74:725-729.

Hall NR, Mc Gillis JP, Spangelo BL, Goldstein AL (1985) Evidence that thymosins and other biologic response modifiers can function as neuroactive immunotransmitters. J Immunol 135:806s-811s.

Johnson HM, Torres BA (1985) Regulation of lymphokiné production by arginine vasopressin and oxytocin: modulation of lymphocyte function by neurohypophyseal hormones. J Immunol 135:773s-775s.

Kelso A, Munck A (1984) Glucocorticoid inhibition of lymphokine secretion by alloreactive T lymphocyte clones. J Immunol 133:784-791.

Scollay R, Bartlett P, Shortman K (1984) T cell development in the adult murine thymus: changes in the expression of the surface antigens Ly-2, L3T4 and B2A2 during development from early precursor cells to emigrants. Immunol Rev 82:79-104.

Snow EC (1985) Insulin and growth hormone function as minor growth factors that potentiate lymphocyte activation. J Immunol 135:776s-778s.

Snyder DS, Unanue ER (1982) Corticosteroids inhibit murine macrophage Ia expression and interleukin 1 production. J Immunol 129:1803-1805.

Stutman O (1978) Intrathymic and extrathymic T cell maturation. Immunol Rev 42:138-184.

Wang SS, Douvan Kulesha I, Winter DP (1979) Synthesis of thymosin α_1. J Am Chem Soc 101:253-254.

Weissman IL, Masuda T, Olive C, Friedberg SH (1975) Differentiation and migration of T lymphocytes. Is Med Sci 11:1267-1269.

Wetzel R, Heyneker KL, Goeddel DV, Jhurani P, Shapiro J, Crea R, Low TLK, Mc Clure JE, Thurman GB, Goldstein AL (1980) Production of biologically active N^{α}-desacetylthymosin α_1 in E. coli through expression of a chemically synthesized gene. Biochemistry 19:6096-6104.

Wybran J (1985) Enkephalins and endorphins as modifiers of the immune system: present and future. Fed Proc 44:92-94.

New Trends in Aging Research
G. Pepeu, B. Tomlinson, C.M. Wischik (eds)
Fidia Research Series, vol. 15
Liviana Press, Padova © 1988

CSF FROM SUBGROUPS OF ALZHEIMER AND PARKINSON PATIENTS CONTAIN ANTIBODIES RECOGNIZING NEURONS IN CHOLINERGIC AND DOPAMINERGIC AREAS IN THE RAT BRAIN

A. McRae-Degueurce, S. Bööj[1], K. Haglid[1], L. Rosengren[1], J.E. Karlsson[1], I. Karlsson[2], A. Wallin[2], L. Svennerholm[2], C.G. Gottfries[2], A. Dahlström[1]

INSERM 259 Bordeaux, France; [1]Institute of Neurobiology, and [2]St Jörgens Hospital, Göteborg, Sweden

INTRODUCTION

This study reports the initial stages of an ongoing investigation to be conducted over several years as a joint effort between the Institute of Neurobiology and the Department of Psychiatry and Neurochemistry at St Jorgen's hospital in Göteborg. The results here presented indicate that, at some stage in the course of pathological events in demented or aging brains, autoimmune mechanisms may come into play. This was, of course, suggested earlier for instance by Ingram et al. (1974) and Mayer et al. (1984), who reported the presence of antineuronal antibodies in the serum of patients with Alzheimer's disease (AD). Also, the amyloid in senile plaques, one of the morphological hallmarks of AD, has been found to be rich in IgG as shown by Ishii and Haga (1976) and as also demonstrated to us by Dr Stam (this volume). If an immunological response occurs in the brain, be it a primary pathogenic or a secondary event, the antibodies should in this case be present not only in the serum but also, and above all, in the

---

Abbreviations: ACh, acetylcholine; AChE, acetylcholine-esterase; AD, Alzheimer's disease; CSF, cerebrospinal fluid; DA, dopamine; MBS, metabisulfate; NA, noradrenaline; PD, Parkinson's disease; SDAT, senile dementia of the Alzheimer type; 5HT, serotonin.

cerebrospinal fluid (CSF) of the diseased patient. The aim of this study was therefore to establish whether the CSF of patients with Parkinson's disease (PD) or AD contains antibodies which recognize specific neuronal populations in the CNS.

The investigation started in 1985, at the meeting of the International Society for Neurochemistry in Riva, Italy, where a poster was presented by Leon et al. (1985); it reported on the death of dopaminergic nerve cells in tissue culture caused by the addition of serum from a PD patient to the culture medium. It was here that Amanda McRae-Degueurce (A.M.D.) and Annica Dahlström (A.D.) met. The latter had worked in Bordeaux for several months together with M. Geffard and his group at the U 259 lab, INSERM and the team had developed a special technique for fixing small transmitter molecules in the central nervous system. A.D. and A.M.D. reasoned as follows: "if serum can do this to dopaminergic nerve cells, what could then CSF do?" A.D. invited A.M.D. to Göteborg where he worked in collaboration with a group of clinicians active in the freezing of samples of CSF from various types of neurological patient for research purpose. When A.M.D. came to Göteborg last year, the ideas were presented to Professor Gottfries and Professor Svennerholm who decided that some CSFs available in the freezer should be tested. When the initial results were available (see below) the immunology/biochemistry group at the Institute of Neurobiology, lead by Dr. Kenneth Haglid, was contacted, and since then it has been actively engaged in the study.

METHODOLOGICAL ASPECTS

The prerequisite for this study is the special perfusion technique, developed by A.M.D. and Michel Geffard (1986), which uses a combination of allyl alcohol at pH 11 and glutaraldehyde (4 or 5%). The mixture fixes small transmitter molecules like dopamine (DA), acetylcholine (ACh) and serotonin (5HT) in the tissue so that they do not diffuse. To demonstrate DA, NA or 5HT with any of the specific rabbit produced antisera against these transmitter molecules, the group in Bordeaux has developed the perfusion mixture so that glutaraldehyde alone can be used. However, to study the localization of ACh, the ad-mixture with allyl alcohol is essential.

This is demonstrated in Figure 1, which shows the presence and localization of NA in the locus coeruleus using the anti-NA antibodies, of 5-HT-immunoreactive neurons in the raphe region, using the anti-5HT antibodies, and also demonstrating a DA-immunoreactive nerve cell in the substantia nigra, using the DA-antiserum. The final figure shows the presence of an ACh-like immunoreactivity in nerve cell bodies of the medial forebrain of the rat.

Our hypothesis, based on the poster of Leon et al. (1985), was that antibodies in the serum used by Leon and coworkers could have a toxic effect on the dopaminergic neurons in the tissue culture. Since earlier attemps to find specific antibodies had failed (e.g. Jonker et al., 1982) we thought that the hypothetically aggressive antibodies might recognize the small transmitter molecule itself, or the transmitter molecule attached to some carrier molecule. As we believed the special perfusion technique would here be useful, we perfused the rat brain with the mixture (5% glutaraldehyde and allyl alcohol). After 15 minutes' postfixation, thorough rinsing in PBS with TRIS-meta-bisulfate (MBS) buffer and sucrose, the brains were frozen and cryostat sectioned at 10 μm. We

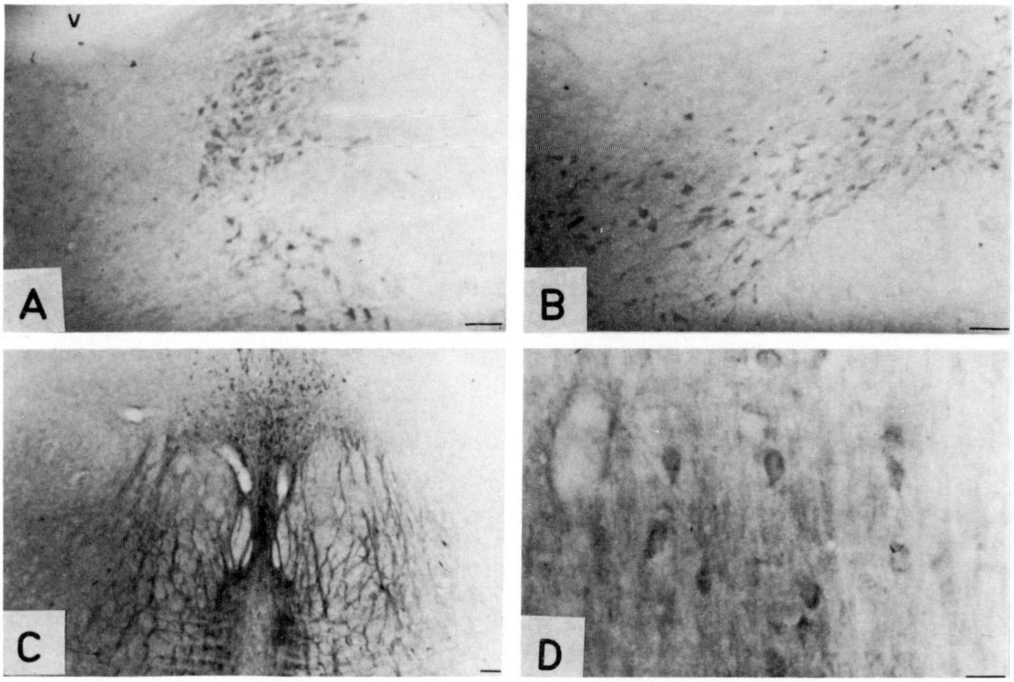

Figure 1 A-D. Photomicrographs of frontal vibratome (50 μm) sections from the same brain following a perfusion of allyl alcohol-glutaraldehyde at pH 12 in a cacodylate buffer. The sections were incubated overnight at 4°C with their respective antibodies and processed for PAP immunocytochemistry. A: Noradrenergic immunoreactive neurons in the locus coeruleus. NA antibody dilution 1/2000. Bar = 100 μm. B: Dopaminergic cell bodies in the pars compacta of the substantia nigra. DA antibody dilution 1/3000. Bar = 100 μm. C: Serotoninergic immunoreactive cell bodies and processes in the raphe dorsalis. 5-HT antibody dilution 1/10,000. Bar = 100 μm. D: Cholinergic immunoreactive cell bodies in the medial septum. ACh antibody dilution 1/1000. Bar = 250 μm.

chose the medial septum or spinal cord for the study of AD patients because of the presence in these areas of cholinergic nerve cell bodies. To study PD patients we cut sections through the mesencephalon to see if substantia nigra neurons could be labeled by the CSF of the patients. As it was essential to compare the picture obtained with CSF and that obtained after labelling DA- or ACh-neurons, neighbouring sections were incubated overnight (at 4°C) *either* with the specific rabbit-produced anti-ACh antiserum or rabbit anti-DA antiserum, *or* with the CSF from AD or PD patients, diluted to a 1:1 ratio. In the next incubation step, biotin-labelled goat-anti-human IgG was used for the CSF-incubated sections, while biotin-labelled goat-anti-rabbit IgG was layered over the sections which were incubated with rabbit-anti-ACh, or rabbit-anti-DA antisera.

The immunocytochemical reaction was then visualized with the avidin peroxidase complex method. The sections were then dehydrated and mounted in Entellan, and examined in a Nikon Optiphot microscope with a bright field condensor.

PARKINSON PATIENTS

When studying the CSF from the PD patients (which were the first CSFs studied) we found that in some of the patients the CSF contained a factor which clearly labelled cell bodies located in the ventral tegmental area of the rat brain (Mc Rae-Degueurce et al., 1986). Some of the patients, however, were negative and failed to show any substance recognizing these cell populations, while others had a weak immunoreaction (Fig. 2). PD is known to be caused by degeneration of the nigro-striatal pathway (see Hornykiewicz, 1977) and our results therefore seemed to indicate that the CSF of the "positive patients" contained a factor which recognized an epitope in neurons in the mesencephalic tectal area of the rat brain. In one patient we obtained CSF on two occasions at a two-year interval studied not only sections from the mesencephalon, but also from the medial forebrain. The first CSF did not show cholinergic cell bodies in the rat basal forebrain, only cells in the ventral tegmental area. However, the CSF removed from the patient two years later presented not only mesencephalic neurons, but also neurons in the basal forebrain, indicating that the disease had progressed.

ALZHEIMER PATIENTS

The etiology of AD is unknown; it may be multifaceted and many transmitter systems may be involved (Price et al., 1986). However, most investigations indicate that cholinergic neurons in the forebrain are involved; their numbers are clearly reduced in AD patients (e.g. Coyle et al., 1983; Mash and Potter, 1983). When the study was extended to AD patients, we therefore tried to ascertain whether the CSF of these patients might contain a factor that recognizes these cholinergic neuron populations in the ventral forebrain, according to the hypothesis of cholinergic involvement in AD. In a subgroup of patients who had a diagnosis of AD/SDAT, on the basis of the DSM III-criteria, we found that the CSF contained a factor which could clearly label neuronal cell bodies located in the ventro-medial septal area, an area known to contain cholinergic nerve cell bodies (Fig. 3A). Some patients' CSFs gave no markage whatsoever, as shown in Figure 3B. Also motor perikaryons in the rat spinal cord were marked (see McRae-Degueurce et al., 1987).

Identification of Labelled Neurons

In order to establish whether the neurons recognized by the CSF factor of the AD patients were indeed cholinergic cell bodies, the following experiment was undertaken. Three consecutive sections of rat forebrain were incubated with 1) the patient's CSF or 2) stained for the ACh-esterase (AChE) (Koelle, 1955) or 3) incubated with the A31-antiserum against ACh. The same cell group is labelled by all three procedures (Fig. 4A-C).

In the three consecutive sections we identify individual neurons. The section in

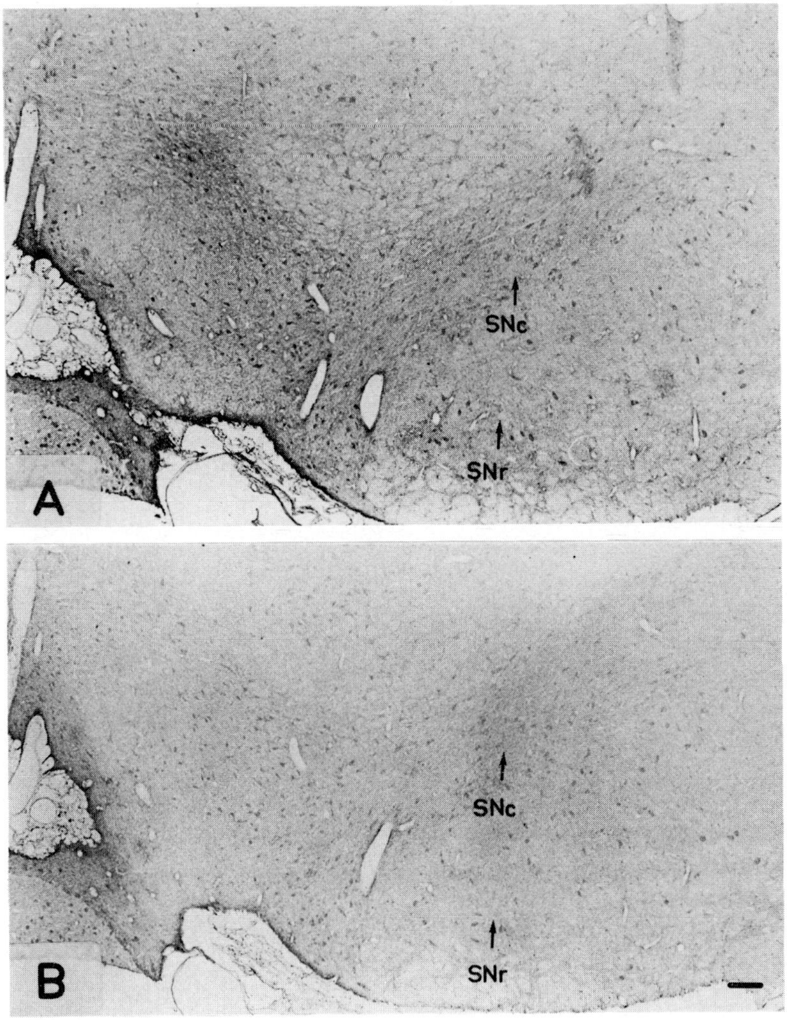

Figure 2. Photomicrographs of frontal cryostat (10 μm) sections of the substantia nigra region following incubation with CSF of Parkinson's patients. A: Immunoreactive neurons are noted in the pars compacta of the substantia nigra following incubation with the CSF from this PD patient. B: The immunocytochemical reaction following incubation with the CSF of this PD patient is weaker than that in A. Biotinylated anti-human IgG was employed as the secondary antibody. Bar = 100 μm.

Figure 4A was incubated with the patient's CSF, the second section (Fig. 4B) was stained for AChE and the third (Fig. 4C) section was stained with the ACh antibody. These sections are about 10 microns thick so there is a chance that the same neuron will be in all three consecutive sections. The arrows indicate neurons that are identified in all three sections. Some neurons can be seen in two consecutive sections (arrows). This

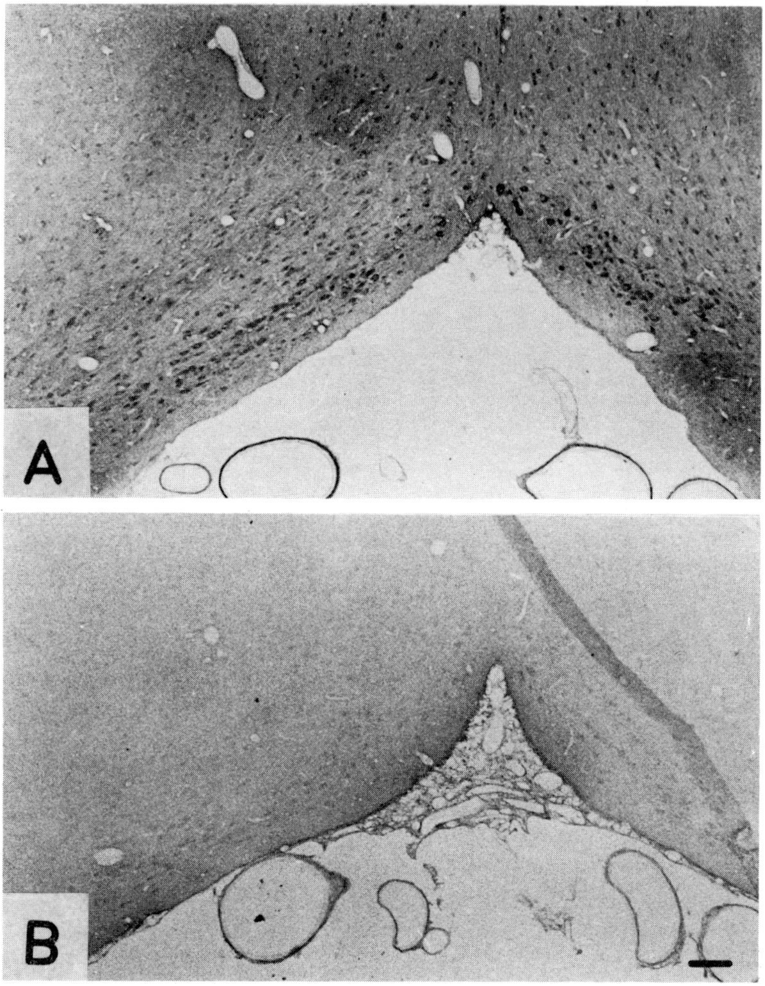

Figure 3. Photomicrographs of frontal cryostat sections of the rodent medial septum region. The brain sections were incubated with the CSF from two AD patients. A: Numerous immunoreactive neurons in the medial septum and diagonal band are noted following incubation with the CSF from this patient. B: With this patient virtually no staining in the medial septum region was observed following incubation CSF. Bar = 100 μm.

identification of neurons suggests that the CSF factor in this particular patient indeed recognized the cholinergic cell bodies in the rat brain.

Attempts to Identify the Recognized Epitope

Based on the hypothesis that the factor in the CSF recognized an ACh-like epitope, the following experiment was performed using sections made through the rat lumbar

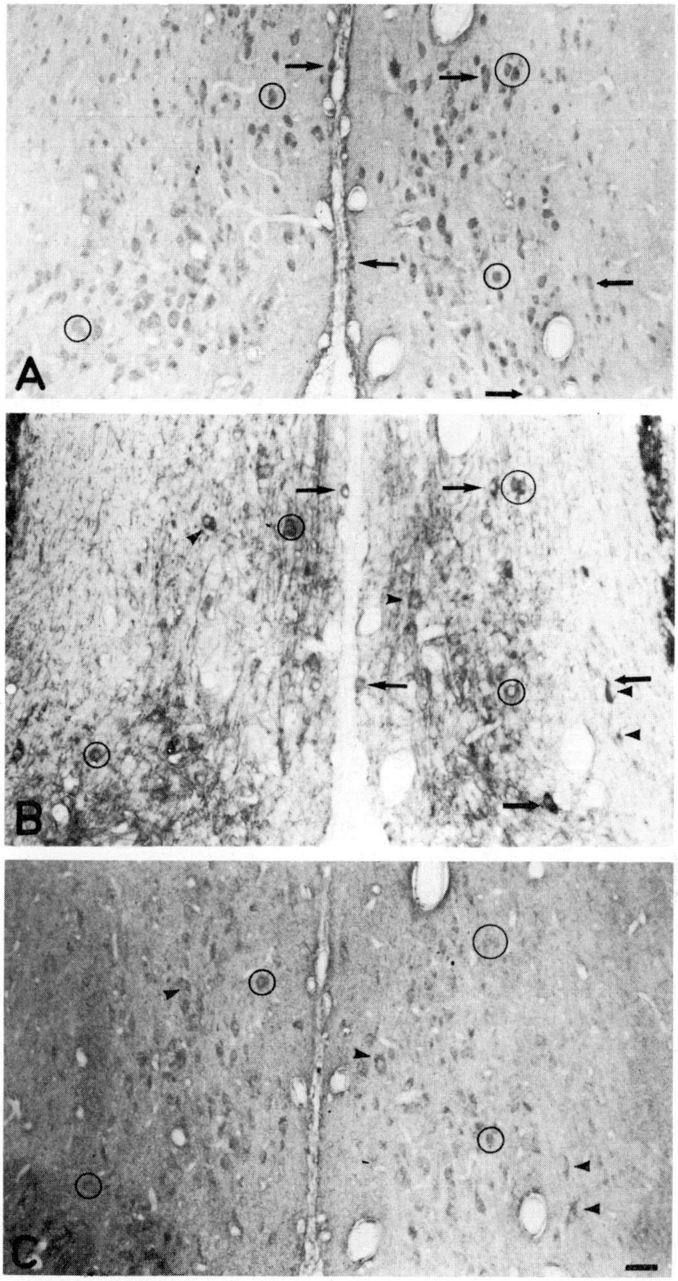

Figure 4. Photomicrographs of consecutive cryostat sections (10 μm) from the medial septum region. (A) Incubated with patient CSF, (B) Stained for acetylcholinesterase. (C) Incubated with ACh antiserum. Neurons (arrows) can be identified in two consecutive sections, A and B; other neurons (encircled) can be seen in all 3 sections. Arrows show neurons seen in sections Band C. Bar = 50 μm.

spinal cord. This tissue was used since the cholinergic motor perikaryons in the ventral horn were clearly labelled by the patient CSF, and since this tissue contains a long segment of homogeneous material to work with. If the hypothesis was correct, the reaction caused by patient CSF, or by the rabbit-ACh antibody, in a crossover incubation schedule would have blocked each other. Alternate sections of spinal cord were first incubated with CSF, or rabbit-anti-ACh antiserum, overnight. The next day they were thoroughly rinsed, and reincubated with the other antibody. Thus the CSF incubated sections were incubated with the ACh-antiserum and sections incubated with the ACh-antiserum were incubated with the CSF. If the CSF recognizes an ACh-like epitope, the first incubation should block these recognition sites so that the antibodies in the second incubation could not bind. After a thorough rinsing the immunocytochemical reaction was performed as before with the avidin-biotin peroxidase technique, the biotin labelled antiserum being chosen to detect the IgG of the second incubation step. Adjacent sections were incubate with a rabbit-ACh antiserum only, or the CSF only.

Figure 5 shows four different sections of the rat spinal cord. In the ventral horn large motor neurons are labelled by the CSF of the patient (Fig. 5A). If a section had been incubated with the anti-ACh antibody prior to incubation with the patient's CSF, large motor neurons would no longer be observed (Fig. 5B). With antibody A43 against ACh, motor neurons can be detected in the spinal cord (Fig. 5D). If, however, the section had been previously incubated with the patient CSF and thereafter incubated with the anti-ACh antibody, there would no longer be any markage over the motor neurons, which instead would appear as light spots in the photograph (Fig. 5C). The results of this experiment indicated that the factor in the patient CSF recognized an ACh-like epitope in the neurons.

Identification of IgG-Subclass

The factor in the CSF was most probably an IgG antibody since it was recognized by the anti-human IgG antisera employed. We decided to try and acertain which IgG subclass was responsible for the recognition of these cholinergic nerve cell bodies in the rat brain. We therefore incubated our CSF from the patient with protein A-sepharose cl 4B-beads. The tubes were then centrifuged and the supernatant I was collected. Of the various IgG subclasses, IgG 3 is the least susceptible to attachment to protein A. Supernatant I therefore probably contains IgG 3. We then eluted the pellet with glycine (O,3M), pH 3, followed by centrifugation and supernatant II collection. This supernatant is assumed to contain the subclass IgG 1 low affinity antibodies. The pellet was further eluted with glycine (O,3M) with MgCl (3M) added, centrifuged and the supernatant III, supposed to contain the subclass IgG 1 high affinity antibodies, was collected. The various supernatant fractions were used to incubate consecutive sections of the medial septum.

Figure 6 shows 3 consecutive sections of the ventro-medial septum area of the rat brain incubated with supernatant I (A), supernatant II (B) or supernatant III (C). It is clearly shown that the highest degree of labeling of the neuronal cell bodies in this area was obtained after incubating with supernatant I which probably contains the IgG 3 fraction. This was further supported by the use of specific anti-human IgG 3-antibodies, which allowed the labelling of sections incubated with whole CSF or with supernatant I.

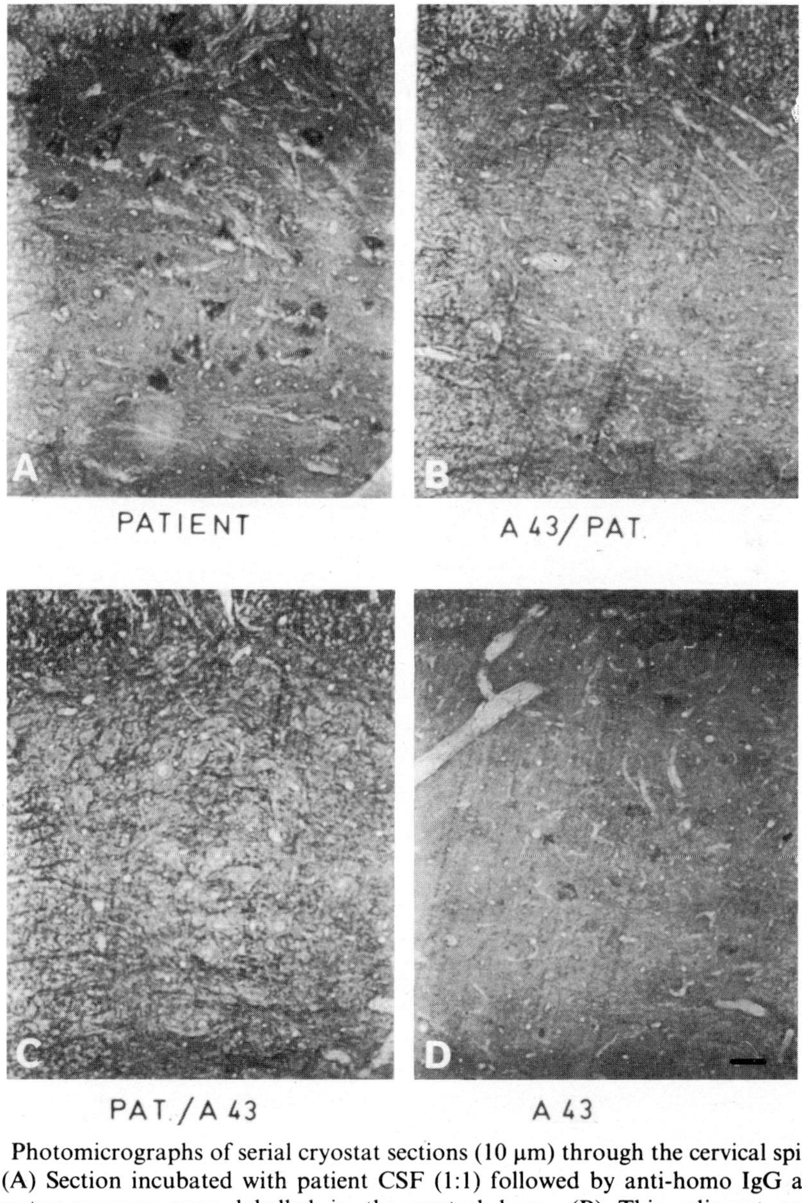

Figure 5. Photomicrographs of serial cryostat sections (10 μm) through the cervical spinal motor neurons. (A) Section incubated with patient CSF (1:1) followed by anti-homo IgG antibodies. Typical motor neurons were labelled in the ventral horn. (B) This adjacent section was preincubated with rabbit anti-ACh antiserum 24 hours prior to incubation with the patient CSF. Biotinylated anti-homo IgG was employed as the secondary antibody. The immunocytochemical reaction of the patient CSF (A) in the spinal motor neurons is totally blocked by the ACh antiserum. (C) Section preincubated with patient CSF 24 h prior to incubation with anti-ACh antiserum. Biotinylated anti-rabbit IgG was employed as the secondary antibody. The immunocytochemical reaction of the anti-ACh antiserum in the ventral horn is totally blocked by the patient CSF (D). (D) Adjacent section incubated with rabbit anti-ACh antiserum. Labeling of the motor neurons is observed in the ventral horn. Bar = 100 μm.

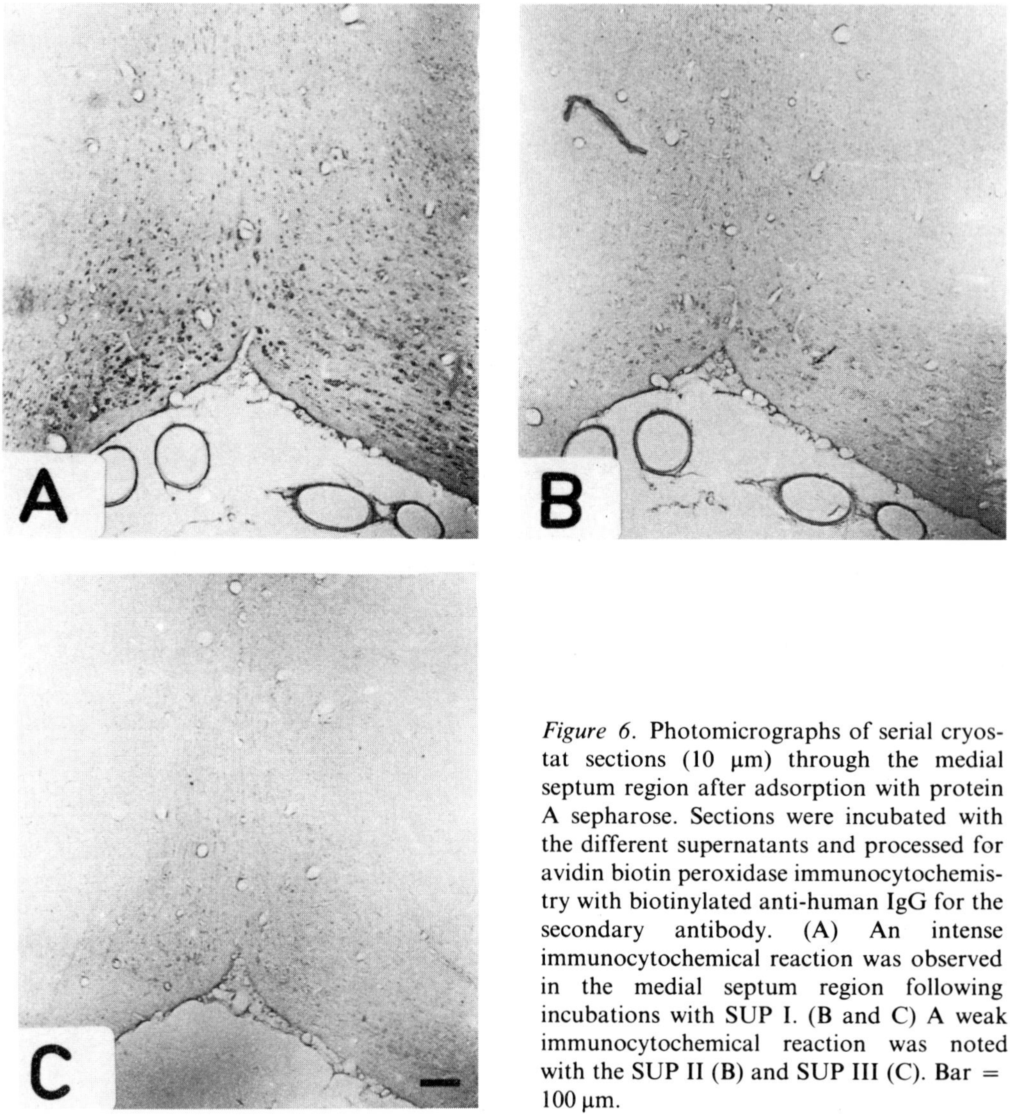

Figure 6. Photomicrographs of serial cryostat sections (10 μm) through the medial septum region after adsorption with protein A sepharose. Sections were incubated with the different supernatants and processed for avidin biotin peroxidase immunocytochemistry with biotinylated anti-human IgG for the secondary antibody. (A) An intense immunocytochemical reaction was observed in the medial septum region following incubations with SUP I. (B and C) A weak immunocytochemical reaction was noted with the SUP II (B) and SUP III (C). Bar = 100 μm.

It is interesting that in this patient the IgG was of subclass 3 because, as stated in the literature, IgG is one of the "aggressive" subclasses of IgG which are present for instance in cases of myasthenia gravis. Therefore, of great interest is the finding that some patients of the AD/SDAT group contain antibodies which recognize cholinergic cell bodies in their CSF. We now intend to continue screening CSFs from various patient groups to see whether we can clinically detect a subgroup with special clinical symptoms which might be correlated with the presence of such neuron-specific antibodies in the CSF. The presence of such antibodies might also give some clue as to the etiology of the disease in the individual patient. PD, in particular AD, is a group of diseases which probably have a multiple etiological origin, and several factors may work simultaneously in the development of dementia in these patients. This observation might provide the paving stone for a specific therapy in certain cases; a therapy directed against the autoimmune mechanisms which clearly play a vital role in certain of these cases.

CONCLUSION

The results here presented indicate that in subgroups of patients with PD and of patients diagnosed as having the AD/SDAT syndrome, the CSF contains IgG type antibodies that recognize mesencephalic or cholinergic neurons in the rat brain. These antibodies can be detected only if a special perfusion technique is used to fix the rat brain, a perfusion mixture which fixes i.a. small transmitter molecules. The antibodies in the CSF of some AD/SDAT patients clearly recognize an ACh-like epitope, since the reaction can be blocked by specific anti-ACh-antisera. The subclass of IgG in one patient investigated was found to be of the IgG 3 subtype. Patients with a strongly immunoreactive CSF (both PD and AD/SDAT-patients) had a high Tourtelotte production number, indicating an intracerebral production of antibodies. These observations may be of great importance in the future for diagnostic, prognostic and therapeutic purposes.

REFERENCES

Coyle JT, Price DL, DeLong MR (1983) Alzheimer's disease: a disorder of cortical cholinergic innervation. Science 219:1184-1190.

Hornykiewicz O (1977) Biogenic amines in the central nervous system. In: Vinken PJ, Bruyn GE (eds): Handbook of clinical neurology, Vol. 29: Metabolic and deficiency diseases of the nervous system. Elsevier, Amsterdam, pp. 459-483.

Ingram CR, Phegan KJ, Blumenthal HT (1974) Significance of an aging-linked neuron binding gamma globulin fraction of human sera. Journal of Gerontology 29:20-27.

Ishii T, Haga S (1976) Immuno-electron microscopic localization of immunoglobulins in amyloid fibrils of senile plaques. Acta Neuropath 36:243-249.

Jonker C, Eikelenboom P, Tavenier P (1982) Immunological indices in the cerebrospinal fluid of patients with presenile dementia of the Alzheimer type. Brit J Psychiat 140:44-49.

Koelle GB (1955) The histochemical identification of acetylcholin- esterase in cholinergic, adrenergic and sensory neurons. J Pharmacol 114:167-184.

Leon A, Dal Toso R, Presti D, Mazzoni S, Vencenzi D, Toffano G (1985) Sera from Parkinsonian patients contain inhibitory activity for development of fetal mesencephalic dopaminergic neurons in culture. J Neurochem (Suppl. 44):S137-(A).

Mash DS, Potter LT (1983) Changes in M1 and M2 muscarine receptors in Alzheimer's disease and aging, and with lesions of cholinergic neurons in animals. Soc Neurosci Abstr 9:582.

Mayer PP, Chughtai MA, Cape RDT (1976) An immunological approach to dementia in the elderly. Age and Ageing 5:164-170.

McRae-Degueurce A, Gottfries C-G, Karlsson I, Svennerholm L, Dahlström A (1986) Antibodies in the CSF of a Parkinson patient recognizes neurons in rat mesencephalic regions. Acta Physiol Scand 126:313-315.

McRae-Degueurce A, Booj S, Haglid K, Rosengren L, Karlsson JE, Karlsson I, Wallin A, Svennerholm L, Gottfries C-G, Dahlström A (1988) CSF from some Alzheimer patients contain antibodies recognizing cholinergic neurons in the rodent central nervous system. In press.

McRae-Degueurce A, Geffard M (1986) One perfusion mixture for immunocytochemical detection of noradrenaline, dopamine, serotonin and acetylcholine in the same rat brain. Brain Research 376:217-219.

Price DL, Struble RG, Whitehouse PJ, Kitt CA, Cork LC, Walker LC, Casanova MF (1986) Alzheimer's disease: a multisystem disorder. In: Martin JB, Barchas JD (eds): Neuropeptides in neurologic and psychiatric disease. New York 200:314.

Section IV

BASIC RESEARCH IN SENILE DEMENTIA

New Trends in Aging Research
G. Pepeu, B. Tomlinson, C.M. Wischik (eds)
Fidia Research Series, vol. 15
Liviana Press, Padova © 1988

SERIAL QUANTITATIVE COMPUTED TOMOGRAPHY (CT) ANALYSIS OF BRAIN MORPHOMETRY IN ADULT DOWN'S SYNDROME AT DIFFERENT AGES

Mark B. Schapiro, Jay S. Luxenberg, Jeffrey A. Kaye, James V. Haxby, Beverly White[1], Angela Moore, Robert P. Friedland and Stanley I. Rapoport

Laboratory of Neurosciences, Section on Brain Aging and Dementia, National Institute on Aging, Clinical Center, Bethesda, MD 20892; and [1]Laboratory of Chemical Biology, National Institute of Diabetes, Digestive and Kidney Diseases, National Institutes of Health, Clinical Center, Bethesda, MD 20892, USA

INTRODUCTION

Data relating Alzheimer's disease to Down's syndrome (DS), a genetic disorder associated with an extra portion of chromosome 21 (q 22.1 band), supports the hypothesis that genetic factors play a role in Alzheimer's disease. First, the incidence of DS is higher in families of Alzheimer's disease patients than in the general population (Heston et al., 1981; Heyman et al., 1983), with a higher number of DS births in families of younger Alzheimer's disease probands. Second, a restriction fragment polymorphism from chromosome 21 segregates with familial Alzheimer's disease (St George-Hyslop et al., 1987). Third, the gene coding for the precursor protein of beta amyloid has been assigned to chromosome 21 (Goldgaber et al., 1987; Tanzi et al., 1987). Fourth, gene dosage measurements have shown that the AD gene is duplicated in patients with sporadic AD (Delabar et al., 1987). Finally, DS adults over 35 years of age present

Abbreviations: DS, Down's syndrome; CT, computed tomography; WISC-R, Wechsler Intelligence Scale Revised; mm, millimeters; cm, centimeters; ANOVA, analysis of variance; ROI, region of interest.

clinical symptoms of, and autopsy neuropathological signs characteristic of, Alzheimer's disease.

Neuropathologic studies indicate that there are many similarities between Alzheimer's disease and DS. Senile (neuritic) plaques and neurofibrillary tangles found in both disorders are ultrastructurally identical (Ohara, 1972), as is the beta amyloid deposited in the senile plaques (Glenner et al., 1984; Masters et al., 1985). These senile plaques and neurofibrillary tangles are found in the same association regions of the neocortex and hippocampus in DS as in Alzheimer's disease, the hippocampus being more severely involved (Burger et al., 1973; Ellis et al., 1974). In support of the neuropathological similarities are neurochemical similarities between DS and Alzheimer's disease, including defects in cholinergic and noradrenergic markers (Yates et al., 1983), accompanied by loss of cells in the nucleus basalis of Meynert and locus coeruleus respectively (Mann et al., 1984; Casanova et al., 1985), as well as defects in somatostatin (Pierotti et al., 1986).

In order to learn more about the functional disturbances in DS, standardized neuropsychologic tests and quantitative computerized assisted transverse tomography (CT) were used in healthy patients with DS. The DS group consisted of 22 young adults aged 19 to 38 years (16 men and 6 women, mean age 26.7 years) and 7 older subjects aged 48 to 63 years (4 men and 3 women, mean age 53.6 years). Three of the older DS subjects (one 63 year-old man; one 55 and one 61 year-old woman) were considered demented. All DS subjects, recruited from family or group homes, had trisomy 21 karyotype. With the exception of two younger and two older subjects none had lived in an institution.

Subjects were carefully screened for primary and secondary brain disease and medical illness following procedures described elsewhere (Schapiro et al., 1986). Complicating features in the young DS adults included: hypothyroidism (2) and functional systolic murmurs (7). In the older DS group, three subjects were hypothyroid (one euthyroid on medication) and three subjects had a functional systolic murmur. None of the other DS subjects had diseases, nor were any taking medication (except thyroid replacement).

NEUROPSYCHOLOGY

Dementia has been diagnosed elsewhere in older DS adults by means of nonstandardized or unsystematic clinical evaluation in autopsy studies (Ropper et al., 1980; Wisniewski et al., 1985) or studies of living DS subjects (Reid et al., 1974; Thase et al., 1982). Of the subjects considered in these studies only 20 to 30% had dementia. However, because the various symptoms of dementia reported in these older DS adults correspond to a late stage of dementia, no detection is made of the disease at its early stages. Moreover, the autopsy studies reported fail to correlate morphometric changes with the diagnosis of dementia. It is therefore possible that a threshold of pathologic changes takes place before clinical symptoms of dementia appear.

Standardized neuropsychologic questionnaires and tests have also been used in the attempt to understand the mental status of older DS adults. Cross-sectional studies have shown that there are neuropsychological variables, depending on the age of the DS adults (Owens et al., 1971; Dalton et al., 1974; Wisniewski et al., 1978; Thase et al.,

1984), although the decline in mental status occurs in subjects over 35 years of age. Longitudinal studies also have demonstrated age related mental declines in older adult DS subjects, but the course of the decline may be prolonged (Dalton et al., 1977; Miniszek et al., 1983).

In our laboratory we therefore attempted to overcome the above-mentioned problems by employing standardized neuropsychologic questionnaires and tests to quantify the mental status of older DS adults.

Neuropsychological Tests

Dementia in Down's syndrome was diagnosed using criteria described elsewhere (Schapiro et al., 1986) (Table 1). The neuropsychological assessment was made using standardized tests. The Peabody Picture Vocabulary Test-Revised (Dunn et al., 1981) was used to assess general intelligence. Visuospatial ability was assessed using the Block Pattern Subtest of the Hiskey Nebraska Test of Learning Aptitude (Hiskey, 1955), the WISC-R Block Design Subtest (Wechsler, 1974), and the Extended Block Design Test (a simplified block design test for low ability subjects, Haxby J, unpublished test). Attention was assessed using forward digit span, object pointing span, and block tapping span (Haxby J, unpublished test). Visual recognition memory was measured with a design span (a test of immediate visual recognition memory for nonrepresentational geometric objects, Haxby J, unpublished test).

Results

Table 2 lists the neuropsychological scores for the young and aged DS groups, with the latter group being subdivided on the basis of the presence or absence of dementia. The mean mental age of the young DS group, as determined by the Peabody Picture Vocabulary Test (Dunn et al., 1981), was 6.5 ± 3.0 (SD) years. For tests of language, visuospatial ability and visual recognition memory, the mean scores of the nondemented group were more similar to the scores of the demented group then to those of the young DS group. There was overlap of one or two individuals in the nondemented group with the young group, but generally no overlap between the demented and young DS groups. On tests of attention, more overlap was present between the nondemented and young groups, though again there was no overlap between the demented and the young groups.

Summary

Our results show significant differences between the demented older DS subjects and the young DS subjects regarding standardized neuropsychological tests for language, visuospatial ability, attention and for memory. However, test scores of the nondemented older group are more similar to the scores of the demented older group than of the young group, although there is some overlap with the young DS group. Indeed, although three of the seven older DS subjects were clearly demented, all seven showed neuropsychological deficits with respect to the young DS group. The deficits found in the nondemented older group may reflect early changes in mental status associated with neuropathological and neurochemical changes that occur in Alzheimer's disease.

Table 1. *Criteria used to diagnose dementia in Down's syndrome*

A. Loss of intellectual abilities severe enough to interfere with social or occupational performance
  1. Loss of skills in everyday life:
     (a) personal hygiene: brushing teeth, combing hair, washing face, bathing, shaving
     (b) eating
     (c) voiding: urine, bowel
     (d) dressing
     (e) running the home: cleaning, shopping, cooking
  2. Loss of vocational skills

B. Memory impairment.

C. At least one of the following:
  1. Impairment of abstract thinking
  2. Impaired judgement: disregard of curfew, playing with fire, disregard of traffic
  3. Other disturbances in higher cortical function:
     (a) aphasia: loss of vocabulary, difficulty with comprehension, echolalia, hesitant speech
     (b) apraxia
     (c) agnosia
     (d) visuospatial difficulty
  4. Personality change
     (a) loss of usual affectionate response to others
     (b) hyperkinetic, impulsive: low frustration level, temper tantrums, irritable, spiteful, obstinate, destructive, demanding, aggressive
     (c) withdrawal: slowness, loss of interest in surroundings, apathy, sudden changes from cheerfulness to sullenness, inattention to vocational tasks, loss of social interests
     (d) automatic movements: rocking, fidgeting with hands, perseveration, stereotypes (speech, motor)
     (e) psychiatric changes: hallucinations (auditory, visual), paranoid delusions, depression

---

D. Supportive evidence for dementia (neurological signs)
  1. Seizures
  2. Gait difficulties: shuffling, incoordination
  3. Release signs: grasp (palmar, plantar), snout, suck, palmomental, glabella
  4. Babinski
  5. Gegenhalten, increased tone
  6. Tremor, myoclonus

It has been suggested that it is paradoxical for 100% of the brains of DS subjects over 35 years of age to present the neuropathological changes associated with Alzheimer's disease (neuritic plaques, neurofibrillary tangles), but for only 20 to 30% of these subjects to be demented (Ropper et al., 1980; Wisniewski et al., 1985). Some authors attribute this discrepancy to the difficulty in diagnosing dementia in mentally

Table 2. *Neuropsychology test scores for young, non-demented aged, and demented aged DS groups*

	Young DS	Non-demented DS	Demented DS
Language			
Peabody picture vocabulary — Test age	6.5. ± 3.0 (22)**	3.6 ± 1.7 (4)*	2.5 ± 0.5 (3)*
Visuospatial			
Hiskey Nebraska Block — Pattern subtest	3.0 ± 1.4 (21)	1.0 ± 1.2 (4)*	0.3 ± 0.6 (3)*
WISC-R block design subtest	7.2 ± 7.1 (21)	2.3 ± 4.5*	0.0 ± 0.0 (3)*
Extended block design test	14.1 ± 1.7 (21)	8.0 ± 5.5	5.0 ± 4.4 (3)*
Attention			
Digit span (score)	13.8 ± 4.8 (20)	13.7 ± 2.1	6.0 ± 3.6 (3)*
Object span (score)	12.1 ± 3.9 (20)	8.3 ± 6.2 (4)	4.7 ± 4.0 (3)*
Block tapping (score)	17.0 ± 5.5 (20)	7.8 ± 6.4 (4)*	6.0 ± 2.6 (3)*
Visual recognition memory			
Design span (score)	4.9 ± 2.1 (20)	2.0 ± 2.2 (4)*	0.7 ± 0.6 (3)*

Number of subjects is shown in brackets. * Differs from mean in young DS with Friedman Test ($p<0.01$).
** Values are means ± S.D.
Differences between mean values in young and old DS groups were compared with a Friedman Test (one-way ANOVA on ranks) ($p<0.05$).

retarded DS subjects (Miniszek, 1983; Reiss et al., 1982), but we believe that the distinction can be made by using specific diagnostic criteria and obtaining an exhaustive clinical history (Schapiro et al., 1986). However, we also found that only a small number of our older DS subjects were demented, despite standardized neuropsychological studies showing a universal reduction in cognitive performance in aged DS, irrespective of the diagnosis of dementia.

Some authors are of the opinion that the densities of senile plaques and neurofibrillary tangles postmortem reflect the severity of dementia in life (Wisniewski et al., 1985); others disagree (Ropper et al., 1980). However, one study showed that even in brains with more than 20 senile plaques and/or neurofibrillary tangles per high power field, only 13 of 28 DS subjects had a history of dementia (Wisniewski et al., 1985). This suggests that an additional factor contributes to the appearance of dementia in older DS subjects who already show measurable decreases during standardized cognitive tests. This factor may be due to an increase in the numbers of neurofibrillary tangles, occurring 10 to 20 years after the appearance of senile plaques (Burger et al., 1973). Alternatively, this paper suggests that the factor is accelerated brain atrophy, which can be demonstrated with studies employing quantitative CT scanning. However, these factors may not be exclusive, as there is a correlation between the density of neurofibrillary tangles and the degree of cell loss in DS (Burger et al., 1973).

COMPUTER ASSISTED TRANSVERSE TOMOGRAPHY (CT)

With CT brain measurements the problems inherent to postmortem studies are obviated. Elsewhere we used quantitative CT to demonstrate that the small brains in young adults with trisomy 21 reflect their smaller stature and smaller cranial vault (Schapiro et al., 1986). We further showed that mental retardation in young DS adults is related to inherent cerebral dysfunction and not to cerebral atrophy (secondary micrencephaly).

Although Alzheimer's disease is accompanied by cerebral cortical atrophy that can be detected with CT (Creasey et al., 1986), it is not known to what extent older demented DS adults have cortical atrophy, because the relation between age and cortical atrophy is the same in nondemented DS subjects as it is in healthy controls (Schapiro et al., 1986). In our laboratory we used quantitative CT, in cross-sectional and longitudinal analyses, to establish whether differences in brain morphology help us to distinguish between dementia and mental retardation in DS adults over 35 years of age.

CT

Non-contrast CT scans were made with an 8800 CT Scanner (General Electric Co., Milwaukee, WI) (Schwartz et al., 1985), for which full width half maximum equalled 1 mm. Serial slices, each 10 mm thick and separated from adjacent slices by 7 mm (center to center), were taken parallel to and from 0 to 110 mm above the inferior orbitomeatal (IOM) line. Analysis was limited to levels 30 to 80 mm above the IOM line.

An image-processing program (CATSEG) allowed the determination of the number of pixels of gray matter, white matter and cerebrospinal fluid (CSF). In addition, regions of interest (ROIs) were outlined around the ventricles and subcortical nuclei. The number of pixels in each ROI was computed. The intracranial surface area was derived with an automatic edge-finding procedure (Schwartz et al., 1985).

The volume of an intracranial structure or tissue category was derived by summing the number of pixels belonging to it in all slices in which it appeared, and by multiplying by pixel area (0.0064 cm^2) and interslice distance (0.7 cm) (5,22). Volumes were expressed in cm^3 or as a percentage of the intracranial volume in the 50 mm horizontal segment.

The rate of change of a volume of an intracranial structure or tissue category in cm^3/yr was derived from the slope of the regression line of that volume (cm^3) on time (yr).

Results

Table 3 lists values for brain measurements in the young and old DS groups, the latter being subdivided on the basis of whether dementia was present or not. No differences were found between the total intracranial volumes or the 7-slice intracranial volumes of the groups, nor were significant differences found between the values of the nondemented older and the young adult DS groups for volume of CSF, white matter, gray matter, gray plus white matter or ventricles, either directly or after normalizing to a 7-slice intracranial volume.

When a comparison was made between the CSF and third ventricular volumes (directly and after normalizing to 7-slice intracranial volume) of demented older and

Table 3. *CT variables for DS groups*

	Young DS (22)	Non-demented DS (4)	Demented DS (3)
Catseg Analysis			
CSF volume (cm^3)	25.5 ± 2.9[a]	18.5 ± 8.2	50.9 ± 6.4[c, d]
White matter volume (cm^3)	311 ± 10	352 ± 43	326 ± 26
Gray matter volume (cm^3)	351 ± 10	315 ± 36	315 ± 25
Gray matter + white matter volume (cm^3)	611 ± 8	673 ± 19	645 ± 50
% CSF volume[b]	3.7 ± 0.4	2.7 ± 1.2	7.5 ± 1.4[c, d]
% White matter volume[b,e]	45.2 ± 1.4	51.7 ± 5.9	47.1 ± 0.8
% Gray matter volume[b,e]	51.1 ± 1.4	45.6 ± 5.0	45.4 ± 0.6[c]
% Gray matter + white matter volume[b]	96.3 ± 0.4	97.3 ± 1.2	92.5 ± 1.4[c, d]
Gray matter/white matter[e]	1.17 ± 0.06	0.95 ± 0.21	0.97 ± 0.01
Roi Analysis			
III ventricle volume (cm^3)	0.61 ± 0.07	0.53 ± 0.17	2.60 ± 0.38[c, d]
R lateral ventricle (cm^3)	8.7 ± 1.0	5.9 ± 2.1	15.1 ± 1.6[d]
L lateral ventricle (cm^3)	11.3 ± 1.4	8.4 ± 3.1	17.1 ± 2.9
Total ventricle volume (cm^3)	20.6 ± 2.4	14.7 ± 5.1	34.8 ± 4.6
Total CSF volume-total ventricle vol (cm^3)	4.9 ± 1.3	3.7 ± 3.2	16.1 ± 2.4[c, d]
% III ventricle volume[b,e]	0.09 ± 0.01	0.07 ± 0.02	0.39 ± 0.08[c, d]
% R lateral ventricle volume[b,e]	1.27 ± 0.16	0.84 ± 0.30	2.23 ± 0.36
% L lateral ventricle volume[b]	1.63 ± 0.20	1.20 ± 0.45	2.33 ± 0.63
% Total ventricle volume[b]	2.99 ± 0.35	2.12 ± 0.73	5.16 ± 1.06
% Total CSF volume-total ventricle vol[b]	0.69 ± 0.19	0.54 ± 0.46	2.37 ± 0.42[c, d]
R/L lateral ventricle volume	-0.24 ± 0.06	-0.32 ± 0.07	-0.11 ± 0.10
Subcortical Nuclei			
R caudate nucleus (cm^3)	2.25 ± 0.15	1.73 ± 0.32	1.70 ± 0.87
L caudate nucleus (cm^3)	2.15 ± 0.13	1.98 ± 0.40	1.57 ± 0.55
R lenticular nucleus (cm^3)	4.58 ± 0.30	5.58 ± 0.25	4.67 ± 0.48
L lenticular nucleus (cm^3)	4.85 ± 0.29	5.58 ± 0.16	4.63 ± 0.20[d]
R thalamus (cm^3)	4.31 ± 0.29	5.08 ± 0.31	4.23 ± 0.58
L thalamus (cm^3)	4.80 ± 0.30	5.10 ± 0.50	4.60 ± 0.68
Cranial Volume			
Total cranial volume	1072 ± 20	1098 ± 39	1055 ± 100
7-slice cranial volume	687 ± 9	691 ± 19	692 ± 45

[a] Mean ± SEM. [b] Normalized to 7-slice cranial volume. [c] Differs from mean in Young DS by Bonferroni T Test ($p<0.05$). [d] Differs from mean in Nondemented DS by Bonferroni T Test ($p<0.05$). [e]Inhomogeneous Variance (Bartlett's Test). Number of subjects shown in brackets. Values are expressed as cm^3, percentage of intracranial volume, or as right/left ratios. Differences between means of young, non-demented aged, and demented aged DS groups were analyzed with a one-way ANOVA. Post hoc comparisons, using Bonferroni t tests, were as follows: young DS vs nondemented aged DS, young DS vs demented aged DS, and nondemented aged DS vs demented aged DS. Homogeneity of variance was ensured by using Bartlett's test. Asymmetry of ventricular volume was calculated as (right-left)/[(right ± left)/2].

Table 4. *Rates of change in CT volumes (cm^3/yr) for DS groups*

	Young DS	Non-demented DS	Demented DS
Catseg analysis			
CSF volume (cm^3/yr)	-1.50 ± 1.02[a] (5)	1.54 ± 0.72 (3)	8.47 ± 0.98[b, c, d] (2)
Gray matter $\pm$ white matter vol (cm^3/yr)	-1.02 ± 3.63 (5)	0.58 ± 9.80 (3)	-8.62 ± 0.25[d] (2)
Roi analysis			
Third ventricle volume (cm^3/yr)	-0.018 ± 0.011 (5)	0.054 ± 0.054 (2)	0.211 ± 0.093 (2)
L lateral ventricle (cm^3/yr)	-0.26 ± 0.20 (5)	-0.56 ± 0.31 (2)	3.88 ± 0.51[b, c, d] (2)
R lateral ventricle (cm^3/yr)	0.08 ± 0.15 (5)	-0.58 ± 0.29 (2)	2.67 ± 0.02[c, d] (2)
L-R lateral ventricle (cm^3/yr)	-0.34 ± 0.20 (5)	0.02 ± 0.02 (2)	1.20 ± 0.49[b] (2)

[a] Mean $\pm$ SEM. [b] Differs from mean in Young DS by Bonferroni t test ($p < 0.05$). [c] Differs from mean in Nondemented DS by Bonferroni t test ($p < 0.05$). [d] Differs from zero with paired t test ($p < 0.1$). Number of subjects shown in brackets. Differences between values of the young and aged groups were analyzed with a one-way ANOVA. Post hoc comparisons, using Bonferroni t tests, were as follows: young DS vs nondemented aged DS, young DS vs demented aged DS, and nondemented aged DS vs demented aged DS. Homogeneity of variance was ensured by using Bartlett's test.

those of the young DS subjects, significantly higher values were found in the former group; demented subjects also had higher values than the nondemented older subjects. Moreover, the absolute right ventricular volume of the demented was larger than that of the nondemented older group. In the demented older subjects, gray matter plus white matter volume, normalized to 7-slice intracranial volume, was significantly less than that of the other two groups, whereas the percentage of gray matter volume and the ratio of gray to white matter volumes was lower than that found in controls. No significant differences were found between the mean asymmetric of ventricles of all the groups.

Table 4 shows the mean rates of changes of brain parameters in cubic centimeters per year, for young and old DS groups, the latter being again subdivided into demented and nondemented groups. The intervals between CT scans were on average 2.7 years in the young DS group and 2.0 years in the old DS group. No differences were observed between the young and nondemented old DS groups for rate of change of CSF volume, gray and white matter volume, ventricular volumes or left-right ventricular differences. Nor did these rates of change differ significantly from zero in either young or nondemented old DS groups (all $p > 0.1$). However, the demented older DS subjects presented a greater rate of change in CSF volume, left ventricular volume and left-right ventricular difference than the young DS group. These rates of change for the right lateral ventricle in the demented old DS group differed significantly from zero; the rates of change for the left lateral ventricle, CSF volume, and gray and white matter volume failed to significantly differ from zero ($p < 0.1$).

Summary

In cross-sectional analysis, our results show that the demented, unlike the non-demented group, had increased CSF and third ventricular volumes with respect to the young DS group. Further, the serial longitudinal studies confirm these increases in the demented DS group and show that they are progressive. Our results suggest that an excessive increase in CSF and ventricular volumes occurs only in older DS subjects who have clinically evident dementia, but not in those without dementia. These volumetric results are in agreement with those reported in qualitative CT studies which also suggest that dementia in older DS subjects is accompanied by cerebral atrophy (Dalton et al., 1977; Lott et al., 1982).

A previous cross-sectional study from our laboratory already showed an increased CSF volume in patients with dementia of the Alzheimer type (DAT) (Creasey et al., 1986). Likewise, this study suggests that the increased CSF volume is due to a loss of gray matter. The lack of volume differences in subcortical nuclei or white matter further suggests that the gray matter loss is mainly cortical. In addition, a serial longitudinal study from our laboratory has shown progressive rates of ventricular enlargement in DAT (Luxenberg et al., 1987) which, together with the results reported here, suggest that rates of ventricular enlargement may be parameters to distinguish between demented and nondemented subjects (whether or not they have DS).

CONCLUSIONS

Our study of DS and aging, using neuropsychological testing and computerized assisted transverse tomography (CT), suggests that a cognitive decline in older DS subjects occurs in two stages; the time interval between them can be as long as 20 years. First, there is a reduction in cognitive performance at standardized neuropsychological tests, and this perhaps reflects the individual's poorer processing skills. There may be a correlation between the reduction and significant accumulations of senile plaques, without there being a marked cell loss or cerebral atrophy. This hypothesis is supported by the lack of change in ventricular volume at CT observed in our nondemented older DS group, with respect to the young DS group. In DS, senile plaques can appear in the fourth decade while dementia appears only in the fifth or sixth decade.

In the second stage, there is an additional loss of overlearned behaviors leading to deterioration in social, occupational and adaptive skills and a characteristic dementia. Concurrently, an accelerated neuronal cell loss and accumulations of neurofibrillary tangles occur and brain atrophy becomes evident, sometimes together with a further accumulation of senile plaques. Atrophy is evidenced by a progressive ventricular dilation, an increased CSF space and loss of gray matter on CT.

Thus, accelerated neuronal loss, in addition to accumulations of senile plaques and neurofibrillary tangles, must be present before a further decline in mental status in DS can result in dementia, as in Alzheimer's disease. In this regard, Ball et al. (1986) found that the brain of a demented 45-year-old adult with trisomy 21 had fewer pyramidal cells in the hippocampal cortex than the brains of five other DS patients without documented dementia, and more neurofibrillary tangles in the hippocampus than four of the other brains.

Elsewhere we demonstrated that mental retardation in young DS subjects is not related to cerebral atrophy (Schapiro et al., 1986). The results here reported suggest that cerebral atrophy and decreased gray matter are present in aged DS subjects with dementia, and that alterations in brain morphometrics measured with CT can provide evidence enabling us to distinguish between dementia and mental retardation in DS. Furthermore, cell counting in the postmortem brain, so as to demonstrate cell loss, not only counting senile plaques and neurofibrillary tangles, may allow us to distinguish between demented and nondemented DS subjects.

REFERENCES

Ball MJ, Schapiro MB, Rapoport SI (1986) Neuropathological relationships between Down syndrome and senile dementia Alzheimer type. In: Epstein C (ed): The Neurobiology of Down Syndrome. Raven Press, New York, pp. 45-58.

Burger PC, Vogel FS (1973) The development of the pathologic changes of Alzheimer's disease and senile dementia in patients with Down's syndrome. Am J Pathol 73:457-476.

Casanova MF, Walker LC, Whitehouse PJ, et al. (1985) Abnormalities of the nucleus basalis in Down's syndrome. Ann Neurol 18:310-313.

Creasey H, Schwartz M, Frederickson H, Haxby JV, Rapoport SI (1985) Quantitative computed tomography in dementia of the Alzheimer type. Neurology 36:1563-1568.

Dalton AJ, Crapper DR (1977) Down's syndrome and aging of the brain. In: Mittler P (ed): Research to Practice in Mental Retardation. University Park Press, Baltimore, pp. 391-400.

Dalton AJ, Crapper DR, Schlotterer GR (1974) Alzheimer's disease in Down's syndrome: visual retention deficits. Cortex 10:366-377.

Delabar JM, Goldgaber D, Lamour Y, et al. (1987) B amyloid gene duplication in Alzheimer's disease and karyotypically normal Down syndrome. Science 235:1390-1392.

Dunn LM, Dunn LM (1981) Peabody Picture Vocabulary Test-Revised. American Guidance Service, Circle Pines, New Mexico.

Ellis WG, McCulloch JR, Corley CL (1974) Presenile dementia in Down's syndrome. Neurology 24:101-106.

Glenner GG, Wong CW (1984) Alzheimer's disease and Down's syndrome: sharing of a unique cerebrovascular amyloid fibril protein. Biochem Biophys Res Commun 122:1131-1135.

Goldgaber D, Lerman MI, McBride OW, Saffiotti U, Gajdusek DC (1987) Characterization and chromosomal localization of a cDNA encoding brain amyloid of Alzheimer's disease. Science 235:877-880.

Heston LL, Mastri AR, Anderson E, White J (1981) Dementia of the Alzheimer type: clinical genetics, natural history and associated conditions. Arch Gen Psychiatry 38:1085-1090.

Heyman A, Wilkinson WE, Hurwitz BJ, et al. (1983) Alzheimer's disease: genetic aspects and associated clinical disorders. Ann Neurol 14:507-515.

Hiskey MS (1955) Hiskey-Nebraska Test of Learning Aptitude. College View Printers, Lincoln, Nebraska.

Lott IT, Lai FL (1982) Dementia in Down syndrome. Ann Neurol 12:210.

Luxenberg J, Haxby JV, Creasey H, Sundaram M, Rapoport SI (1987) Rate of ventricular enlargement in dementia of the Alzheimer type (DAT) correlates with rate of neuropsychological deterioration. Neurology 37:1135-1140.

Mann DMA, Yates PO, Marcyniuk B (1984) Alzheimer's presenile dementia, senile dementia of Alzheimer type and Down's syndrome in middle age form an age related continuum of pathological changes. Neuropath Appl Neurobiol 10:185-207.

Masters CL, Simms G, Weinmann NA, Multhaup G, McDonald BL, Bayreuther K (1985) Amyloid plaque core protein in Alzheimer's disease and Down's syndrome. Proc Natl Acad Sci USA 82:4245-4249.

Miniszek NA (1983) Development of Alzheimer disease in Down syndrome individuals. Am J Ment Defic 87:377-385.

Ohara PT (1972) Electron microscopic study of the brain in Down's syndrome. Brain 95:681-684.

Owens D, Dawson JC, Losin S (1971) Alzheimer's disease in Down's syndrome. Am J Ment Def 75:605-612.

Pierotti AR, Harmar AJ, Simpson J, Yates CM (1986) High-molecular-weight forms of somatostatin are reduced in Alzheimer's disease and Down's syndrome. Neuroscience Letters 63:141-146.

Reid AH, Aungle PG (1974) Dementia in ageing mental defectives: a clinical psychiatric study. J Ment Defic Res 18:15-23.

Reiss S, Leviton GW, Szyszko J (1982) Emotional disturbance and mental retardation: diagnostic overshadowing. Am J Ment Defic 86:567-574.

Ropper AH, Williams RS (1980) Relationship between plaques, tangles, and dementia in Down syndrome. Neurology 30:639-644.

Schapiro MB, Haxby JV, Grady CL, Rapoport SI (1986) Cerebral glucose utilization, quantitative tomography, and cognitive function in adult Down syndrome. In: Epstein CJ (ed): The Neurobiology of Down Syndrome. Raven Press, New York, pp. 89-108.

Schwartz M, Creasey H, Grady CL, et al. (1985) Computed tomographic analysis of brain morphometrics in 30 healthy men, aged 21 to 81 years. Ann Neurol 17:146-157.

St George-Hyslop PH, Tanzi RE, Polinsky RJ, et al. (1987) The genetic defect causing familial Alzheimer's disease maps on chromosome 21. Science 235:885-890.

Tanzi RE, Gusella JF, Watkins PC, et al. (1987) Amyloid B protein gene: cDNA, mRNA distribution, and genetic linkage near the Alzheimer locus. Science 235:880-884.

Thase ME, Tigner R, Smeltzer DJ, Liss L (1984) Age-related neuropsychological deficits in Down's syndrome. Biol Psychiatry 19:571-585.
Thase ME, Liss L, Smeltzer DJ, Maloon J (1982) Clinical evaluation of dementia in Down's syndrome: a preliminary report. J Ment Defic Res 26:239-244.
Wechsler D (1974) Wechsler Intelligence Scale for Children-Revised. Psychological Corporation, New York.
Wisniewski KE, Howe J, Williams DG, Wisniewski HM (1978) Precocious aging and dementia in patients with Down's syndrome. Biol Psychiatry 13:619-627.
Wisniewski KE, Wisniewski HM, Wen GY (1985) Occurrence of neuropathological changes and dementia of Alzheimer's disease in Down's syndrome. Ann Neurol 17:278-282.
Yates CM, Simpson J, Gordon A, et al. (1983) Catecholamines and cholinergic enzymes in pre-senile and senile Alzheimer-type dementia and Down's syndrome. Brain Res 280:119-126.

New Trends in Aging Research
G. Pepeu, B. Tomlinson, C.M. Wischik (eds)
Fidia Research Series, vol. 15
Liviana Press, Padova © 1988

A NEW PROTEIN IN ALZHEIMER AND OTHER NEURODEGENERATIVE DISEASES UBIQUITIN

Pierluigi Gambetti, Valeria Manetto, Massimo Tabaton, Paul Mulvihill, Victor A. Fried[1], Harry T. Smith[1], Lucila Autilio-Gambetti and George Perry

Division of Neuropathology, Institute of Pathology,
Case Western Reserve University, Cleveland, Ohio, USA; and
[1]Department of Biochemistry, St Jude Children's Research Hospital,
Memphis, Tennessee, USA

Eighty years after Alois Alzheimer's original description, the pathogenesis of Alzheimer disease (AD) remains elusive. A major difficulty encountered in postulating a convincing pathogenetic mechanism is the complexity of the pathologic changes (Mann, 1985; Tomlinson et al., 1968). These include:

— selective loss of neurons;

— focal deposition of amyloid in vessels and in cerebral parenchyma associated with degeneration of neurites forming neuritic plaques (NP);

— selective impairment of neurotransmitter systems; and

— presence of neuronal cytoplasmic inclusions, in particular the neurofibrillary tangle (NFT), made of bundles of paired helical filaments (PHF) (Wisniewski et al., 1976).

Abbreviations: Ab, antibody; AD, Alzheimer disease; kDa, kilodalton; GVD, granulovacuolar degeneration; mAb, monoclonal antibody; MAP, microtubule-associated protein; MAP2, microtubule-associated protein 2; NFH, high molecular weight neurofilament protein subunit; NFM, medium molecular weight neurofilament protein; NF, neurofilament; NFT, neurofibrillary tangle; NP, neuritic plaque; PHF: paired helical filament; PSP, progressive supranuclear palsy; Ub, ubiquitin.

Attempts have been made to establish whether and how these diverse changes are related. The deficit of neurotransmitter systems might be explained on the basis of preferential loss of corresponding neuronal populations (Tomlinson et al., 1970); in turn, the loss of neurons may be secondary to the damage of neurites at the NP or to the formation of NFT. Amyloid deposits and degeneration of neurites forming the NP may also be associated lesions. While reasonable explanations can be given for the impairment of neurotransmitter systems and loss of neurons, the origin of the amyloid deposit and the mode of formation of the NFT as well as the relation between these two events remain elusive.

PHF COMPOSITION

The fast advances made in establishing the nature and origin of amyloid (Glenner and Wong, 1984a; 1984b; Masters et al., 1985; Goldgaber et al., 1987; Kang et al., 1987) contrast with the slow pace in establishing the nature and mode of formation of NFT. Because of difficulties in the purification and solubilization of NFT (Selkoe, 1986), investigators have relied largely on immunochemical techniques to identify the components of these inclusions. Two mirror approaches have been pursued:

1. search for normal antigens recognized by antibodies (Abs) to PHF; and
2. search for Abs raised to known antigens that cross-react with PHF.

Using these techniques, it has been shown that insoluble phosphorylated determinants of a set of microtubule-associated proteins (MAP), the tau proteins, are present in NFT (Brion et al., 1985; Kosik et al., 1986; Grundke-Iqbal et al., 1986; Wood et al., 1986) along with epitopes of neurofilaments (NF) (Autilio-Gambetti et al., 1983), the high molecular weight MAP2 (Kosik et al., 1984) and other epitopes not yet identified. Tau proteins are thought to be a prominent component of PHF as virtually all the tested antisera and monoclonal antibodies (mAb) to tau react with the PHF. In contrast, PHF are recognized by few Abs to phosphorylated epitopes of the high and medium molecular weight subunits of NF (NFH and NFM). Some of these Abs have been reported to cross-react with tau proteins (Ksiezak-Reding et al., 1987; Nukina et al., 1987); however, others unquestionably do not (Gambetti et al., 1988; Sternberger, personal communication). Also, only a few Abs to MAP2 cross-react with PHF (Kosik et al., 1984). Antibodies to PHF have been obtained that do not cross-react with tau, MAP2, NF or any identified antigen (Perry et al., 1987a), and the possibility has been raised that these Abs recognize antigens unique to PHF. Finally, Alz 50, a mAb to a 68 kDa protein present in AD (Wolozin et al., 1986), also decorates PHF (Tabaton et al., in press).

Thus, during the past few years consistent evidence for the presence in PHF of epitopes from the following proteins has been obtained: tau proteins, MAP2, NFH protein, Alz 50 antigen and other unidentified components. None of these proteins have been isolated from PHF and sequenced; therefore, it is not known whether they are present in PHF as fragments or in their entirety. The possibility still exists that PHF components share epitopes with, but are different from, tau, NFH and MAP2. More recently, one of us, G. Perry, and coworkers (1987b), and Mori et al. (1987), independently reported that ubiquitin (Ub) epitopes are present in PHF. Mori et al.

succeeded in extracting and sequencing fragments from fractions enriched in PHF, providing evidence that at least a large portion of the Ub molecule is present in PHF.

UBIQUITIN

Ub is a highly conserved 8.5 kDa protein present in all eukaryotic cells (Goldstein et al., 1975). The unparalleled degree of phylogenetic conservation of Ub lead early investigators to suspect that it plays a vital role in cells. More recent studies have shown that Ub forms conjugates with selected cytoplasmic and nuclear proteins by means of covalent isopeptide bonds between its C-terminal carboxy group and free amino groups of proteins (Finley and Varshavsky, 1985). Ub-conjugated proteins may undergo degradation to yield free amino acids and functional Ub as end products (Finley and Varshavsky, 1985). This Ub system offers an alternative to the long-known lysosomal pathway of proteolysis. The existence of Ub conjugates that are not rapidly degraded suggests that Ub may also serve nonproteolytic functions. For example, in conjugates with histones, Ub has been thought to regulate gene expression and repair (Goldknopf and Busch, 1977; West and Bonner, 1980); in conjugates with membrane receptors, Ub may modulate cell to cell interaction (Siegelman et al., 1986; St John et al., 1986; Yarden et al., 1986). Moreover, Ub itself can also act as a protease under appropriate conditions (Fried et al., 1987). When Ub forms conjugates, its conformation and antigenic properties change. Thus, mAbs that recognize conformational forms of Ub unique to certain conjugates have been obtained.

Synthesis and protein conjugation of Ub increase significantly in cells exposed to heat-shock or other stress conditions known to alter *de novo* synthesized proteins (Bond and Schlesinger, 1985), and Ub has recently been shown to be a heat-shock protein (Bond and Schlesinger, 1986). Moreover, cellular proteins altered in the course of various stress conditions are ubiquitinated more rapidly than native proteins (Dice, 1987). The Ub system is thought to play a role in preventing or limiting cell damage caused by abnormal proteins (Bond and Schlesinger, 1985). In heat shock and aging there is an increase in stable, high molecular weight Ub conjugates present in cytoskeletal fractions (Carlson et al., 1987). Thus, the Ub system may be involved in the regulation of the cytoskeleton following stress (Collier and Schlesinger, 1986). Although the Ub and heat-shock protein systems have been studied extensively only in non-neuronal cells, it is likely that they operate similarly in neurons. The presence in PHF of a protein with such diverse roles as Ub is intriguing.

UBIQUITIN IN ALZHEIMER DISEASE

We used ten antisera and eight mAbs (St John et al., 1986) raised to artificial Ub conjugates to investigate the presence and distribution of Ub epitopes in brain tissue obtained at autopsy from patients with AD and from neurologically normal individuals of various ages, including age-matched controls. Unfixed frozen sections were used for immunofluorescence. Bouin's or paraformaldehyde fixed tissue was used to obtain paraffin sections for light microscopy and vibrotome sections for electron microscopy.

Vibratome sections were heat treated in order to obtain immunoreaction with the Ub Abs we used.

All antisera and five of the eight mAbs intensely immunostained brain tissue of patients with AD. NFT were intensely immunostained and the perikarya of a few scattered neurons with no detectable NFT showed various degrees of diffuse immunostaining (Fig. 1). A dense meshwork of thin cell processes, probably neuronal, was also intensely immunostained. This meshwork was especially prominent in the hippocampal cortex but could be seen throughout the neocortex. In the hippocampus and other areas, small, rounded structures in the neuropil were intensely immunostained (Fig. 2). Amyloid in NP and in vessels was not immunostained. The nucleus was diffusely and weakly immunostained by the mAbs in some neurons regardless of the presence of NFT in the perikaryon. With the exception of the occasional nuclear staining, the pattern of immunoreaction in paraffin sections from AD brains was similar to that of Abs to tau. However, in double immunofluorescence preparations there was not a complete overlapping in the staining of NFT by these two Abs.

The immunostaining by Ub Abs in control tissues appeared to be age related. Immunostaining was detected only in brains from individuals over 70 years of age, and it was present in scattered NFT and in neurites regardless of their association with neuritic plaques. No immunostaining was seen in brains of younger individuals.

At the ultrastructural level, PHF were immunodecorated in intact tissue as well as

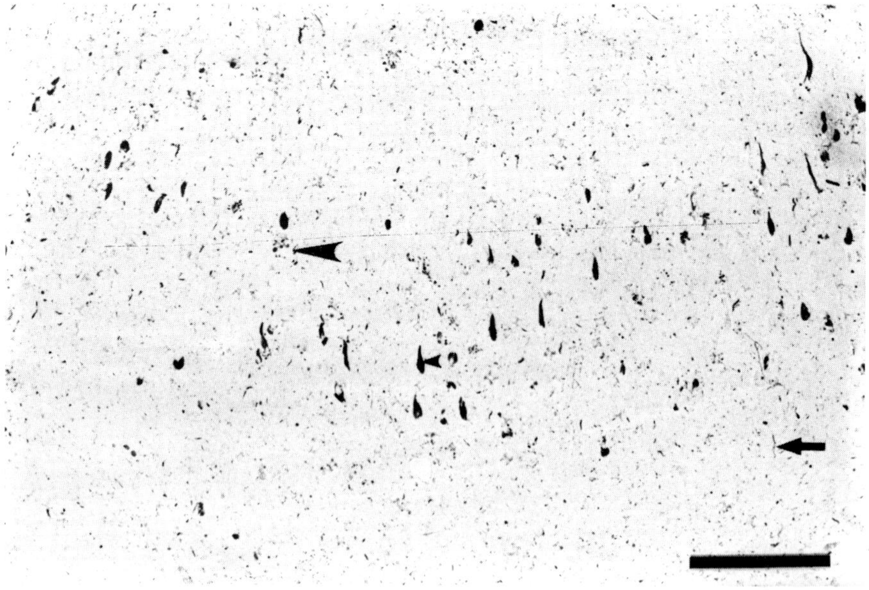

Figure 1. Neurofibrillary tangles (small arrowhead), altered neurites (arrow) and neuritic plaques (large arrowhead) show intense immunostaining with an immunoaffinity purified antiserum to ubiquitin in a brain from a patient with Alzheimer disease. Peroxidase-antiperoxidase. Light micrograph. Scale bar = 250 μm.

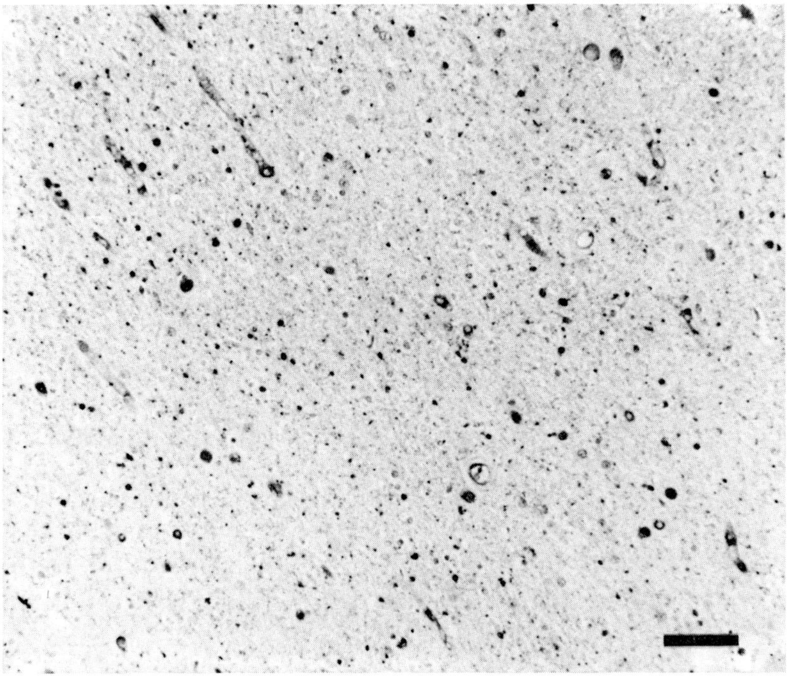

Figure 2. "Dot-like" structures throughout the white matter of Alzheimer disease were immunostained with antibodies to ubiquitin. Light micrograph. Scale bar = 50 μm.

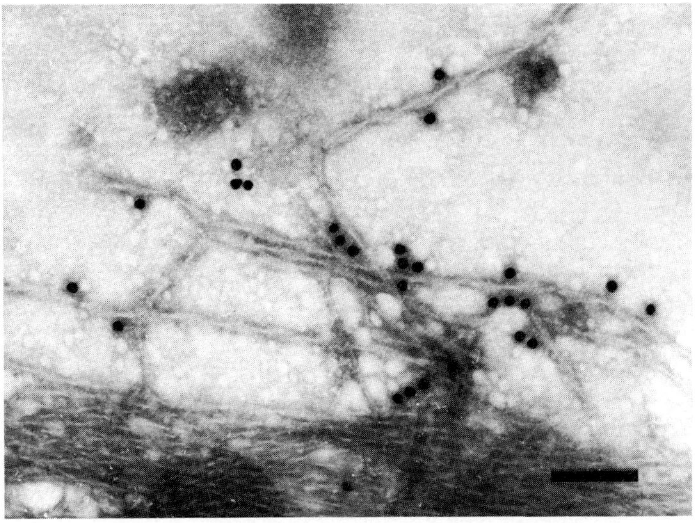

Figure 3. Isolated PHF treated with sodium dodecyl sulfate to extract soluble components are immunodecorated by immunoaffinity purified antiserum to ubiquitin. Electron micrograph. Scale bar = 01. μm.

following isolation and treatment with the ionic detergent SDS to remove soluble components (Fig. 3). Thus, Ub in PHF is either present in an SDS-insoluble form or is conjugated to an SDS-insoluble acceptor protein. Immunoblot and immunodot analysis confirmed that Ub Ab reacted with SDS-insoluble fractions known to be enriched in PHF, as did Abs raised to PHF.

The finding of Ub in PHF raises several questions, one of which is whether Ub is the previously unidentified component recognized by Abs raised to PHF.

UBIQUITIN IS RECOGNIZED BY mAbs ANTIBODIES RAISED TO PHF

Mori et al. (1987) showed that a mAb raised to PHF recognizes Ub. We examined several mAbs (Wang et al., 1984) and antisera raised to PHF to assess and characterize their cross-reactivity with Ub (Perry et al., 1987c). One of five antisera and two of three mAbs raised to PHF recognized Ub. These two sets of Ub Abs showed a similar pattern of immunostaining of AD tissues. However, all Abs to Ub raised with PHF as immunogen immunoreacted with AD tissues on frozen, unfixed sections and recognized free Ub on blots, whereas the mAbs to Ub tested did not. Analysis of tryptic fragments of Ub showed that the epitopes recognized by the two mAbs to PHF reside within residues 50-65 and 64-76 of Ub (Perry et al., 1987c). Mori et al. (1987), after peptidase digestion of a PHF fraction, purified and sequenced two peptides that correspond to residues 11-26 and 34-48 of Ub. Collectively, these data provide evidence that most of the Ub molecule is present in PHF.

UBIQUITIN IN OTHER NEURODEGENERATIVE DISEASES

NFT are not the only neuronal inclusions common to AD and aging; further, AD is not the only disease characterized by the presence of distinct fibrillary inclusions in the neuronal cytoplasm. Thus, a second question that was raised is whether Ub is present also in other neuronal inclusions of AD or other degenerative conditions.

Hirano bodies (Hirano et al., 1968), paracrystalline structures made of sheets of 6-10 nm filaments containing actin and actin-binding proteins (Goldman, 1983; Galloway et al., 1987b, c), and granulovacuolar degeneration (GVD), a non-filamentous inclusion reported to contain tubulin epitopes (Price et al., 1986), are two neuronal inclusions commonly seen in AD. In Pick disease and progressive supranuclear palsy (PSP), two rarer dementing illnesses of advanced age, neurons also contain abnormal filamentous structures, the Pick body and NFT of PSP (Schoene, 1985). These differ from NFT of AD in that they are made of straight rather than helical filaments (Takauchi et al., 1984; Tellez-Nagel and Wisniewski, 1973) and do not form during normal aging (Tomlinson and Corsellis, 1984). Despite these differences, Pick bodies and the NFT of PSP share antigenic determinants with PHF of AD, and tau proteins seem to be a major constituent of all these inclusions (Perry et al., 1987d; Tabaton et al., 1988). Lewy bodies, the hallmark of Parkinson disease, share only a few antigenic determinants with the NFT of AD and were shown not to contain tau proteins

(Galloway et al., 1987a); they are also not commonly observed during normal aging (Tomlinson and Corsellis, 1984).

We used the same Abs to Ub to immunostain tissues obtained at autopsy from two cases each of Pick, Parkinson disease and PSP. Two cases of AD with a relatively large number of Hirano bodies and GVD in the hippocampus were also examined. Lewy bodies were immunostained by all the antisera and with the same mAb that reacted with the NFT of AD (Fig. 4). In addition to the Lewy bodies, numerous neurites were also immunostained in the substantia nigra and locus coeruleus, two regions containing Lewy bodies. Pick bodies and NFT of PSP immunoreacted with all mAbs to PHF that recognize Ub but with only one of the eight mAbs to Ub (Manetto et al., 1988); fewer neurites were immunostained in these two diseases. No immunoreaction was seen in Hirano bodies and GVD; control tissues from the same regions showed no immunostaining. Ultrastructural immunocytochemistry demonstrated that both immunoaffinity-purified antisera and the mAbs to Ub decorated the fibrillary component of each of the reacting inclusions. As in NFT, the Ub Abs decorated the amorphous material interspersed among the straight filaments of the Pick bodies and of the NFT of PSP. On the contrary, only the fibrillary component at the edge of the Lewy body was decorated, while there was no reaction with the amorphous core (Fig. 5).

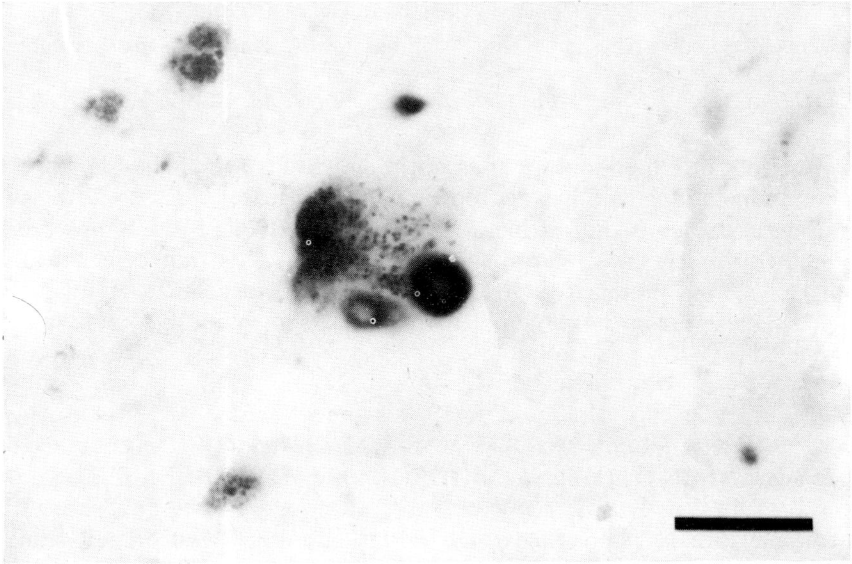

Figure 4. Two Lewy bodies in the locus coeruleus of a patient with Parkinson disease are imunostained by the antiserum to ubiquitin. The periphery of the body is more intensely immunostained. The scattered immunostained structures are probably neuronal cell processes. Light micrograph. Scale bar = 25μm.

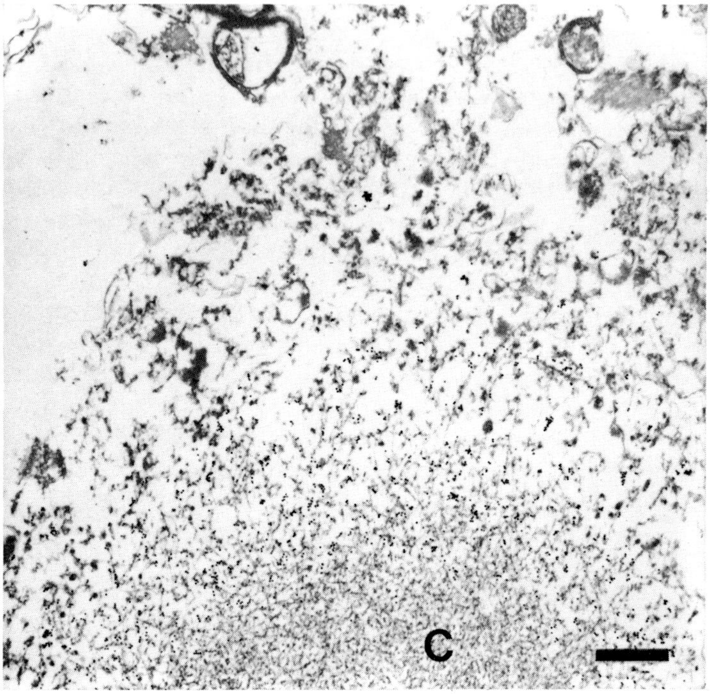

Figure 5. Electron micrograph of a Lewy body immunodecorated with an antiserum to ubiquitin. The filaments in the outer region of the inclusion but not the denser core are immunodecorated. C = core. Scale bar = 0.5 μm.

The presence of Ub epitopes is thus not a unique feature of the PHF in AD; it is shared by the inclusions of other neurodegenerative diseases, such as Lewy bodies of Parkinson disease, Pick bodies of Pick disease, and NFT of PSP. Ub, however, is not indiscriminately present in all neuronal inclusions, as we did not detect it in Hirano bodies and GVD. The presence of Ub does not seem to be dependent on the presence of tau proteins; Ub is present in Lewy bodies which were shown not to contain tau epitopes (Galloway et al., 1987a).

ROLE OF UBIQUITIN IN ALZHEIMER DISEASE AND IN OTHER NEURODEGENERATIVE DISEASES

The significance of the presence of Ub in PHF and other fibrillary inclusions can be speculated on the basis of available knowledge of the function of ubiquitin in cells under normal and pathological conditions. It has been reported that following heat shock the rate of protein degradation decreases while stable high molecular weight Ub-conjugates are increased (Carlson et al., 1987). It has been suggested that the increase of stable high molecular weight Ub conjugates is the result of the saturation of the Ub-mediated proteolytic system due to an increased amount of altered proteins (Carlson et al., 1987; Speiser and Etlinger, 1983). The failure of the Ub-mediated proteolytic system might be responsible for the abundance of Ub in insoluble and highly stable cellular inclusions observed in our studies. Other explanations for the presence of Ub in intracellular inclusions that contain cytoskeletal proteins cannot be excluded. For example, it has recently been reported that in several cell lines Ub is associated with the microtubule network (Murti et al., 1988). Therefore, the presence of Ub in intracellular inclusions could result from reorganization of preexisting Ub-conjugates that are normally associated with the cytoskeleton (Murti et al., 1988). Whatever the mechanism for the presence of Ub in intracellular inclusions, it is likely to be shared by different degenerative diseases, such as Alzheimer, Parkinson, Pick, PSP, and other conditions. At the same time, ubiquitination of intracellular inclusions is selective. At this writing, all the cellular inclusions that have Ub also contain cytoskeletal proteins, but not all inclusions that contain cytoskeletal proteins appear to be ubiquitinated. It is thus likely that some, but not all, cytoskeletal proteins are Ub acceptors.

ACKNOWLEDGEMENTS

Supported by the National Institutes of Health Grant AG 00795, the David S. Ingalls Fund, the Gertrude Dominik Memorial Fund and the American Health Assistance Foundation. Dr. Manetto is a recipient of a fellowship from the Britton Fund.

REFERENCES

Autilio-Gambetti L, Gambetti P, Crane RC (1983) Paired helical filaments: relatedness to neurofilaments shown by silver staining and reactivity with monoclonal antibodies. In: Katzman R (ed): Biological Aspect of Alzheimer's disease. Banbury Report 15. Cold Spring Harbor Laboratory, New York, pp. 117-124.

Bond U, Schlesinger MJ (1985) Ubiquitin is a heat shock protein in chicken embryo fibroblasts. Mol Cell Biol 5:949-956.

Bond U, Schlesinger MJ (1986) The chicken ubiquitin gene contains a heat shock promoter and expresses an unstable mRNA in heat-shock cells. Mol Cell Biol 6:4602-4610.

Brion JP, van den Bosch de Aguilar P, Flament-Durand J (1985) Senile dementia of the Alzheimer type. In: Traber J and Gispen WH (eds): Advances in Applied Neurological Science, Vol. 2. Springer-Verlag, Berlin, pp. 164-174.

Carlson N, Rogers S, Rechsteiner M (1987) Microinjection of ubiquitin: Changes in protein degradation in Hela cells subjected to heat-shock. J Cell Biol 104:547-555.

Collier NC, Schlesinger MJ (1986) The dynamic state of heat shock proteins in chicken fibroblasts. J Cell Biol 103:1495-1507.

Dice JF (1987) Molecular determinants of protein half-lives in eukaryotic cells. FASEB J 1:349-357.

Finley D, Varshavsky A (1985) The ubiquitin system: Functions and mechanisms. Trends Biochem Sci 10:343-346.

Fried VA, Smith HT, Hildbrandt E, Weiner K (1987) Ubiquitin has intrinsic proteolytic activity: Implications for cellular regulation. Proc Natl Acad Sci USA 84:3685-3689.

Galloway P, Grundke-Iqbal I, Autilio-Gambetti L, Gambetti P, Perry G (1987a) Neuronal Cytoskeletal involvement in Lewy body formation. J Neuropathol Exp Neurol 46:374 (Abstract).

Galloway P, Perry G, Gambetti P (1987b) Hirano body filaments contain actin and actin-associated protein. J Neuropathol Exp Neurol 46:185-199.

Galloway P, Perry G, Kosik K, Gambetti P (1987c) Hirano bodies contain tau protein. Brain Res 403:337-340.

Gambetti P, Autilio-Gambetti L, Manetto V, Perry G (1988) Composition of paired helical filaments of Alzheimer disease as determined by specific probes. In: Finch C and Davies P (eds): Banbury Report 27, The Neurochemistry of Aging. Cold Spring Harbor, NY, pp. 309-320.

Glenner GG, Wong CW (1984a) Alzheimer's disease: Initial report of the purification and characterization of a novel cerebrovascular amyloid protein. Biochem Biophys Res Commun 120:885-890.

Glenner GG, Wong CW (1984b) Alzheimer's disease and Down's syndrome: Sharing of a unique cerebrovascular amyloid fibril protein. Biochem Biophys Res Commun 122:1131-1135.

Goldgaber D, Lerman MI, McBride OW, Saffiotti U, Gajdusek DC (1987) Characterization and chromosomal localization of a cDNA encoding brain amyloid of Alzheimer's disease. Science 235:877-880.

Goldknopf IL, Busch H (1977) Isopeptide linkage between nonhistone and histone 2A polypeptides of chromosomal conjugate protein A24. Proc Natl Acad Sci USA 74:864-868.

Goldman JE (1983) The association of actin with Hirano bodies. J Neuropathol Exp Neurol 42:146-152.

Goldstein G, Scheid M, Hammerling U, Boyse EA, Schlesinger DH, Niall HD (1975) Isolation of a polypeptide that has lymphocyte-differentiating properties and is probably represented universally in living cells. Proc Natl Acad Sci USA 72:11-15.

Grundke-Iqbal I, Iqbal K, Tung YC, Quinlan M, Wisniewski HH, Binder LI (1986) Abnormal phosphorylation of the microtubule associated protein tau in Alzheimer cytoskeletal pathology. Proc Natl Acad Sci USA 83:4913-4917.

Hirano A, Dembitzer HM, Kurland LT, Zimmerman HM (1968) The fine structure of some intraganglionic alterations. J Neuropathol Exp Neurol 27:167-182.

Kang J, Lemaire HG, Unterbeck A, Salbaum JM, Masters CL, Grzeschik KH, Beyreuther K, Malthaup G, Muller-Hill B (1987) The precursor of Alzheimer's disease amyloid A4 protein resembles a cell-surface receptor. Nature 325:733-736.

Kosik KS, Duffy LK, Dowling MM, Abraham C, McCluskey A, Selkoe DJ (1984) Microtubule-associated protein 2: Monoclonal antibodies demonstrate the selective incorporation of certain epitopes into Alzheimer neurofibrillary tangles. Proc Natl Acad Sci USA 81: 7941-7945.

Kosik KS, Joachim CL, Selkoe DJ (1986) The microtubule-associated protein is a major antigenic component of paired helical filaments. Proc Natl Acad Sci USA 83:4044-4048.

Ksiezak-Reding H, Dickson DW, Davies P, Yen S-H (1987) Recognition of tau epitopes by anti-neurofilament antibodies that bind to Alzheimer neurofibrillary tangles. Proc Natl Acad Sci USA 84:3410-3414.

Manetto V, Perry G, Tabaton M, Mulvihill P, Fried VA, Smith HT, Gambetti P, Autilio-Gambetti L (1988) Ubiquitin is associated with abnormal cytoplasmic filaments characteristic of neurodegenerative diseases. Proc Natl Acad Sci USA 85:4501-4505.

Mann DMA (1985) The neuropathology of Alzheimer's disease: A review with pathogenetic, aetiological and therapeutic considerations. Mech Ageing Dev 31:213-255.

Masters CL, Simms G, Weinman NA, Multhaup G, McDonald BL, Beyreuther K (1985) Amyloid plaque core protein in Alzheimer disease and Down syndrome. Proc Natl Acad Sci USA 82:4245-4249.

Mori H, Kondo J, Ihara I (1987) Ubiquitin is a component of paired helical filaments in Alzheimer's disease. Science 235:1641-1644.

Murti KG, Smith HT, Fried VA (1988) Ubiquitin is a component of the microtubule network. Proc Natl Acad Sci USA 85:3019-3023.

Nukina N, Kosik KS, Selkoe DJ (1987) Recognition of Alzheimer paired helical filaments by monoclonal neurofilament antibodies is due to crossreaction with tau protein. Proc Natl Acad Sci 84:3415-3419.

Perry G, Friedman R, Kang DH, Manetto V, Autilio-Gambetti L, Gambetti P (1987a) Antibodies to the neuronal cytoskeleton are elicited by Alzheimer paired helical filament fractions. Brain Res 420:233-242.

Perry G, Friedman R, Shaw G, Chau V (1987b) Ubiquitin is detected in neurofibrillary tangles and senile plaque neurites of Alzheimer disease brain. Proc Natl Acad Sci USA 86: 3033-3036.

Perry G, Mulvihill P, Manetto V, Fried V, Smith H, Grundke-Iqbal I, Iqbal K, Autilio-Gambetti L, Gambetti P (1987c) Ubiquitin epitopes in Alzheimer paired helical filaments: a study with monoclonal antibodies to ubiquitin and paired helical filaments. J Cell Biol 105:203.

Perry G, Stewart D, Friedman R, Manetto V, Autilio-Gambetti L, Gambetti P (1987d) Filaments of Pick's bodies contain altered cytoskeletal elements. Am J Pathol 127:559-568.

Price DL, Altschuler RJ, Struble RG, Casanova MF, Cork LC, Murphy DB (1986) Sequestration of tubulin in neurons in Alzheimer's disease. Brain Res 385:305-310.

Schoene WC (1985) Degenerative diseases of the central nervous system. In: Davis RL, Robertson DM (eds): Textbook of Neuropathology, Chapter 15. Williams & Wilkins, Baltimore, pp. 788-823.

Selkoe DJ (1986) Altered structural proteins in plaques and tangles: What do they tell us about the biology of Alzheimer's disease? Neurobiol Aging 7: 425-432.

Siegelman M, Bond MW, Gallatin WM, St John T, Smith HT, Fried VA, Weissman IL (1986) Celle surface molecule associated with lymphocyte homing is a ubiquitinated branched-chain glycoprotein. Science 231:823-829.

Speiser S, Etlinger JD (1983) ATP stimulated proteolysis in reticulocyte extracts by repressing an endogenous protease inhibitor. Proc Natl Acad Sci USA 80:3577-3580.

St John T, Gallatin WM, Siegelman M, Smith HT, Fried VA, Weissman IL (1986) Expression cloning of a lymphocyte homing receptor cDNA: Ubiquitin is the reactive species. Science 231:845-850.

Tabaton M, Perry G, Autilio-Gambetti L, Manetto V, Gambetti P (1988) Influence of neuronal location on antigenic properties of neurofibrillary tangles. Ann Neurol, 23:604-610.

Tabaton M, Whitehouse PJ, Perry G, Davies P, Autilio-Gambetti L, Gambetti P (1988) The antigen recognized by the monoclonal antibody ALZ-50 is associated with abnormal filaments in Alzheimer disease and progressive supranuclear palsy. Ann Neurol in press.

Takauchi S, Hosomi M, Marasigan S, Sato M, Hiyashi S, Miyoshi K (1984) An ultrastructural study of Pick bodies. Acta Neuropathol (Berl) 64: 344-348.

Tellez-Nagel I, Wisniewski HM (1973) Ultrastructure of neurofibrillary tangles in Steele-Richardson-Olszewski syndrome. Arch Neurol 29:324-327.

Tomlinson BE, Blessed G, Roth M (1968) Observation on the brains of nondemented old people. J Neurol Sci 7:331-356.

Tomlinson BE, Blessed G, Roth M (1970) Observations on the brains of demented old people. J Neurol Sci 11:205-242.

Tomlinson BE, Corsellis JAN (1984) Ageing and the dementias. In: Adams JH, Corsellis JAN, Dunchen LW (eds): Greenfield's Neuropathology (4th ed). Wiley & Sons, NY, pp. 951-1025.

Wang GP, Grundke-Iqbal I, Kascsak RJ, Iqbal K, Wisniewski HM (1984) Alzheimer neurofibrillary tangles: Monoclonal antibodies to inherent antigen(s). Acta Neuropathol (Berl) 62:268-275.

West MHP, Bonner WM (1980) Histone 2b can be modified by attachment of ubiquitin. Nucleic Acids Res 8:4671-4680.

Wisniewski HM, Narang HK, Terry RD (1976) Neurofibrillary tangles of paired helical filaments. J Neurol Sci 27:173-181.

Wood JG, Mirra SS, Pollock NJ, Binder LF (1986) Neurofibrillary tangles of Alzheimer disease share antigenic determinants with the axonal microtubule-associated protein tau. Proc Natl Acad Sci USA 83:4040-4043.

Wolozin BL, Pruchinicki A, Dickson DW, Davies P (1986) A neuronal antigen in the brains of Alzheimer patients. Science 232:648-650.

Yarden Y, Escobedo JA, Kuang WJ, Yang-Feng TL, Daniel TO, Tremble PM, Chen EY, Ando ME, Harkins RN, Francke U, Fried VA, Ullrich A, Williams LT (1986) Structure of the receptor for platelet-derived growth factor helps define a family of closely related growth factor receptors. Nature 323:226-232.

New Trends in Aging Research
G. Pepeu, B. Tomlinson, C.M. Wischik (eds)
Fidia Research Series, vol. 15
Liviana Press, Padova © 1988

MULTIPLE BIOCHEMICAL DISTURBANCES IN BRAINS FROM PATIENTS WITH ALZHEIMER DEMENTIA

C.G. Gottfries

Department of Psychiatry and Neurochemistry,
Gothenburg University, St. Jörgen's Hospital, S-422 03
Hisings Backa, Sweden

INTRODUCTION

Several reports have shown changes in brains from patients with Alzheimer's disease (AD) and patients with *senile dementia of the Alzheimer type* (SDAT). Investigations have focused on neurotransmitter disturbances in gray matter (Reisberg, 1983). Some authors consider the cholinergic disturbance important, while others have shown that disturbances of monoamine neurotransmitters are also of importance (Gottfries et al., 1983; 1986; Hardy et al., 1985).

Changes in white matter have been studied less. There are, however, neuropathological investigations (Brun and Gustafson, 1978) reporting white matter degeneration in brains from demented patients, not only in those with cerebrovascular disorders but also in patients with AD/SDAT. Neurochemical investigations of white matter have also revealed reduced concentrations of myelin components (Gottfries et al., 1985; Svennerholm et al., 1987).

The aim of this study is to report on biochemical disturbances in brains from patients with AD/SDAT, studying them in relation to the clinical diagnosis of dementia.

Abbreviations: ACh, Acetylcholine; AD, Alzheimer's disease; CAT, Choline-acetyl transferase; CSF, Cerebrospinal fluid; CT, Computer tomography; CVD, Cerebrovascular disorder; DA, Dopamine; 5-HIAA, 5-hydroxyindolacetic acid; HMPG, 3-methoxy 4-hydroxyphenylglycol; 5-HT, 5-hydroxytryptamine; HVA, Homovanillic acid; MAO-A, Monoamine oxidase-A; MAO-B, Monoamine oxidase-B; NA, Noradrenaline; NMR, Nuclear magnetic resonance; SDAT, Senile dementia of Alzheimer type.

The data presented here are reported on in part elsewhere (Gottfries et al., 1986; Oreland and Gottfries, 1986; Regland et al., 1987).

THE CLASSIFICATION OF DEMENTIAS

The criteria generally used to classify the different types of dementia are rather superficial and not very systematic. As shown in Figure 1, the dementia syndrome is divided into different categories depending on the diagnostic description. Dementia is a syndrome with evidence of decline in memory and thinking, sometimes also a deterioration in emotional functions. This deterioration can be severe enough to impair daily living. Some add that only when the syndrome appears in individuals with "clear" consciousness can a reliable diagnosis be established, otherwise the concept pseudodementia must be introduced. In some textbooks dementia is also defined as a longstanding (at least six months) or irreversible disorder. Dementia may also be defined as a syndrome which is global although memory and thinking are considered the most important guidelines. Here our definition of dementia is based upon the syndrome being considered a decline in intellectual and emotional functions irrespective of the etiology, the age of onset, the course or the extent of the disorder.

There is still controversy as to whether mental impairment in the elderly is a quantitative disorder in which the normal aging process is accelerated, the dementia

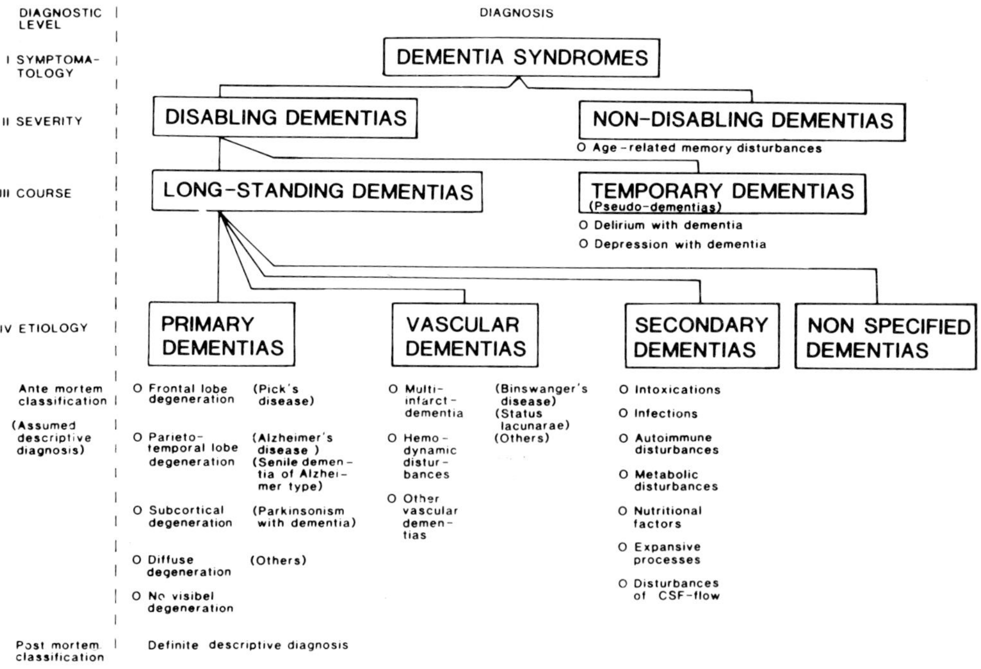

Figure 1. Classification of dementias.

appearing when reserves are exhausted and compensatory mechanisms fail. The concept of *senile benign forgetfulness* cannot be separated from that of cognitive impairment due to normal aging. Now data are available indicating that in subjects over 60 years of age an involution process takes place in the brain, causing atrophy and biochemical disturbances in neurotransmitter functioning. The idea of an involution process is in line with that there is a continuity between normal aging and dementia (Gottfries, 1986).

The group of dementias called primary degenerative disorders includes the quantitatively important group, *senile dementia*. As neuropathologists have found senile plaques and fibrillary tangles (Alzheimer lesions) in brains from patients with senile dementia, this group has been named SDAT. SDAT has an insidious onset and is progressing gradually, in subjects over 65 years of age. From a clinical point of view, it is heterogeneous. The diagnosis is made through exclusion: when no other etiology can be found, the condition is called senile dementia. From a clinical standpoint the concept of SDAT is impractical because the diagnosis cannot be confirmed until a post mortem investigation has been made. If the concept SDAT is used, a group of dementias with an unknown etiology must also be introduced.

In some studies patients with AD are sampled together with patients with SDAT to form an Alzheimer dementia group. From a scientific viewpoint this appears unwise because, clinically speaking, the AD group is more homogenous than the SDAT group.

Investigations made on families in Scandinavia (Sjögren et al., 1952; Sourander and Sjögren, 1970) have shown that AD and SDAT behave like two separate disorders. Also biochemical investigations have shown results indicating that early onset dementia (AD) and late onset dementia (SDAT) should be considered separate entities (Gottfries et al., 1983; Rossor et al., 1984; Bråne et al., 1988).

MATERIAL AND METHODS

Twenty-two brains from patients who died of somatic disorders with no history of neurological or psychiatric disease were used as control material. The macroscopic examination of the brain revealed no pathological disorders and microscopic investigation of the hippocampus and the cortex from the frontal lobe, showed a number of senile plaques that could reasonably be attributed to normal aging. Fibrillary tangles were not found in the cortical areas and were only occasionally present in the hippocampus.

Twenty-one brains from patients with AD/SDAT were investigated at autopsy. The clinical diagnoses were made according to the DSM III and the final diagnosis was made in accordance with macroscopic findings at the autopsy and histological investigation of the frontal cortex and the hippocampus. Fibrillary tangles and senile plaques were seen in numbers consistent with the diagnosis of AD/SDAT. The criterion used to distinguish between AD and SDAT was whether the onset of dementia occurred in subjects before or after the age of 65 years.

In the brains from the controls and those from the demented patients, different nuclei and areas were dissected by following anatomical landmarks. The tissue used for biochemical investigation was deep-frozen to -80° Celsius. While deep-frozen, the tissue samples were ground into a powder homogenate from which tissue subsamples were taken and then delivered to different laboratories for chemical analyses. Through a particular cooperation between neurochemical laboratories in Sweden, it was possible to determine several biochemical variables in one and the same brain sample. We here present data from determinations of 5-hydroxytryptamine (5-HT), 5-hydroxyindolacetic acid (5-HIAA), noradrenaline (NA), 3-methoxy 4-hydroxyphenylglycol (HMPG), dopamine (DA), homovanillic acid (HVA), and choline-acetyl transferase (CAT) in the hippocampus (for methods used, see Gottfries et al., 1983 and Gottfries et al., 1986). In the cingulate cortex and putamen the imipramine binding sites were ascertained (for details, see Marcusson et al., 1987). In white matter phospholipids, cholesterol, cerebrosides and sulfatides were ascertained (for methods used, see Svennerholm et al., 1987). Gangliosides were also ascertained in the caudate nucleus (for details, see Svennerholm et al., this issue). Monoamine oxidase was ascertained in the caudate nucleus and the white matter (for details, see Oreland and Gottfries, 1986).

We also report the vitamin B-12-levels in serum from 158 demented patients who are still alive. This group of patients with "clinically diagnosed dementia" was subdivided into a control group (n = 16), a group with cerebrovascular dementia (CVD) (n = 54), a group with AD (n = 35), a group with SDAT (n = 56) and a group of patients with dementia and confusion (n = 10) (for details see Regland et al., 1988).

RESULTS

In the controls significant negative correlations were found between 5-HT in the caudate nucleus and age, between NA in the hippocampus and age and between DA in the hippocampus and age. No significant correlations were however found between age and the monoamine metabolites indicating that although the active amines decrease in the 60 to 90 years age group there is no coincidental decrease in the metabolites (Table 1).

In the hippocampus several significantly reduced concentrations of biochemical variables were found in the AD/SDAT group with respect to the controls (Table 2 and Fig. 2). The CAT activity was significantly reduced — it was about half that of the

Table 1. *The product moment correlation (r) between age and biochemical variables in brains from patients with normal aging*

Age	Nucleus caudatus		Hippocampus	
	r	n	r	n
5-HT	-0.60***	22	-0.04	22
5-HIAA	-0.06	22	0.22	22
NA	0.20	22	-0.70***	22
HMPG	0.29	22	0.31	22
DA	-0.24	22	0.58***	22
HVA	-0.34	22	-0.15	22

*** = $p < 0.005$; n = number of cases

controls. It was, however, also evident that there were significant reductions in the 5-HT and 5-HIAA concentrations in the AD/SDAT patients — they were 3/5 that of the

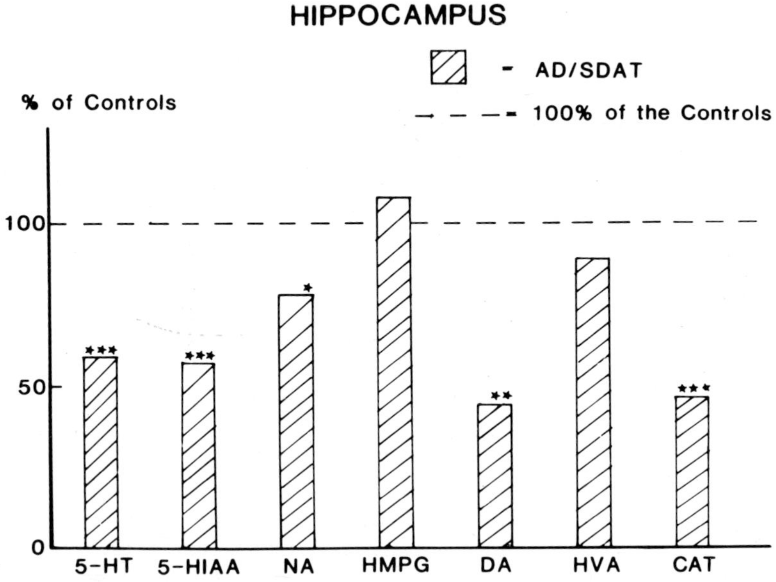

Figure 2. Biochemical disturbances in the hippocampus. The dotted line, mean of the controls (n=21); columns, the concentrations in different biochemical variables in brains from patients with AD/SDAT (n=19-20). Asterisks indicate significant group differences according to Student's t-test. (* = $p<0.05$, ** = $p<0.01$, *** = $p<0.005$).

Table 2. *Neurochemical variables in brains from controls and from patients with AD/SDAT dementia*

	Hippocampus					
	Controls			AD/SDAT		
	n	M	SD	n	M	SD
5-HT nmol/g	21	0.30	0.14	19	0.18***	0.09
5-HIAA nmol/g	21	288	115	19	164***	69
NA nmol/g	21	0.11	0.04	19	0.09*	0.04
HMPG nmol/g	21	0.36	0.16	20	0.39	0.17
DA nmol/g	21	0.13	0.11	19	0.06**	0.07
HVA nmol/g	21	1.8	0.7	20	1.6	1.3
CAT μkat/kg protein	21	488	329	19	223***	206

Group differences according to Student's t test.
* = $p<0.05$, ** = $p<0.01$, *** = $p<0.005$; n = number of cases; M = mean; SD = standard deviation.

controls. NA was reduced in the group of patients with dementia but the end metabolite, HMPG, was not reduced. DA was significantly reduced when the AD/SDAT group was compared to the controls but the metabolite HVA was not significantly reduced in the dementia group.

As seen in Figure 3, the presynaptic marker for the 5-HT system, the imipramine binding sites, were found to be significantly reduced in the cingulate cortex and the putamen (for details see Marcusson et al., 1987).

As is evident in Table 3, the monoamine oxidase-B (MAO-B) activity was significantly increased in the white matter of demented patients with respect to that of the controls. The monoamine oxidase-A (MAO-A) activity had not changed.

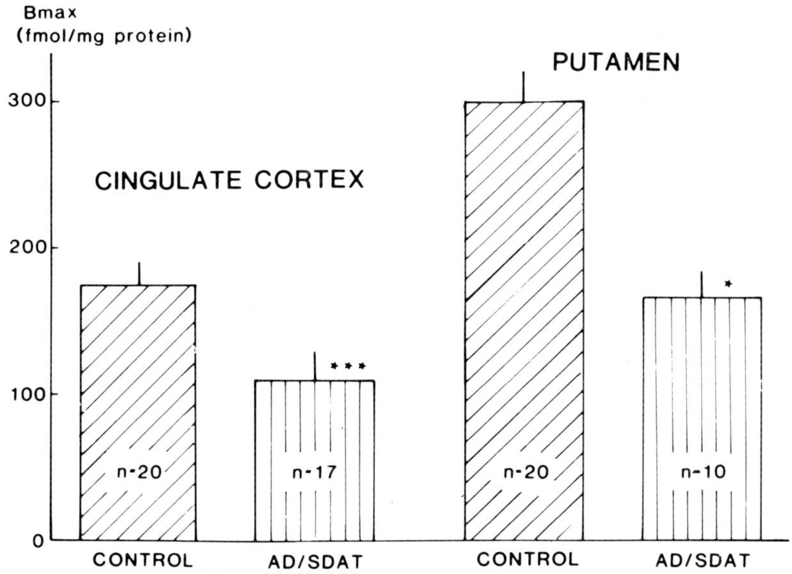

Figure 3. 5-HT-sensitive imipramine binding to post-mortem cingulate cortex and putamen from a control group and patients with AD/SDAT (for details, see Marcusson et al., 1987).

Table 3. *MAO activities (μkat/kg/prot) in white matter from age-matched controls and patients with AD/SDAT*

	Controls		AD/SDAT	
	n	M SD	n	M SD
MAO-A	13	2.86 ± 0.64	9	3.18 ± 0.87
MAO-B	15	7.43 ± 1.91	13	12.53 ± 6.56***

Group differences according to Student's t test, *** = $p < 0.05$; n = number of cases; M = mean; SD = standard deviation.

When investigating white matter from centrum semiovale it was evident that in the group of AD/SDAT patients there were significant reductions in the myelin components phospholipids, cholesterol, cerebrosides and sulfatides as is shown in Table 4 and Figure 4.

Table 4. *Levels of myelin components in white matter in a group of controls and a group of patients with AD/SDAT*

	Controls			AD/SDAT		
	n	M	SD	n	M	SD
Phospholipids						
neutral (μmol/g)	17	75.9	9.2	13	57.1***	11.3
acidic (μmol/g)	17	21.1	2.6	13	15.9***	3.6
Cholesterol (μmol/g)	17	112.0	16.2	13	84.3***	20.2
Cerebrosides (μmol/g)	17	39.5	6.4	13	28.2***	5.4
Sulfatides (μmol/g)	14	15.9	4.0	13	10.0***	2.6

Group differences according to Student's t test, *** = $p < 0.005$; n = number of cases; M = mean; SD = standard deviation.

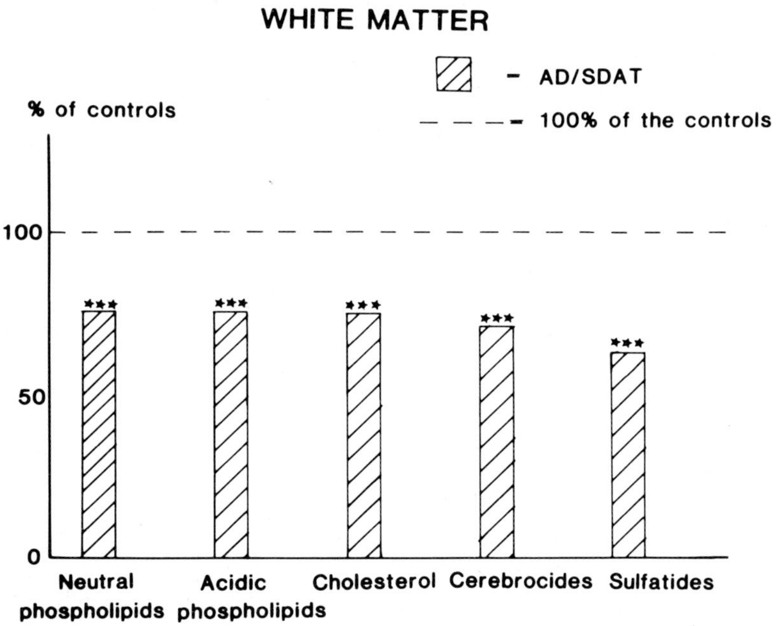

Figure 4. Myelin components in white matter from a control group (n = 17) and a group of patients with AD/SDAT (n = 13). The dotted line is 100% of the mean of the controls and the columns are the concentrations found in the AD/SDAT brains; asterisks indicate significance of difference according to Student's t test (*** = $p < 0.005$).

The results of the investigation of vitamin-B-12 in groups of patients with clinically diagnosed dementia are shown in Figure 5. The figure shows that no controls (n = 16) had vitamin-B-12 levels under the vitamin-B-12 distribution values considered normal at our laboratory (lower limit 130 pmol/l). Five (9%) of the 54 patients with CVD and

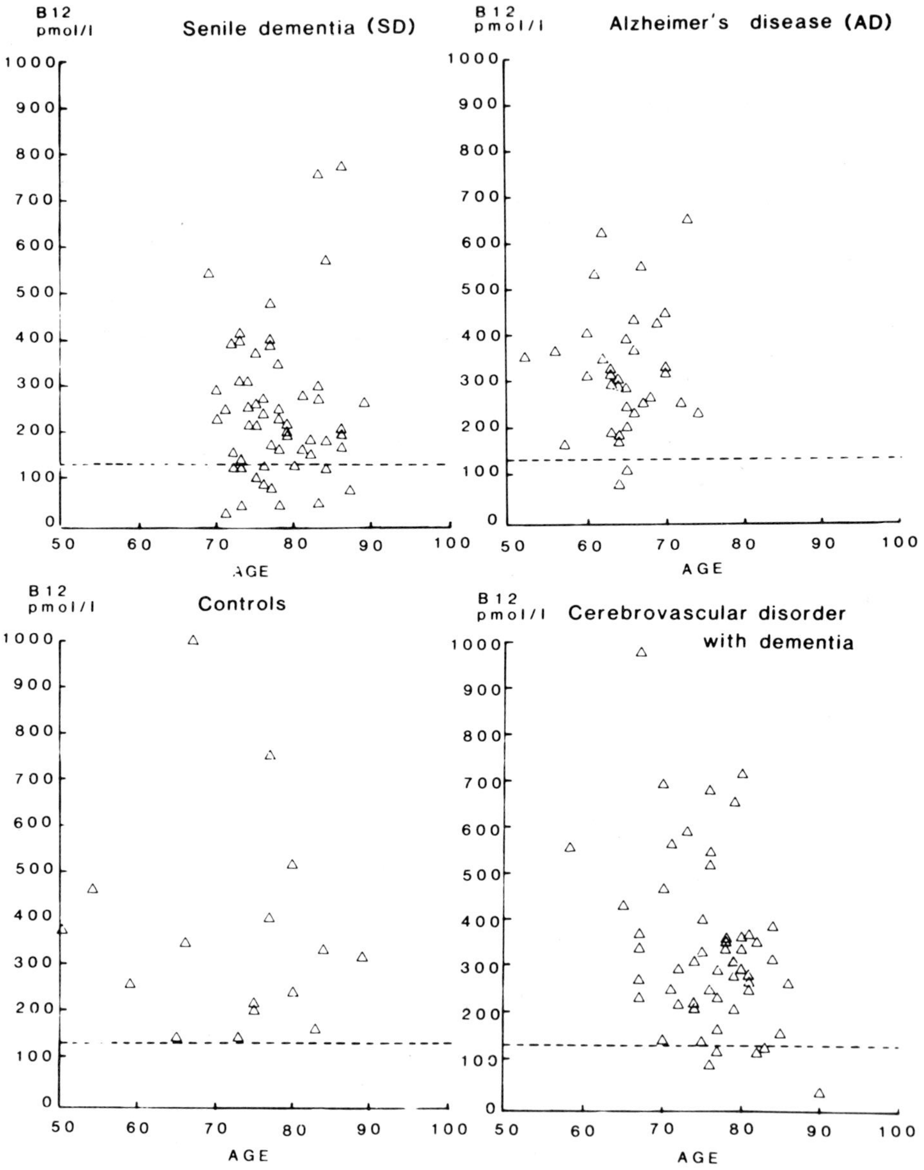

Figure 5. Vitamin B12 in pmol/l in a control group (n = 16) and three groups of patients with organic dementia (senile dementia n = 56, Alzheimer's disease n = 35, cerebrovascular disorder with dementia n = 54). The dotted line, lower limit for vitamin B12 (130 pmol/l).

dementia and two (6%) of the 35 patients with the early onset AD had vitamin-B-12 levels below the lower limit. In the group of 55 patients with a clinical diagnosis of SDAT, 14 (23%) had vitamin-B-12 levels under the lower limit.

DISCUSSION

As is evident from the investigation of brains from patients with normal aging, reduced concentrations of active amines are present in the brains of aged patients although these patients showed no signs of cognitive impairment. It is interesting that although the active amines are reduced, the end metabolites of the monoamine metabolism are not reduced. This may indicate that in the normally aged brain there is a neuron loss, reflected as a reduced concentration of the active amines. The remaining neurons, however, seem to be able to speed up their metabolism so that the release and the concentration of the end metabolites is maintained at a normal level. This may be a compensatory mechanism of the neuron. In patients with AD/SDAT this compensatory mechanism does not seem to function, at least where the 5HT-metabolism is concerned.

It is evident that in the Alzheimer demented brains there are multiple disturbances. In the gray matter the reduced CAT activity indicates a severe loss of cholinergic neurons or a severely disturbed acetylcholine (ACh) metabolism. There is, however, also a significantly reduced activity in the serotonin systems, which is reflected not only by reduced concentrations of 5-HT and 5-HIAA but also by reduced imipramine binding sites in cortical areas and putamen. To some extent catecholaminergic systems are also disturbed.

MAO-B is increased in gray as well as in white matter (Oreland and Gottfries, 1986). As is evident in Table 3, a rather high increase was found in MAO-B in white matter. As shown by Oreland et al. (1980) the increased MAO-B activity seems to reflect an invasion of extra neuronal tissue. The MAO-B activity may be considered a marker for gliosis of the brain. A white matter disturbance is also reflected by a significant reduction in myelin components in centrum semiovale.

Our findings show that in AD/SDAT brains the biochemical disturbances are not restricted to the cholinergic system. It is evident that in gray matter monoaminergic systems are also disturbed. Moreover, the neuropeptides e.g. somatostatin and P substance are also reduced (Reisberg, 1983).

Pathological changes are, however, not only restricted to gray matter. In white matter rather severe changes are found. Significantly reduced concentrations of myelin components indicate a degeneration of white matter. This is in line with neuropathological findings described by Brun (1983), Brun and Englund (1985) and by computed tomography (CT)-scan- and nuclear magnetic resonance (NMR)-findings (de Leon et al., 1985; Erkinjuntti et al., 1987).

The multiple disturbances found in brains from patients with AD/SDAT may be given different interpretations. One is that the recorded findings are of secondary type and of no etiological importance. A more fundamental disturbance in the brain metabolism is to be found beyond the disturbed neurotransmitter functions. As yet we do not know the nature of this fundamental disturbance. It is assumed that the etiological factors may be aluminum intoxication, viral infection, hypoxemia or autoimmune disorders.

The fact that the recorded biochemical changes in the brain are of secondary type does not mean that they are of no pathogenetic importance. In fact, in some studies we have shown that the disturbed neurotransmitter function in the brain of AD/SDAT patients as reflected by reduced cerebro-spinal fluid (CSF) metabolites can be correlated to behavioural disturbances (Bråne et al., 1988).

Another interpretation of the multiple changes in Alzheimer brains is that the clinical delimitation of AD/SDAT dementias does not correspond to etiologically homogenous groups.

In fact our clinical investigation of surviving patients with dementia indicates that a more careful and improved diagnostic methodology may improve the clinical possibilities of delimiting dementia groups. As is evident from the investigation of vitamin-B-12 levels, new subgroups can be formed when a clinical diagnosis of SD or SDAT is made. It is evident that 23% of the patients in this group had pathologically low concentrations of vitamin-B-12. The further study of this group showed that they had low concentrations of pepsinogen in serum, indicating atrophic gastritis. In previous investigations it was shown that MAO in platelets are increased in patients with AD/SDAT, although no valid explanation for this finding has been proposed. However, here we discovered that the group of clinically diagnosed SDAT patients with low vitamin-B-12 levels also had high MAO platelet activity (Regland et al., 1988). None of the patients with low vitamin-B-12 levels had anemia but it is known that patients with pernicious anemia have platelets with a short survival time. It is also known that platelets with a short survival time have an increased MAO activity.

It is therefore clear that demented patients with a clinical diagnosis of SD or SDAT with low vitamin-B-12 levels, should rather be diagnosed as having secondary dementia due to vitamin-B-12 deficiency without being anemic.

Any progress made in the field of dementia research will of course depend upon further studies of the biochemistry of the brain. It is, however, equally important to make progress in the clinical diagnosis of dementia. Homogenous dementia groups must be formed to enable us to interpret the biochemical findings and to formulate treatment strategies and to perform pharmacological treatment studies.

ACKNOWLEDGMENTS

This study was supported by grants from the Lundbeck Foundation, the Hjalmar Svensson Research Fund, the Swedish Medical Research Council, the Söderström-Königska Foundation and the Greta and Johan Kock Foundation.

REFERENCES

Bråne G, Gottfries CG, Karlsson I, Parnetti L, Svennerholm L (1988) Monoamine metabolites in CSF correlated to psychological variables in demented patients. Submitted.

Brun A (1983) An overview of light and electron microscopic changes. In: Reisberg B (ed): Alzheimer's disease. The Free Press, New York and London, pp. 37-47.

Brun A, Englund E (1985) A white matter disorder in dementia of the Alzheimer type: A pathoanatomical study. Ann Neurol 19:253-262.
Brun A, Gustafson L (1978) Limbic lobe involvement in presenile dementia. Arch Psychiatr Nervenkr 226:76-93.
Erkinjuntti T, Ketonen L, Sulkava R, Vuorialho M, Palo J (1987) CT in the differential diagnosis between Alzheimer's disease and vascular dementia. Acta Neurol Scand 75:262-270.
Gottfries CG (1986) Nosological aspects of differential typology of dementia of Alzheimer type. In: Dimensions in aging. Academic Press, London, pp. 207-219.
Gottfries CG, Adolfsson R, Aquilonius SM, Carlsson A, Eckernäs SM, Nordberg A, Oreland L, Svennerholm L, Wiberg Å, Winblad B (1983) Biochemical changes in dementia disorders of Alzheimer type (AD/SDAT). Neurobiol Aging 4:261-271.
Gottfries CG, Karlsson I, Svennerholm L (1985) Senile dementia - A "white matter" disease? In: Gottfries CG (ed): Normal Aging, Alzheimer's disease and senile dementia. Aspects on etiology, pathogenesis, diagnosis and treatment. Éditions de l'Université de Bruxelles, Bruxelles, pp. 111-118.
Gottfries CG, Bartfai T, Carlsson A, Eckernäs SÅ, Svennerholm L (1986) Multiple biochemical deficits in both gray and white matter of Alzheimer brains. Prog Neuro Psychopharmacol and Biol Psychiat 10:405-413.
Hardy J, Adolfsson R, Alafuzoff I, Bucht G, Marcusson J, Nyberg P, Perdahl E, Wester P, Winblad B (1985) Review. Transmitter deficits in Alzheimer's disease. Neurochem Int 7:545-563.
De Leon MJ, George AE, Ferris SH, Christman D, Gentes CI, Miller JD, Fowler J, Reisberg B, Wolf AP (1985) CT, PET and NMR brain imaging in aging and Alzheimer's disease. In: Gottfries CG (ed): Normal Aging, Alzheimer's disease and senile dementia. Aspects on etiology, pathogenesis, diagnosis and treatment, pp. 199-202.
Marcusson JO, Alafuzoff I, Bäckström IT, Ericson E, Gottfries CG, Winblad B (1987) 5-HT sensitive (^{3}H) imipramine binding of protein nature in the human brain II: Effect of normal aging and dementia disorders. Brain Res 425:137-145.
Oreland L, Fowler CJ, Carlsson A, Magnusson (1980) Monoamine oxidase-A and-B activity in the rat brain after hemitransection. Life Sci 26:139-146.
Oreland L, Gottfries CG (1986) Brain and platelet monoamine oxidase in aging and in dementia of Alzheimer's type. Progr Neuropsychopharmacol Biol Psychiatry 10:533-540.
Regland B, Gottfries CG, Oreland L, Svennerholm L (1988) Low S-B12 levels related to high MAO activity in platelets. A clue for etiology to senile dementias? Acta Psychiatr Scand, in press.
Reisberg B (1983) Alzheimer's disease. The standard reference, The Free Press, New York.
Rossor MN, Iversen LL, Reynolds GB, Mountjoy CQ, Roth M (1984) Neurochemical characteristics of early and late onset types of Alzheimer's disease. Brit Med J 288:961-964.
Sjögren T, Sjögren H, Lindgren AGH (1952) Morbus Alzheimer and morbus Pick. A genetic, clinical and patho-anatomical study. Acta Psychiatr Neurol Scand, Suppl. 82.
Sourander P, Sjögren H (1970) The concept of Alzheimer's disease and its clinical implications. In: Wolstenholme GEW, O'Connor M (eds): Alzheimer's disease and related conditions. Churchill, London, pp. 11-36.
Svennerholm L, Gottfries CG, Karlsson I (1987) Neurochemical changes in white matter of patients with Alzheimer's disease. Proceedings of the NATO-conference "Multidisciplinary approach to myelin diseases", Plenum Press, in press.
Svennerholm et al., this volume.

New Trends in Aging Research
G. Pepeu, B. Tomlinson, C.M. Wischik (eds)
Fidia Research Series, vol. 15
Liviana Press, Padova © 1988

CONTINGENT NEGATIVE VARIATION (CNV) AND RELATED COMPONENTS IN PATIENTS WITH INITIAL IDIOPATHIC PRESENILE COGNITIVE DECLINE AND PRESENILE ALZHEIMER-TYPE DEMENTIA

R. Zappoli, A. Versari, G. Arnetoli, M. Paganini, A. Battaglia[1], S. Costantini[1] and S. Porcú[2]

Second Neurological Institute, University of Florence;
[1]Medical Department Farmitalia, Carlo Erba, Milano; and
[2]DASRS Department of Aerospace Medicine,
Neuropsychophysiology Group, Pomezia, Roma, Italy

The aim of the present study was to examine possible differences in magnitude and latency of some contingent negative variation (CNV) components (post-S1 N1, P2, P3; early CNV; N1200; late pre-S2 CNV; CNV resolution) and reaction time (RT) between a group of twenty selected right-handed very healthy subjects (10 young adults and 10 presenile subjects, mean age respectively 28.3 and 59.6), a group of 10 patients with initial presenile cognitive decline (PICD), and 7 patients affected by early stages of presenile Alzheimer-type dementia (PAD). All these subjects were tested with a simple warned RT paradigm: S1 (click) - 2 sec - S2 (2 sec TV-screen presentation of black/white checkerboard around a central fixation point) - motor response to interrupt S2. Rare unpredictable distracting stimuli during S1-S2 interval were administered for CNV distraction and rebound effect examination. Before CNV complex measurements, all patients underwent CT-scan, EEG spectral analysis and a battery of psychometric tests. Some patients were examined also with NMR. In all patients CT-scan showed no evidence of focal lesions. Only one of the PICD patients had a moderate diffuse cerebral atrophy; all the other patients of this group had CT-scan in the normal limits for age. All PAD patients showed a more or less severe diffuse cortical-subcortical atrophy at CT-scan and NMR examinations. CNV complex, a sort of mosaic of components related to different neuro-psychophysiological functions already sufficiently known,

Abbreviations: CNV, contingent negative variation; RT, reaction time; PICD, initial presenile cognitive decline; PAD, presenile Alzheimer-type dementia.

were recorded with a TC of 5.5 sec from Fz (or F3, F4), C3, Cz, C4, P3, Pz, P4 and sometimes also from Oz referred to linked mastoid electrodes. Electro-oculogram (EOG), RT and stimuli were also recorded. EEG and each artifact-free S1-S2 response were analyzed by B.A.S.I.S.-E.P.M. (OTE-Biomedica) and Brain Electrical Activity Mapping (B.A.S.I.S.-Brain Surveyor) systems.

In comparison with the younger subjects, in the presenile group a significant mean amplitude reduction of N1 to S1 was measured at all recording sites. A significant young-presenile difference was observed also in P3 to S1 mean latencies which were longer in the presenile group at all leads. The main age effects on CNV activity were found in the early and late component (O-wave and P-wave) which resulted in a significant decrease in the older subjects especially in centro-parietal areas. A progressive amplitude reduction only in frontal leads between O-wave and P-wave with the lowest point being reached in the latter was characteristic in the presenile group. Furthermore, presenile subjects showed relatively flat CNV waveshapes of low amplitude and, as a whole, this group performed a little worse than young persons. This finding suggests that the statistically significant changes of post-S1 EPRs and CNV activity recorded in our presenile subjects without appreciable deficits of behavioural and mental performances, could be signs of early stages of brain involutional processes related to minimal and subclinical decrement of orienting, attentiveness and response preparation capabilities.

Reduced amplitude of some CNV components and longer RT were recorded in PICD and especially in PAD patients compared to controls. All the patients, as a whole, performed much worse than the normal subjects (Zappoli et al., 1986). Particularly relevant in the subjects with PICD was the significant reduction in all leads of the late CNV component (preparatory of P-wave). This phenomenon may be indicative of a difficulty in sustaining a sufficient level of attention and preparation essential to respond properly to imperative signals. In all PAD patients the CNV activity on the whole was practically non-existent. The lack of CNV activity in this group of patients probably depends on their inability to recognize the warning significance of the first signal (S1), and so they responded with enormous delay only to the second imperative signal which means they were not waiting for S2. PAD patients therefore had highly significant prolonged RTs compared to the other two groups of subjects. Significant negative correlation both in PICD and PAD patients was observed in fronto-central areas especially between the P component and RT: the smaller the P component, the longer the RT. Four of the 7 PAD patients presented very large PINVs in several of the averaged 8 trial blocks.

On the whole, the differences in CNV activity and related performances between PICD and PAD patients appeared to be essentially quantitative rather than qualitative and such phenomenon might make one presume that the CNV changes observed in PICD patients may be precursor signs of a real progressive presenile dementia. A prolonged follow-up study with neuroradiological, neurochemical, neuropsychological, laboratory and clinical examinations of these patients with a mild cognitive deficit will be able to confirm (or not) the suspicion of an early stage of primary presenile dementia. The data collected until now seem to prove that the mentioned significant CNV/RT changes may provide a potentially useful neurophysiological discriminator of normal and pathophysiological brain functioning and may facilitate the diagnosis of early stages of presenile dementia. Furthermore, this investigation will supply normative data for evaluating psychogeriatric drugs in the treatment of PICD and PAD patients.

Full publication of these findings is in preparation.

ACKNOWLEDGEMENTS

This study was supported in part by a Ministry of Public Education Research Grant, 1985.

REFERENCES

Zappoli R, Arnetoli G, Paganini M, Versari A, Battaglia A, Grignani A, Porcú S (1986) CNV activity and RT in patient with presenile idiopathic cognitive decline and presenile Alzheimer-type dementia: A preliminary report. Riv It EEG Neurofisiol Clin 9:233-250.

Section V

PLASTICITY AND THERAPEUTIC POSSIBILITIES

New Trends in Aging Research
G. Pepeu, B. Tomlinson, C.M. Wischik (eds)
Fidia Research Series, vol. 15
Liviana Press, Padova © 1988

GENETIC MESOTELENCEPHALIC DOPAMINE DEFICIENCY IN WEAVER MUTANT MICE: REINSTATEMENT OF NEURONAL CONNECTIVITY BY SOLID GRAFTS OF FOETAL MESENCEPHALON

Lazaros C. Triarhou[1,3], Walter C. Low[2,3] and Bernardino Ghetti[1,3]

[1]Department of Pathology, Division of Neuropathology,
[2]Department of Physiology and Biophysics, and
[3]Program in Medical Neurobiology,
Indiana University School of Medicine,
Indianapolis, IN 46223, USA

INTRODUCTION

A genetic deficit of the mesotelencephalic dopamine (DA) projection system has been identified in weaver mutant mice (Schmidt et al., 1982; Triarhou et al., 1986). The neostriatal DA deficiency is 75% relative to control values, and it is accompanied by a 27% DA deficiency in the olfactory tubercle and a 77% DA deficiency in the frontal cortex (Schmidt et al., 1982).

At the time when striatal DA concentration in weaver mutants is at its peak level, i.e., on postnatal day 20 (Schmidt et al., 1982), the overall incidence of junctional synapses formed by DA afferents in the weaver striatum is found to be decreased with respect to that seen in the normal striatum; further, the proportion of axosomatic contacts in the striatum of weaver homozygotes is double than that found in controls (Triarhou et al., 1988).

Our recent studies point to substantial neuronal losses in all groups of the mesencephalic DA cell system (Ghetti et al., 1987): by three months of age, homozygous

Abbreviations: DA, dopamine; TH, tyrosine hydroxylase.

weaver mutants display a 56% DA cell deficit in the retrorubral nucleus (area A8), a 69% DA cell deficit in the substantia nigra (area A9), and a 26% DA cell deficit in the ventral tegmental area (area A10). Such losses of DA cell bodies account for the DA deficiency found in the telencephalic terminal fields normally receiving DA innervation from these cells.

Primordial neural tissues can be grafted successfully to the brain of developing, adult or aged recipient animals (Björklund and Stenevi, 1984). One of the applications of intracerebral neural implants is the replacement of lost cell populations and the re-establishment of severed neuronal connexions. Such use is particularly meaningful in conditions characterised by focal loss of a selective group of neurones, as is the case in striatal DA denervation associated with the loss of mesencephalic DA neurones.

Attempts to reconstruct the damaged nigrostriatal pathway by neural transplants have proven fruitful in experiments carried out in rats (reviewed in Björklund and Stenevi, 1984; Olson, 1986). Those animals had been rendered DA deficient by local injection of 6-hydroxydopamine into the ventral midbrain, as originally described by Ungerstedt (1968). Grafts of foetal ventral mesencephalon have been shown to counteract anatomical (Björklund and Stenevi, 1979; Perlow et al., 1979; Freund et al., 1985; Mahalik et al., 1985), physiological (Wuerthele et al., 1981; Strömberg et al., 1985), biochemical (Schmidt et al., 1982; Freed et al., 1983) and behavioural (Björklund and Stenevi, 1979; Perlow et al., 1979; Björklund et al., 1981; Dunnett et al., 1981) deficits resulting from the depletion of striatal DA stores.

Foetal mesencephalic grafts have been implanted into the recipient brain either as solid blocks of tissue (Björklund and Stenevi, 1979; Perlow et al., 1979) or in the form of dissociated cell suspensions (Schmidt et al., 1981). Implants have been grafted to three different brain sites:

— intracerebroventricularly, adjacent to the medial aspect of the caudate-putamen complex (Perlow et al., 1979);

— directly onto the surface of the caudate-putamen complex, which had previously been exposed by removal of the overlying cortex (Stenevi et al., 1976); and

— intraparenchymally to the striatal substance (Björklund et al., 1980).

Each of these approaches has its own advantages and may be more or less useful in addressing particular issues. For example, intraventricular grafts are bathed into cerebrospinal fluid, which may enhance their survival. However, placement of the graft and reinnervation of the striatum cannot be directed very precisely. Intracavitary grafts can be placed on selected areas of the host neostriatum, but surgical procedures are more invasive, as a neocortical cavity is created; nevertheless, they are useful for experimental purposes, as they make separation of graft and host tissues relatively easy. Intraparenchymal cell suspensions have the potential for better survival in comparison with solid grafts. However, once placed into the recipient striatum, it is difficult to separate graft from host cellular elements without having previously resorted to labeling techniques.

Graft survival and growth has been documented in genetically normal hosts, which are subsequently rendered pathological through surgical-chemical manipulation (cf. Brundin et al., 1986). Since the ultimate goal of such experimentation is to use neural transplants to counteract naturally occurring diseases, it is obvious that experimental models with spontaneously occurring neurodegenerative disorders may be particularly valuable in developing knowledge on graft survival and graft-host tissue interrelationships. The weaver mutant mouse offers a valuable model for investigating graft-host interactions in a system characterised by genetically determined striatal DA deficiency.

In an attempt to reconstruct the defective pathway, grafts of foetal ventral mesencephalon were taken from genetically normal mice and implanted intracerebrally into adult weaver mutants. Donor tissue was placed either into the lateral ventricle or into a surgical cavity overlying the dorsal neostriatum of the recipients.

INTRAVENTRICULAR GRAFTS

Histological evidence for survival of grafted DA neurones in the genetically abnormal environment was initially obtained from experiments with intracerebroventricular grafting (Triarhou et al., 1986), and in the series donor tissue was taken from the ventral mesencephalic flexure of normal embryos at 14-15 days of gestation and was implanted stereotaxically into the lateral cerebral ventricle of 2 to 3 month-old weaver mutants. Transplant recipients were allowed survival times of 1 to 2 months after grafting. Following transcardial perfusion with aldehydes, brain tissues were processed for histology and for immunocytochemical staining according to the unlabeled antibody PAP method (Sternberger et al., 1970). Immunopositivity for tyrosine hydroxylase (TH) and immunonegativity for DA β-hydroxylase were taken as evidence for the dopaminergic nature of grafted cells. Surviving transplants contained approximately 100-800 TH immunoreactive neurones. Reinnervation of the caudate-putamen complex by TH immunoreactive fibres was observed to a depth of 250 μm.

INTRACAVITARY GRAFTS

Longer survival times of 4 to 5 months were allowed in the animals that had received grafts into a neocortical cavity (Triarhou et al., 1987). In this series, donor tissue obtained from the ventral mesencephalic flexure of normal embryos at gestational days 14-15 was implanted into a surgical cavity overlying the dorsal striatum of 2 to 4 month-old weaver recipients; the cavity had been produced 2 to 4 weeks prior to grafting, following the delayed cavity transplantation protocol of Stenevi et al. (1976). Brain tissues were processed for light and electron microscopic immunocytochemistry; pre-embedding immunolabeling of tissue slices was carried out *en bloc* with an antiserum to TH.

Grafts contained an estimated 100-1,000 TH immunoreactive neurones (Fig. 1). Under the electron microscope, TH immunoreactive cell bodies were readily recognised in the transplants. The somata of grafted TH immunoreactive neurones received synaptic input from unlabeled axon terminals. TH immunolabeled dendrites in the grafts were also invested by unlabeled axon terminals, which contained sphaeroid or flattened synaptic vesicles. Such axodendritic synapses were predominantly asymmetrical, characterised by the presence of a thick postsynaptic membrane density (Fig. 2).

The aim of this part of the study was to examine the ability of grafts for long-term survival and the form of connectivity established by graft deriving DA afferents in the

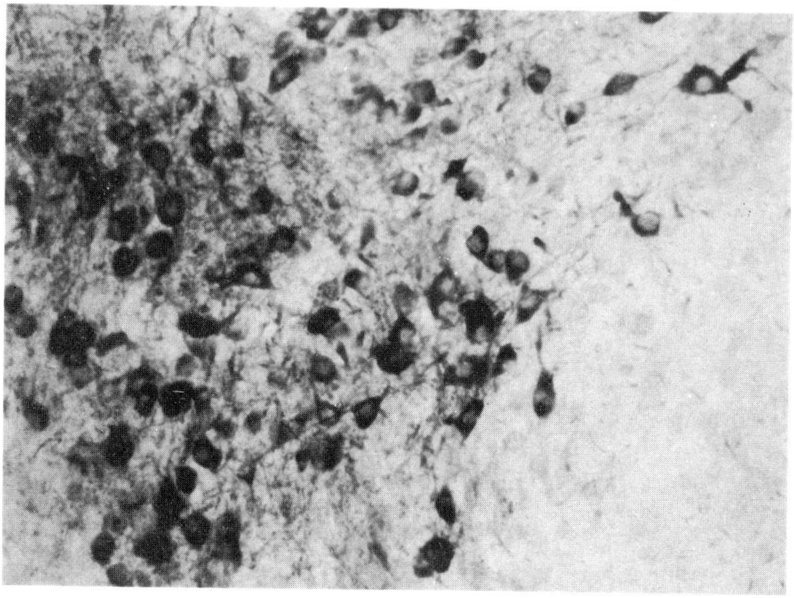

Figure 1. TH immunoreactive cell bodies and processes in a ventral mesencephalic graft transplanted to the caudate-putamen complex of a weaver mutant mouse, 4.5 months after transplantation. ×280.

host neostriatum. Animals were selected for quantitative ultrastructural examination of the striatum on the basis of

— rotational asymmetry tests following administration of methamphetamine, in which mutants with grafts exhibited a circling preference away from the grafted side (Low et al., 1987), and

— histological evidence for extensive reinnervation of the dorsal striatum by TH immunoreactive fibres. The depth of reinnervation of the host striatum reached 1,000 μm at 4-5 months after transplantation (Fig. 3). Reinnervation occurred to a similar extent in the rostrocaudal direction. Occasionally, TH immunoreactive axons formed pericellular baskets around unlabeled striatal neurones.

Under the electron microscope, TH immunoreactive nerve terminals were readily found in the grafted striatum. The percentages that corresponded to non-junctional (70%) and junctional symmetrical (28%) contacts markedly contrasted with the respective percentages in the non-grafted side (91% and 9%). Percentages in the grafted striatum did not only indicate a reinstatement of the connectivity observed in 20-day-old weaver mutants (83% and 16%), but further approximated the corresponding percentages found in normal animals (73% and 26% respectively). The majority of synaptic contacts were made with dendritic spines and shafts (Fig. 4). The proportion of contacts with axons and perikarya appeared somewhat increased in relation to the normal situation. On several occasions, multiple TH immunoreactive nerve terminals were found to contact the soma of the same striatal neurone (Fig. 5).

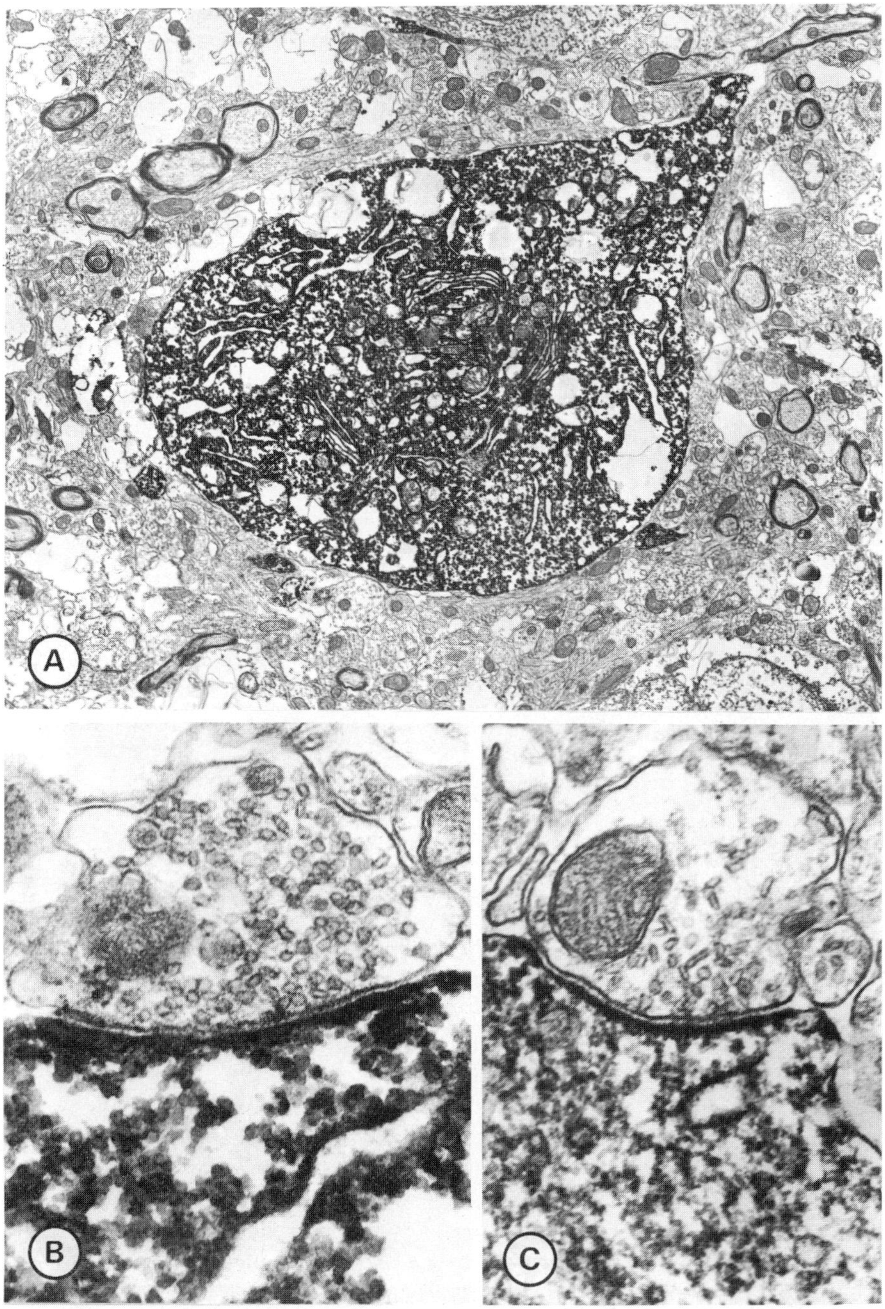

Figure 2. (A) Part of a grafted TH immunopositive neurone, 4.5 months after transplantation. x6,480. (B,C) Afferent synapses formed by unlabeled axon terminals on somata of grafted, TH immunoreactive neurones. × 62,000.

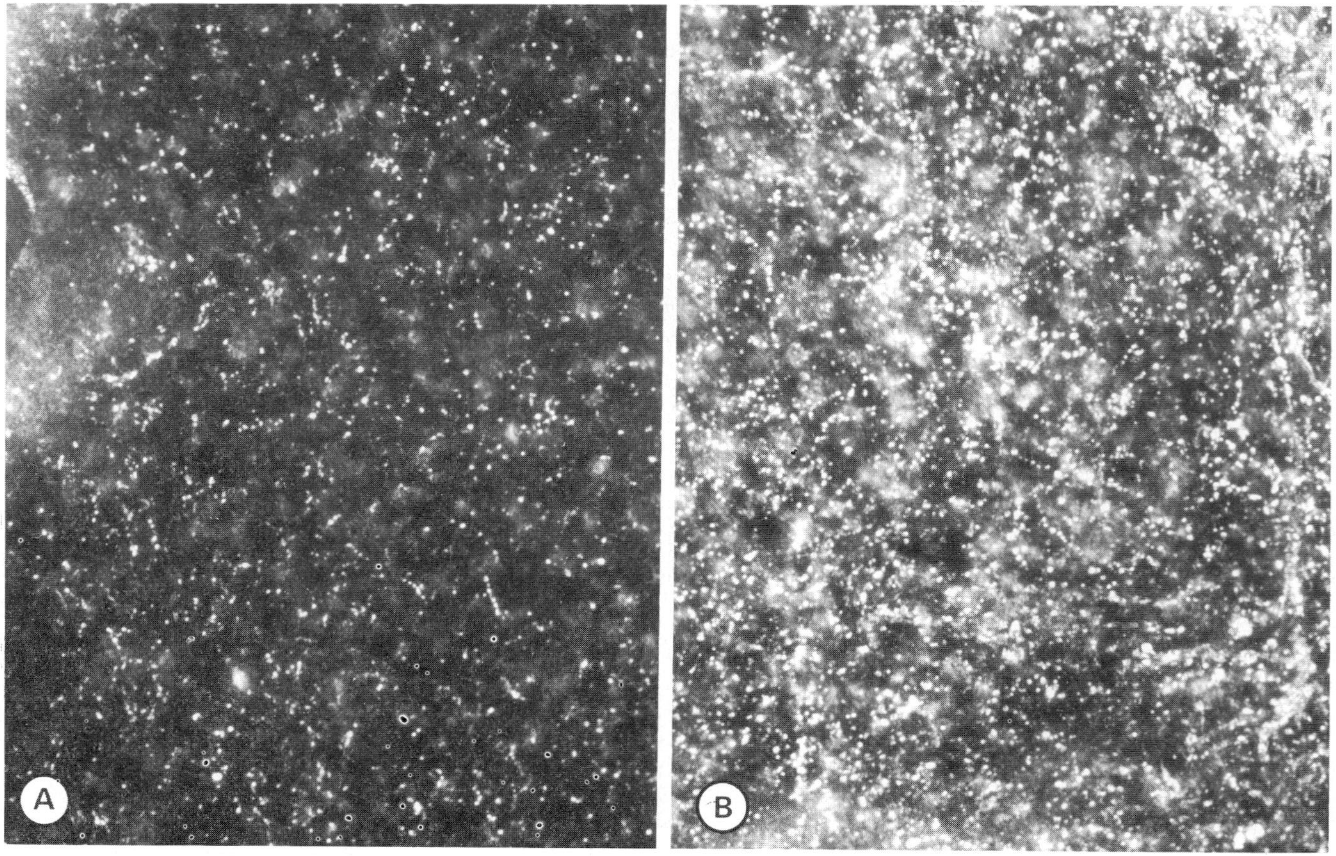

Figure 3. (A) TH immunoreactivity in the DA depleted, non-grafted caudate-putamen complex of a weaver mutant mouse. (B) Reinnervation of the dorsal caudate-putamen complex of the recipient weaver mutant by TH immunoreactive fibres from the graft. Dark-field illumination. ×450.

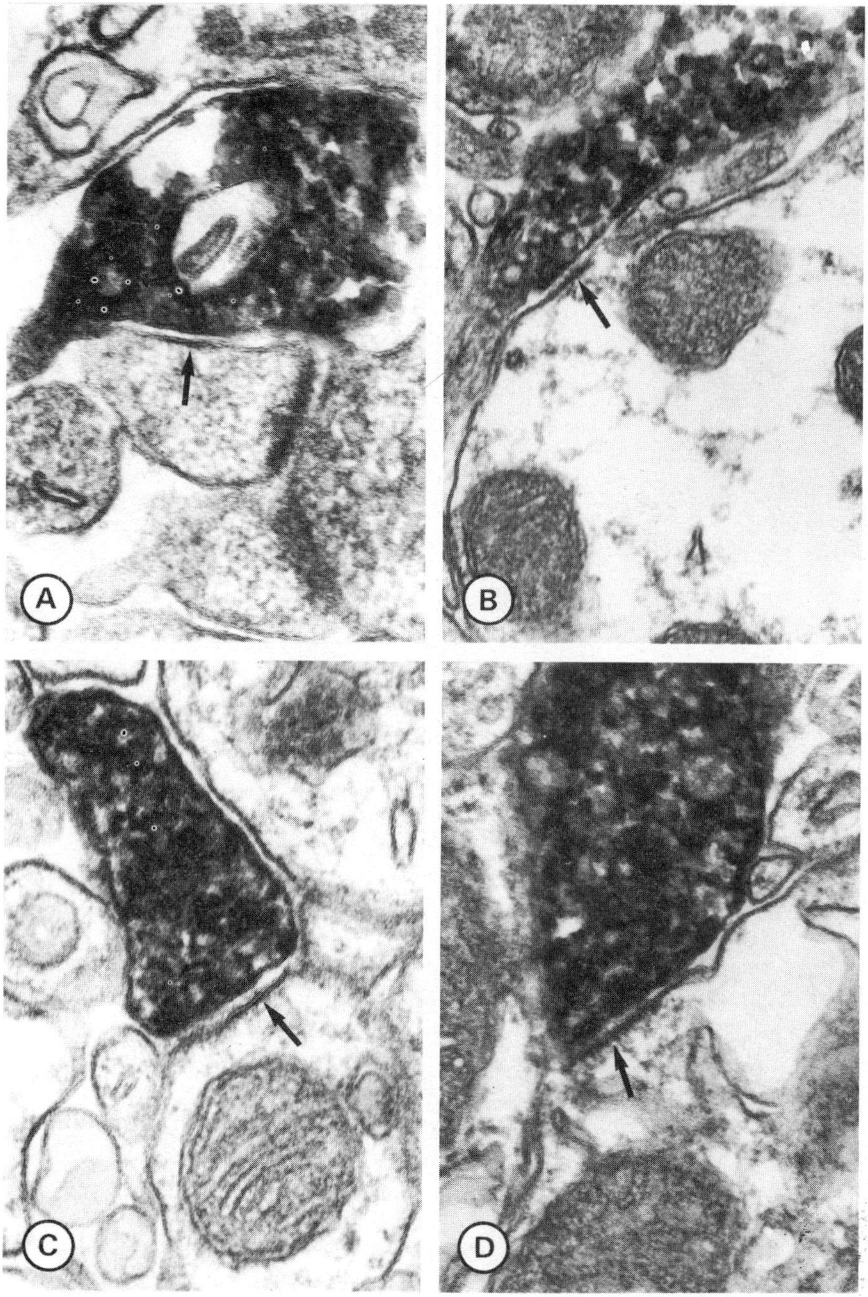

Figure 4. (A) Axospinous synapse formed by a TH nerve terminal in the grafted striatum of a weaver mutant mouse. ×120,000. (B-D) Axodendritic synapses formed by TH immunoreactive nerve terminals in the grafted striatum of a weaver mutant mouse. (B) ×88,000. (C) ×108,000. (D) ×100,000.

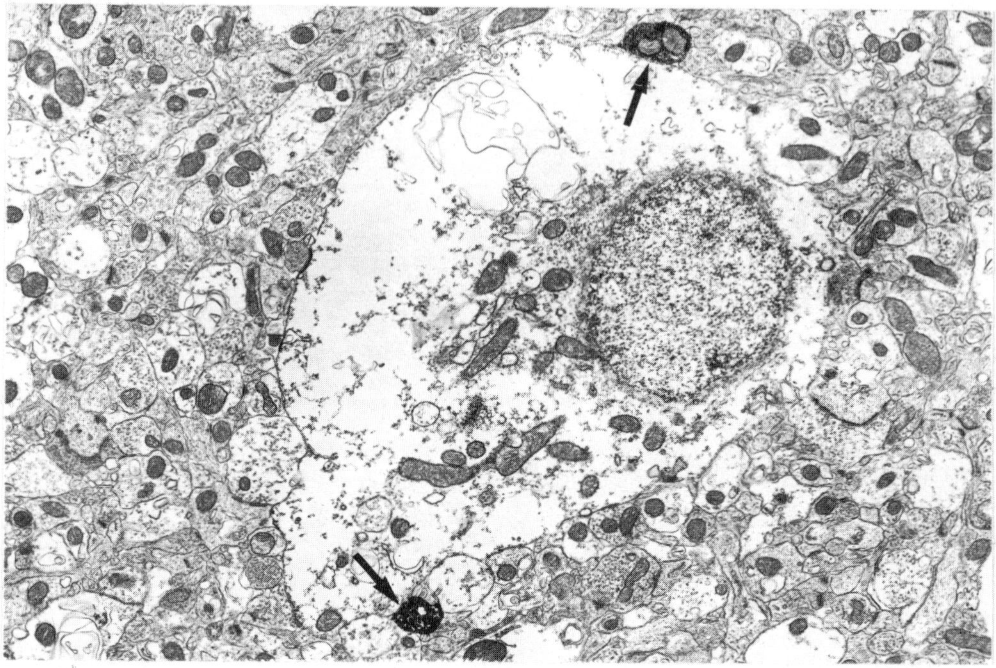

Figure 5. Two TH immunoreactive nerve terminals contacting the soma of the same striatal neurone in a recipient weaver mutant mouse. x7,600.

CONCLUSIONS

Our findings support the following conclusions:

1. The environment of the recipient weaver mutants allows the survival and axonal growth of genetically normal DA neurones (Triarhou et al., 1986).

2. The striatal neurones of weaver mutants are receptive to synaptic investment by DA afferents originating in the grafts. A certain degree of anatomical immaturity may be indicated by the increased incidence of axosomatic contacts (Triarhou et al., 1987), which is a morphological feature of the nigrostriatal anlage (Specht et al., 1981); nevertheless, the fact that the majority of synapses are formed on normal cellular sites indicates a connexional selectivity during reinnervation.

3. The reinnervation of the weaver striatum is functional, as suggested by behavioural tests of rotational asymmetry (Low et al., 1987).

4. Intracerebral grafting of DA neurones may be used effectively to overcome mesotelencephalic DA deficiency of genetic origin.

ACKNOWLEDGEMENTS

We thank Dr. C.D. Nordschow of the Department of Pathology for support; Ms.

C.J. Alyea and Ms. R. Funkhouser of the Department of Pathology for technical help; and Mr. J. Demma of the Department of Medical Illustrations for skilful assistance with photomicrography. This research was supported in part by USPHS grant RO1-NS14426 (B.G.).

REFERENCES

Björklund A, Stenevi U (1979) Reconstruction of the nigrostriatal dopamine pathway by intracerebral nigral transplants. Brain Res 177: 555-560.

Björklund A, Stenevi U (1984) Intracerebral neural implants: Neuronal replacement and reconstruction of damaged circuitries. Ann Rev Neurosci 7: 279-308.

Björklund A, Schmidt RH, Stenevi U (1980) Functional reinnervation of the striatum in the adult rat by use of intraparenchymal grafting of dissociated cell suspensions from the substantia nigra. Cell Tissue Res 212: 39-45.

Björklund A, Stenevi U, Dunnett SB, Iversen SD (1981) Functional reactivation of the deafferented neostriatum by nigral transplants. Nature (Lond) 289: 497-499.

Brundin P, Isacson O, Gage FH, Prochiantz A, Björklund A (1986) The rotating 6-hydroxydopamine-lesioned mouse as a model for assessing functional effects of neuronal grafting. Brain Res 366:346-349.

Dunnett SB, Björklund A, Stenevi U, Iversen SD (1981) Behavioural recovery following transplantation of substantia nigra in rats subjected to 6-OHDA lesions of the nigrostriatal pathway: I. Unilateral lesions. Brain Res 215: 147-161.

Freed WJ, Ko GN, Spoor HE, Morihisa JM, Wyatt RJ, Hoffer BJ, Neihoff DL, Kuhar MJ, Olson L (1983) Normalization of spiroperidol binding in the denervated rat striatum by homologous substantia nigra transplants. Science 222: 937-939.

Freund TF, Bolam JP, Björklund A, Stenevi U, Dunnett SB, Powell JF, Smith AD (1985) Efferent synaptic connections of grafted dopaminergic neurons reinnervating the host neostriatum: A tyrosine hydroxylase immunocytochemical study. J Neurosci 5: 603-616.

Ghetti B, Norton J, Triarhou LC (1987) Neuroanatomical definition of the mesostriatal dopamine deficit in weaver mutant mice. Neuroscience 22:S783.

Low WC, Triarhou LC, Kaseda Y, Norton J, Ghetti B (1987) Functional innervation of the striatum by ventral mesencephalic grafts in mice with inherited nigrostriatal dopamine deficiency. Brain Res 435: 315-321.

Mahalik TJ, Finger TE, Strömberg I, Olson L (1985) Substantia nigra transplants into denervated striatum of the rat: Ultrastructure of graft and host interconnections. J Comp Neurol 240: 60-70.

Olson L (1986) On the use of transplants to counteract the symptoms of Parkinson's disease: Background, experimental models, and possible clinical applications. In: Cotman CW (ed): Synaptic Plasticity. Guilford Press, New York, pp. 485-505.

Perlow MJ, Freed WJ, Hoffer BJ, Seiger Å, Olson L, Wyatt RJ (1979) Brain grafts reduce motor abnormalities produced by destruction of nigrostriatal dopamine system. Science 204: 643-647.

Schmidt MJ, Sawyer BD, Perry KW, Fuller RW, Foreman MM, Ghetti B (1982) Dopamine deficiency in the weaver mutant mouse. J Neurosci 2: 376-380.

Schmidt RH, Björklund A, Stenevi U (1981) Intracerebral grafting of dissociated CNS tissue suspensions: A new approach for neuronal transplantation to deep brain sites. Brain Res 218: 347-356.

Schmidt RH, Ingvar M, Lindvall O, Stenevi U, Björklund A (1982) Functional activity of substantia nigra grafts reinnervating the striatum: Neurotransmitter metabolism and [14C]-2-deoxy-D-glucose autoradiography. J Neurochem 38: 737-748.

Specht LA, Pickel VM, Joh TH, Reis DJ (1981) Fine structure of the nigrostriatal anlage in fetal rat brain by immunocytochemical localization of tyrosine hydroxylase. Brain Res 218: 49-65.

Stenevi U, Björklund A, Svendgaard N-A (1976) Transplantation of central and peripheral monoamine neurons to the adult rat brain: Techniques and conditions for survival. Brain Res 114: 1-20.

Sternberger LA, Hardy PH Jr, Cuculis JJ, Meyer HG (1970) The unlabeled antibody-enzyme method of immunohistochemistry. Preparation and properties of soluble antigen-antibody complex (horseradish peroxidase-antihorseradish peroxidase) and its use in identification of spirochetes. J Histochem Cytochem 18: 315-333.

Strömberg I, Johnson S, Hoffer B, Olson L (1985) Reinnervation of dopamine-denervated striatum by substantia nigra transplants: Immunohistochemical and electrophysiological correlates. Neuroscience 14: 981-990.

Triarhou LC, Norton J, Ghetti B (1988) Synaptic connectivity of tyrosine hydroxylase immunoreactive nerve terminals in the striatum of normal, heterozygous, and homozygous weaver mutant mice. J Neurocytol 17: 221-232.

Triarhou LC, Low WC, Ghetti B (1986) Transplantation of ventral mesencephalic anlagen to hosts with genetic nigrostriatal dopamine deficiency. Proc Natl Acad Sci USA 83: 8789-8793.

Triarhou LC, Low WC, Ghetti B (1987) Synaptic investment of striatal cellular domains by grafted dopamine neurons in weaver mutant mice. Naturwissenschaften 74:591-593.

Ungerstedt U (1968) 6-Hydroxydopamine induced degeneration of central monoamine neurons. Eur J Pharmacol 5: 107-110.

Wuerthele SM, Freed WJ, Olson L, Morihisa J, Spoor L, Wyatt RJ, Hoffer BJ (1981) Effect of dopamine agonists and antagonists on the electrical activity of substantia nigra neurons transplanted into the lateral ventricle of the rat. Exp Brain Res 44: 1-10.

New Trends in Aging Research
G. Pepeu, B. Tomlinson, C.M. Wischik (eds)
Fidia Research Series, vol. 15
Liviana Press, Padova © 1988

THE SEROTONERGIC AND DOPAMINERGIC SYSTEMS IN THE AGED RAT BRAIN AS STUDIED BY IMMUNOHISTOCHEMISTRY WITH ANTIBODIES TO SEROTONIN AND DOPAMINE. PRELIMINARY OBSERVATIONS

Harry W.M. Steinbusch, Jan G. Wolters, Mariëlle G.P.A. Van Luijtelaar and [1]Jeroen A.D.M. Tonnaer

Department of Pharmacology, Free University, Amsterdam, and
[1]Department of CNS Pharmacology, Organon Int. BV.,
Oss, The Netherlands

INTRODUCTION

Until recently aging of neurotransmitter systems was studied mainly by behavioral (Collier et al., 1987) and clinical (McGeer et al., 1976; Beck, 1978) observations and biochemical techniques (Algeri et al., 1983; Allen et al., 1983; Morgan, 1987) in animals and humans. Cell counts of neurons in certain brain nuclei, as e.g. the substantia nigra, gave additional information about changes in the aging as well as the pathological brain (McGeer and McGeer, 1980; Mann et al., 1984; Marcyniuk et al., 1986; Herregodts et al., 1987). Normal aging has been characterized neurochemically among others by a decrease of the cholinergic and monoaminergic transmission. It is well known that the dopamine transmitter system is involved in Parkinson's disease, and that the acetylcholine and serotonin transmitter systems play a role in Alzheimer's disease (Adolfson et al., 1979; Hardy et al., 1985; Cross et al., 1983; Herregodts et al., 1987).

The scope of the present study is to add morphological data to the knowledge of aging processes in the rat brain as far as the 5-HT and the DA systems are concerned.

Abbreviations: Da_i, dopamine-immunoreactive; $5HT_i$, serotonin-immunoreactive.

Using immunohistochemistry with antibodies to 5-HT and to DA we compared the presence and distribution of 5-HT-immunoreactive ($5HT_i$) and dopamine-immunoreactive (DA_i) structures in brains of young adult and aged rats.

MATERIALS AND METHODS

A large number of young adult (2 months; 160-180 gr b.wt.) and eight aged (28 months or older; 300 and more gr b.wt.) male rats were used. Four old rats were used for studying serotonin- and four for dopamine-immunohistochemistry. The animals were anesthetized with sodium pentobarbital (Nembutal, 24 mg/kg) and perfused through the ascending aorta.

Tissue Preparation

For *serotonin-immunocytochemistry*, the blood was washed out with ice-cold, oxygen-enriched, Ca^{2+}-free Tyrode's buffer (for 2 min) followed by 500 ml of a mixture of ice-cold 4% (w/v) paraformaldehyde, 0.05% (v/v) glutaraldehyde and 0.2% picric acid in 0.1 M sodium phosphate buffer (pH 7.4) at a pressure of 90 mm Hg for about 20 min. Brains were quickly removed and immersed in fixative without glutaraldehyde at 4°C for 120 min.

For *dopamine-immunocytochemistry*, the blood was removed with a brief preperfusion with Krebs-Ringer buffer (without $CaCl_2$ and glucose, but including 1% sodiummetabisulfite; final pH 5.6, aerated for 30 min with carbogen), at room temperature, followed by 500 ml freshly made icecold 5% glutaraldehyde and 1% sodiummetabisulfite in 0.05 M cacodylate buffer (pH 7.3) for 5 min. The 1% sodiummetabisulfite was added to the fixative 30 min prior to perfusion. Brains were postfixed in the same fixative for 30-60 min at 4°C.

Immunohistochemical Procedures

The brains were cut on a Vibratome or a freeze microtome. For obtaining freeze microtome sections, the brains were rinsed in 20% sucrose dissolved in 0.1 M sodium phosphate buffer (pH 7.4) for at least 1 day. Free floating frozen microtome sections were collected in Tris-buffered saline (TBS).

The sections were used for immunohistochemistry according to the peroxidase-antiperoxidase procedure.

For *serotonin-immunohistochemistry*, the frozen microtome sections (35 μm thickness) were first washed with TBS, TBS containing 0.5% Triton X-100 (TBS-T) and TBS-T at room temperature for 3 × 10 min resp. They were then incubated with rabbit anti-5-HT serum diluted in TBS-T for 40 hrs at 4°C at a dilution of 1:2500. Details about the specificity and sensitivity of antibodies to serotonin have been published elsewhere (Steinbusch et al., 1986; 1988; Steinbusch and Tilders, 1987). Hereafter, the sections were washed alternately with TBS-T, TBS and TBS-T for 3 × 10 min.

Sections were incubated with goat-antirabbit IgG (Fc-specific) diluted 1:60 with TBS-T for 2 hrs and washed alternately in TBS-T, TBS and TBS-T for 3 × 10 min at room temperature. They were then treated with rabbit peroxidase-antiperoxidase complex diluted 1:600 with TBS-T for 1 hr at room temperature and washed for 10 min in TBS and finally for 2 × 10 min in 0.05 M Tris-HCL (pH 7.6). Hereafter, the sections were incubated with 0.05% (w/v) diaminobenzidine dissolved in Tris-HCL containing H_2O_2 (0.01%). The sections were mounted on glass slides coated with chrome alum gelatine and dried. They were postfixed in 2% glutaraldehyde; diluted in Tris-HCL for 10 min; dehydrated in five steps of alcohol (70%, 90%, 96%, 100%, 100%) and xylol, 2 min each step, and lastly mounted in Entellan.

For *dopamine-immunohistochemistry*, the brains were cut either on a Vibratome or on a freeze microtome. For the Vibratome the brains were cut immediately into 50 µm thick sections which were collected in TBS first transferred to 20% sucrose including 1% sodiummetabisulfite over the night. Before incubation the sections were pretreated with 1% sodiumborohydride and 1% sodiummetabisulfite in TBS for 30 min to reduce double bounds introduced by the glutaraldehyde fixation. Hereafter the sections were washed in TBS-T, TBS and TBS-T for 3 × 10 min resp. The sections were incubated free floating with rabbit anti-dopamine serum diluted 1:2000 in Tris buffered saline including 0.5% Triton X-100 and 1% sodiummetabisulfite for two nights at 4°C. To enhance the immunoprecipitation product we used a DAB-Nickel intensification by which the dopamine-antiserum can be used at a dilution of 1:8000. The best results were obtained with the Vibratome.

RESULTS AND DISCUSSION

In this immunohistochemical study, using antibodies to 5-HT and dopamine, the localization and distribution of serotonin and dopamine-immunoreactive cell bodies and the density of serotonergic and dopaminergic fibers in the forebrain of young adult (2 months old) and aged (28 months or older) rats were compared.

As to the *serotonergic system*, the changes we observed in several brain structures of aged rats consist mainly of spider-like fiber clusters (30-60 µm), which are not present in young adult rats (Figs. 1 and 2). In addition, varicosities are less regular in shape, morphology and distribution throughout the 5-HT innervated regions. We might consider these changes as the main signs of degeneration of the 5-HT system, particularly visible in all layers of the frontoparietal cortex, the caudate-putamen complex, the medial preoptic region and the intermediolateral cell column of the spinal cord. In certain forebrain regions additionally a decrease of serotonergic fibers was noticed, e.g. in the cortex, striatum and hippocampus. The number of $5HT_i$ neurons in the nucleus raphe dorsalis (B7), the nucleus centralis superior (B8), and in and around the lemniscus medialis (B9) is not reduced in the aged rat (see Fig. 3). This seems consistent with the 5-HT innervation pattern in the aged rat forebrain, which shows changes in morphological sense, but is only slightly reduced.

The *dopaminergic system* in the brain of the aged rat showed a slight decrease in the number of dopaminergic fibers in most forebrain regions, known to receive a dopaminergic innervation. We did not observe highly degenerated varicose fibers as seen in the serotonergic system. A conspicuous decrease in dopamine (DA) innervation was demonstrated in the aged endopiriform nucleus, the primary olfactory cortex and dorsal cortex. The area of the prefrontal and entorhinal cortex as well as the caudate-putamen

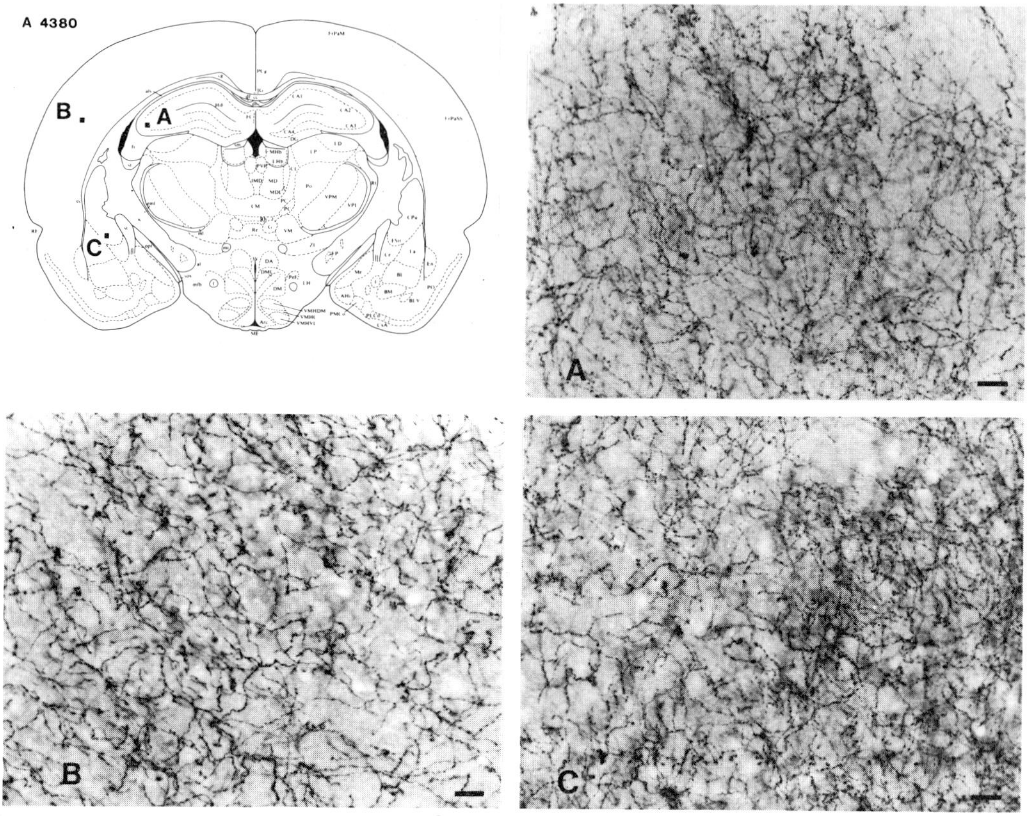

Figure 1. Photomicrographs of serotonin-immunoreactive fibers in the young adult rat brain. A. hippocampus; B. cortex; C. caudate-putamen complex. (Bars:10μ).

complex were equally densely innervated in young and aged rats (Figs. 4 and 5). As to the number of dopaminergic cell bodies there are few differences between young and old rats. Only in the substantia nigra pars reticulata of aged rats a slight loss of dopaminergic neurons was found (Fig. 6).

These data indicate that aging results in a local and mainly morphologically defined degeneration of the serotonergic system, whereas the dopaminergic system shows a more global decline in quantity and intensity of immunostaining. It is known that both serotonergic as well as dopaminergic cell bodies send their axons to a whole variety of different forebrain regions. Retrograde tracing studies have shown that these cell bodies can send collaterals to various brain regions. The local degeneration of the serotonergic system in some forebrain regions and the absence of similar changes in the dopaminergic system might indicate the appearance of an intraneurotoxic compound, possibly specific for the serotonergic system, having no effect on the dopaminergic system. Alternatively, a diminished production at high age of neurotrophic factors, critical for the support and maintenance of innervating serotonergic neurons, may be hypothesized to result in a

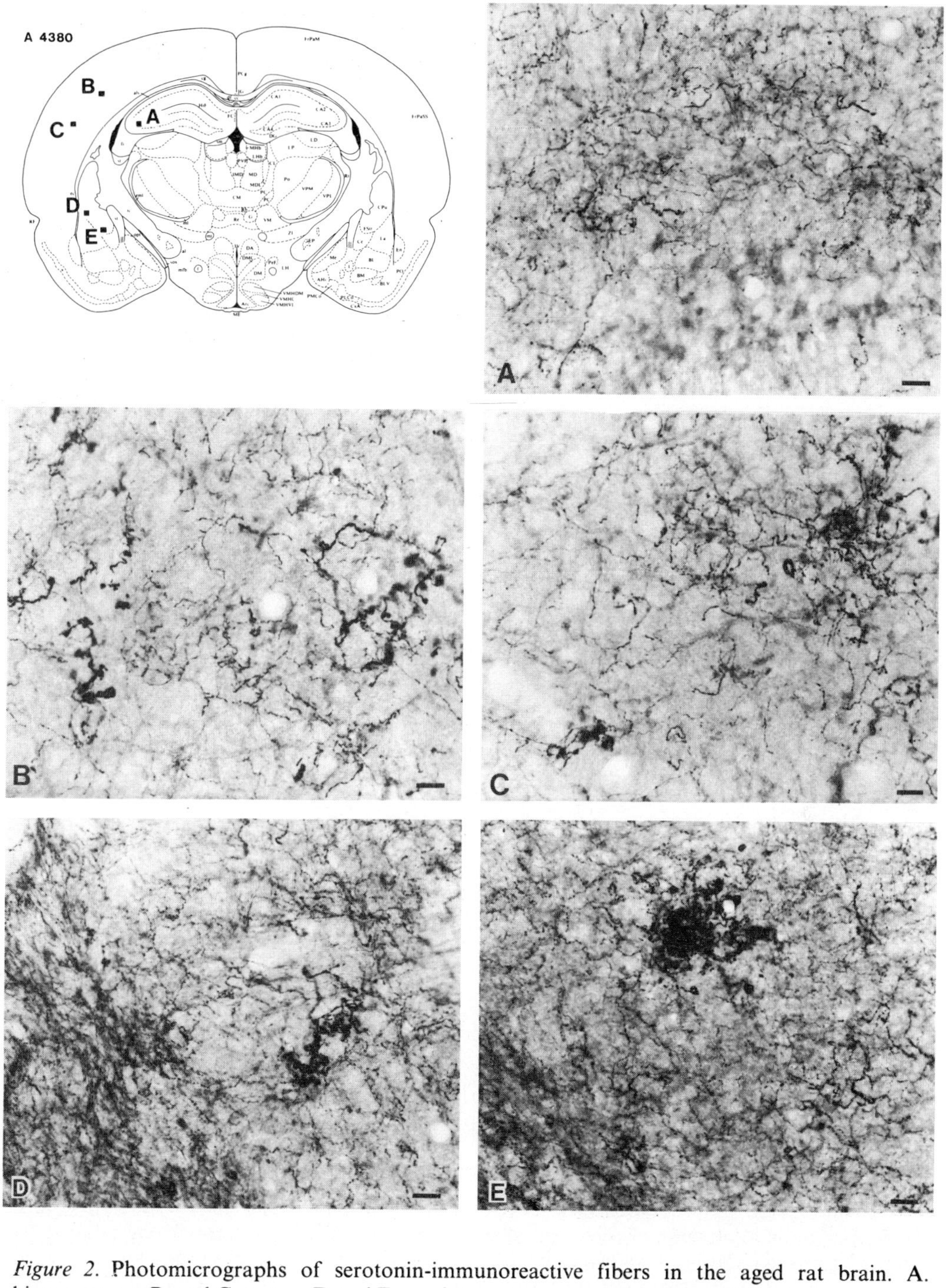

Figure 2. Photomicrographs of serotonin-immunoreactive fibers in the aged rat brain. A. hippocampus; B. and C. cortex; D and E. caudate-putamen complex. (Bars:10μ).

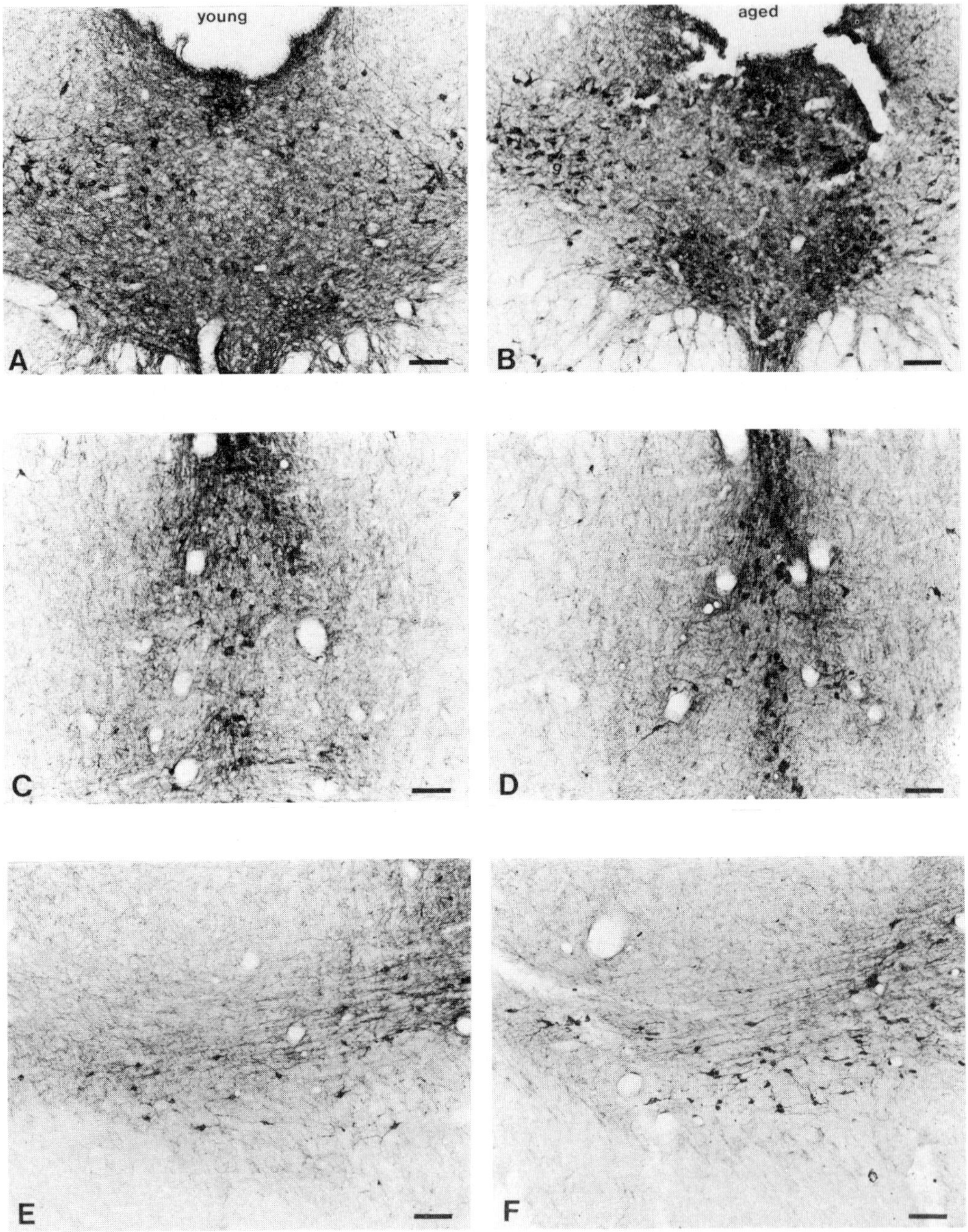

Figure 3. Photomicrographs of serotonin-immunoreactive cell bodies in the young adult (left) and the aged (right) rat brain showing the distribution of serotonergic cells in the nucleus raphe dorsalis (A and B), the nucleus centralis superior (C and D) and the B9 cell group in the ventral tegmentum (E and F) (Bars:50μ).

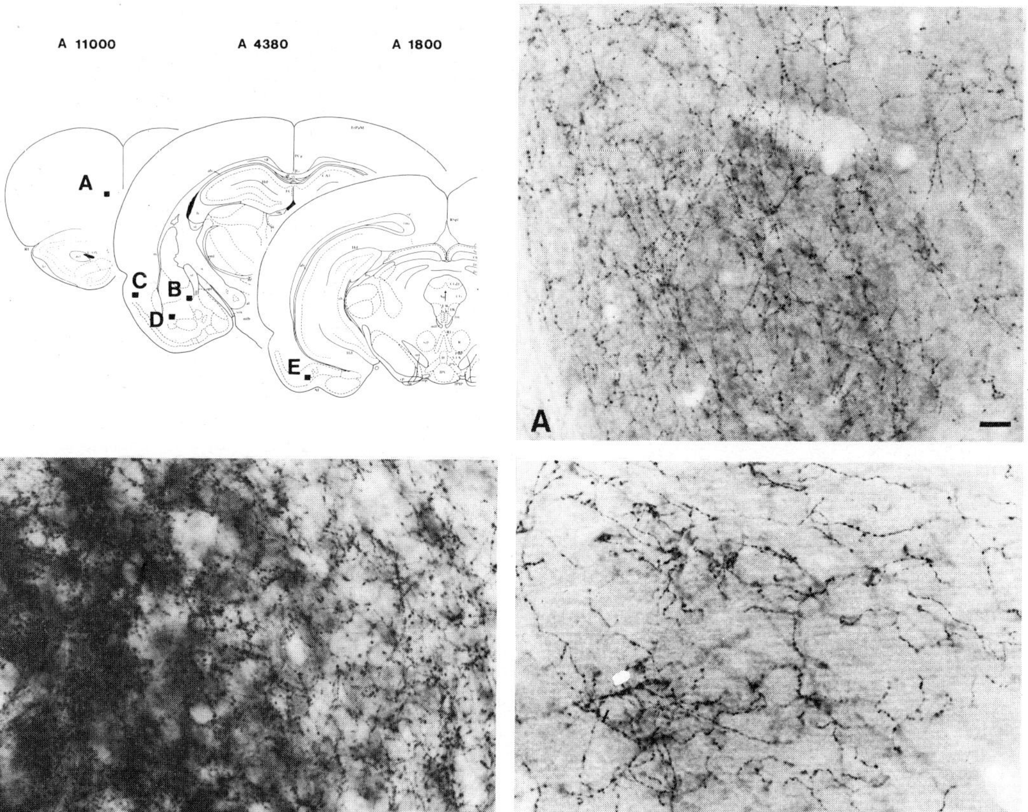

Figure 4. Photomicrographs of dopamine-immunoreactive fibers in the young adult rat brain. A. prefrontal cortex; B. central amygdaloid nucleus; C. primary olfactory cortex; D. basolateral amygdaloid nucleus; E. entorhinal cortex. (Bars:10μ).

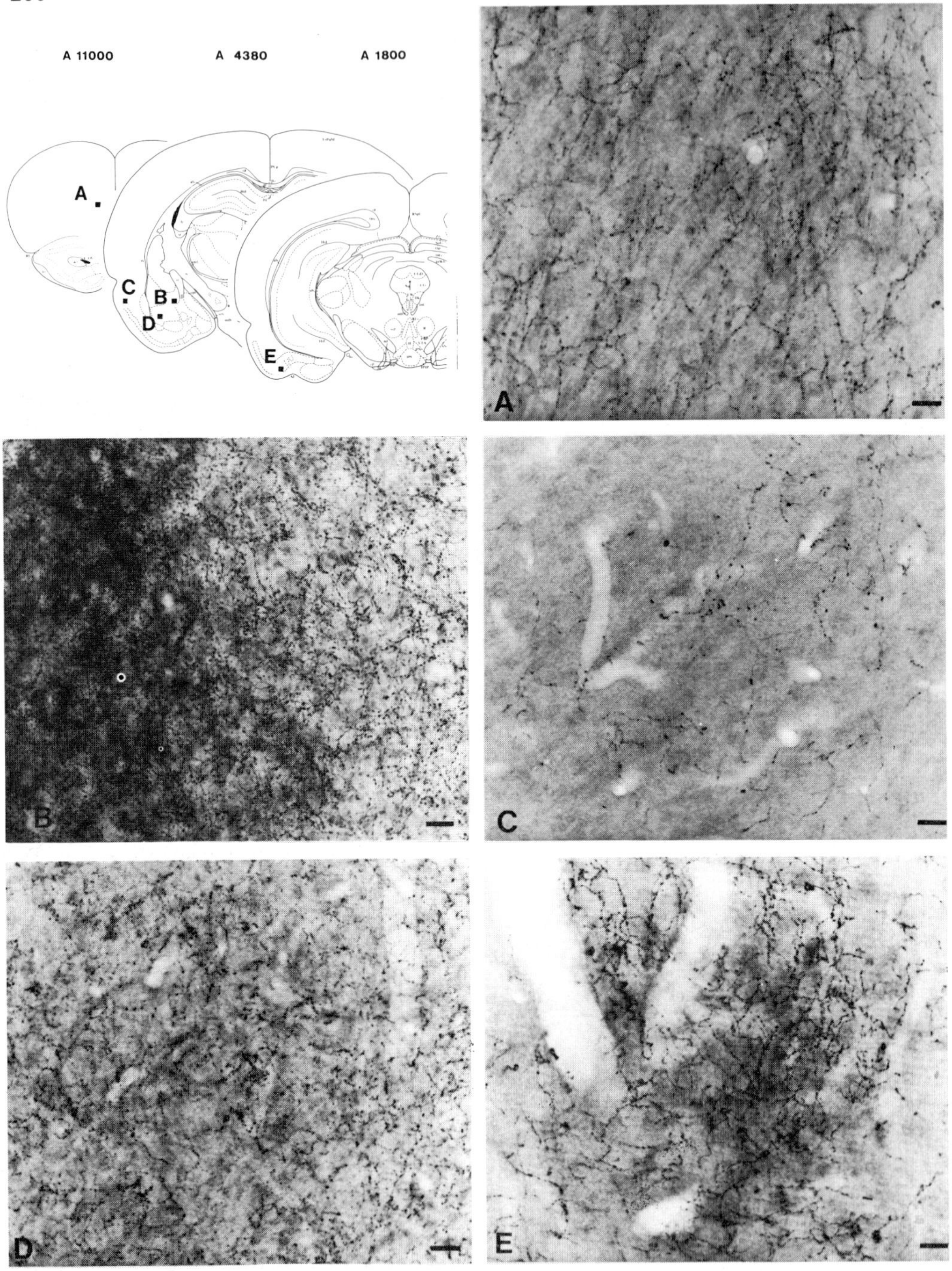

Figure 5. Photomicrographs of dopamine-immunoreactive fibers in the aged rat brain. A. prefrontal cortex; B. central amygdaloid nucleus; C. primary olfactory cortex; D. basolateral amygdaloid nucleus; E. entorhinal cortex. (Bars:10μ).

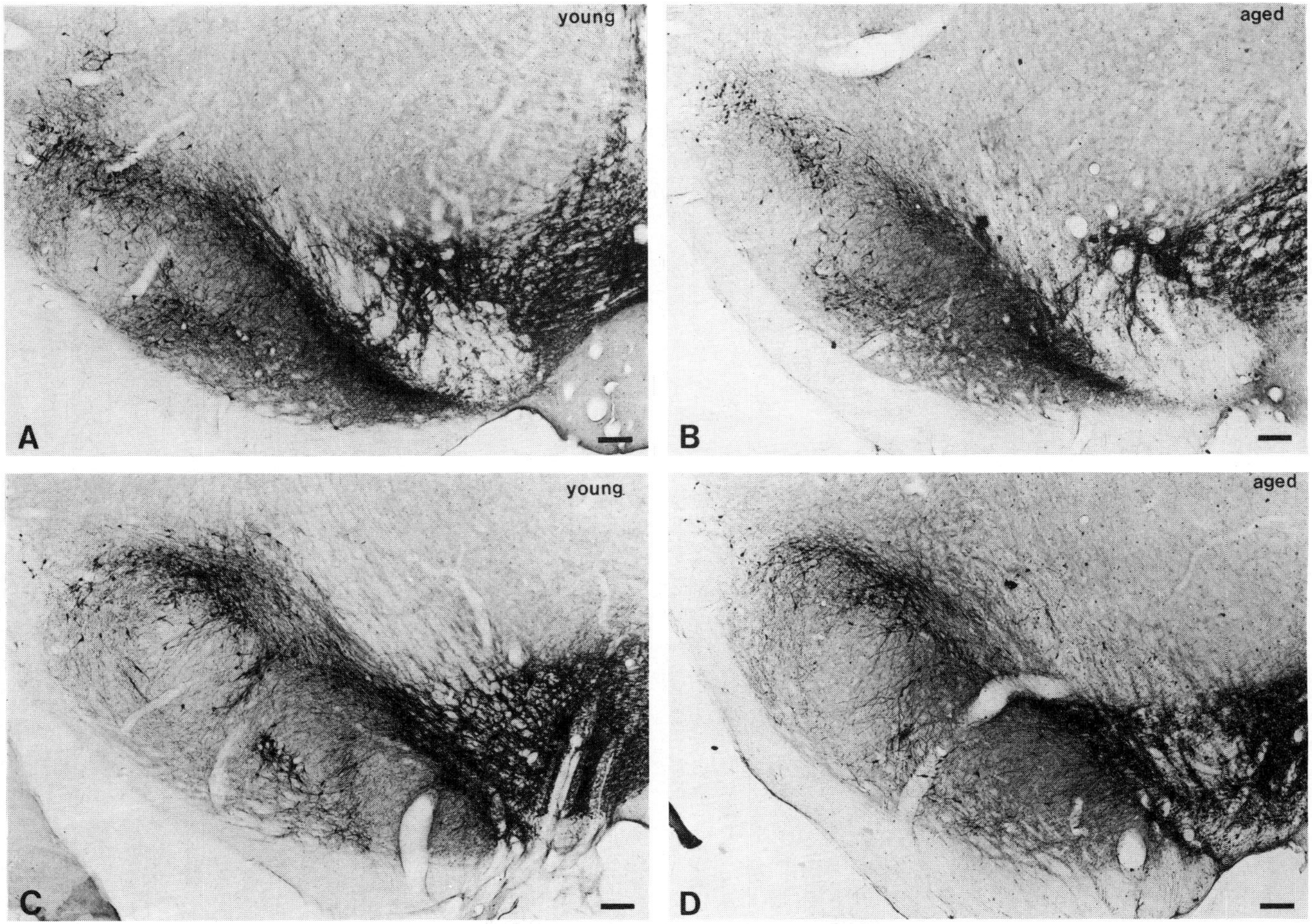

Figure 6. Photomicrographs of dopamine-immunoreactive cell bodies in the young adult (left) and the aged (right) rat brain showing the distribution of dopaminergic cells in the substantia nigra and ventral tegmental area (Bars: 50 μm).

retrograde degeneration of particular serotonergic afferents. The disappearance of a subpopulation of dopaminergic neurons in the substantia nigra suggests a higher vulnerability of these cells to age-related compromising processes.

Conclusively, we assume that serotonergic and dopaminergic systems in the aged rat brain are declining in a different and system-specific way.

ACKNOWLEDGEMENTS

This work was supported by Grant 900-552-072 from the Netherlands Foundation for Medical Research (MEDIGON). We want to thank John G.J.M. Bol for excellent technical assistance, and Henk Nordsiek for processing the photomicrographs.

REFERENCES

Adolfsson R, Gottfries C-G, Roos B-E, Winblad B (1979) Changes in the brain catecholamines in patients with dementia of the Alzheimer type. Br J Psychiatry 135:216-223.

Algeri S, Calderini G, Toffano G, Ponzio F (1983) Neurotransmitter alterations in aging rats. In: Samuel D, Algeri F, Gershon S, Grimm VE, Toffano G (eds): Aging of the Brain. Raven Press, New York, pp. 227-243.

Allen SJ, Benton JS, Goodhardt MJ, Haan EA, Sims NR, Smith CCT, Spillane JA, Bowen DM, Davison AN (1983) Biochemical evidence of selective nerve cell changes in the normal ageing human and rat brain. J Neurochem 41: 256-265.

Beck CHM (1978) Functional implications of changes in the senescent brain. A review. Can J Neurol Sci 5: 417-424.

Collier TJ, Gash DM, Sladek JR jr (1987) Norepinephrine deficiency and behavioural senescence in aged rats. Transplanted locus coeruleus neurons as an experimental replacement therapy. In: Azmitia EC and Björklund A (eds): Cell and tissue transplantation into the adult brain. Ann NY Acad Sci, Vol. 95, pp. 396-403.

Cross AJ, Crow TJ, Johnson JA, Joseph MH, Perry EK, Perry RH, Blessed G, Tomlinson BE (1983) Monoamine metabolism in senile dementia of Alzheimer type. J Neurol Sci 60:383-392.

Goldstein M, Lieberman A, Calne DB, Thorner MO (eds) Ergot compounds and brain function: neuroendocrine and neuropsychiatric apsects. Advances in biochemistry and psychopharmacology. Vol 23, Raven Press, New York, pp. 305-314.

McGeer PL, McGeer EG, Suzuki JS (1976) Aging and extrapyramidal function. Arch Neurol 34:33-35.

Hardy J, Adolfsson R, Alafuzoff I, Bucht G, Marcusson J, Nyberg P, Perdahl E, Wester P, Winblad B (1985) Transmitter deficits in Alzheimer's disease. Neurochem Int 7:545-563.

Herregodts P, Cras P, Bruyland M, Michotte Y, Martin JJ, Ebinger G (1987) Degeneration of the serotonergic system in Alzheimer's disease. Clin Neurol Neurosurg 89 (2):20-21.

Mann DMA, Yates PO, Marcyniuk B (1984) Alzheimer's presenile dementia, senile dementia of Alzheimer's type and Down's syndrome in middle age form an age related continuum of pathological changes. Neuropathol Appl Neurobiol 10:185-207.

Marcyniuk B, Mann DMA, Yates PO (1986) Loss of nerve cells from the locus coeruleus in Alzheimer's disease is topographically arranged. Neurosci Lett 64:247-252.

Morgan DG (1987) The dopamine and serotonin systems during aging in human and rodent brain. A brief review. Prog Neuropsychopharmacol Biol Psychiatry Vol 11:153-157.

Steinbusch HWM, De Vente J, Schipper J (1986) Immunocytochemistry of monoamines in the central nervous system. In: Panula P, Päivärintä H, Soinila S (eds): Neurohistochemistry Today, Neurology and Neurobiology. Vol. 16, Alan R. Liss Inc, New York, pp. 75-106.

Steinbusch HWM, Tilders FJH (1987) Immunohistochemical techniques for light-microscopical localization of dopamine, noradrenaline, adrenaline, serotonin and histamine in the central nervous system. In: Steinbusch H.W.M. (ed): Monoaminergic Neurons: Light Microscopy and Ultrastructure. IBRO Handbook Series: Methods in the Neurosciences, Vol. 10, Wiley, Chichester, pp. 125-166.

Steinbusch HWM, Wouterlood FG, De Vente J, Bol JGJM, Berkenbosch F (1988) Immunohistochemical localization of monoamines and cyclic nucleotides. Their application in quantitative immunofluorescence studies and tracing monoaminergic neuronal connections. Acta Histochem, suppl. 25:85-106.

New Trends in Aging Research
G. Pepeu, B. Tomlinson, C.M. Wischik (eds)
Fidia Research Series, vol. 15
Liviana Press, Padova © 1988

COMPENSATORY EVENTS THAT ACCOMPANY LESION OF CHOLINERGIC CELLS IN NUCLEUS BASALIS: THERAPEUTIC IMPLICATIONS

Jacqueline de Belleroche, Ian M. Gardiner, Laurence J. Reed, Francoise H. Harlow and Philippa Lamb

Department of Biochemistry, Charing Cross and Westminster Medical School, Fulham Palace Road, London, W6 8RF, U.K.

INTRODUCTION

There are a number of neurodegenerative conditions that affect the elderly such as Alzheimer's disease (AD) in which selective populations of neurones are at risk, e.g. the nucleus basalis of Meynert (NBM) in the basal forebrain in AD. The selective vulnerability appears to be influenced by the ageing process in view of the late onset of these conditions. Although extensive studies have been made on the nature of the morphological and transmitter deficits that occur, the subsequent effects on the functional properties of the brain are largely unexplored. Recent biochemical and morphological evidence shows that the nervous system is capable of enormous plasticity in response to lesions even in the aged brain (Cotman and Nieto-Sampedro, 1984). We have preliminary evidence (described below) to indicate that compensatory events develop after neuronal lesion which may prove a valuable basis for targeting drug treatment. A knowledge of the time course of these events may prove useful in defining the temporal window over which appropriate treatments may be most beneficial.

In this study we have concentrated on documenting the changes that occur in the cerebral cortex following cholinergic deafferentation, which is typical of Alzheimer's disease. Although only one of the components is affected in Alzheimer's disease, the cholinergic system is clearly associated with deficits in memory, cholinergic antagonists themselves causing memory loss. We have found that the response to lesion is dynamic and hence optimal treatment is likely to depend on the course of development of the disease, and the same treatment will not work at all stages. Other transmitters implicated in the pathology of Alzheimer's disease are noradrenaline, 5-hydroxytryptamine, gamma-aminobutyric acid (GABA), somatostatin and glutamate. The latter is proving to be a likely candidate for a role in memory processing (Maragos et al., 1987) since recently glutamate antagonists of the NMDA subclass have been shown to impair learning and long-term potentiation (Morris et al., 1987). The study of the dynamic changes occurring in these transmitter systems is also merited in future studies.

MODELS OF NEURODEGENERATIVE CONDITIONS

A number of experimental animal models of neurodegenerative disorders have been developed in which a discrete lesion of specific brain nuclei is made, e.g. lesion of nucleus basalis, to investigate the effect of the cholinergic deafferentation of cerebral cortex typical of AD. The latter procedure produces a rapid decline in *five* markers of the cholinergic system in cerebral cortex, i.e. choline acetyltransferase (ChAT), acetylcholinesterase (AChE), high affinity choline uptake (HACU), muscarinic receptors (mAChR) and the depolarisation-induced release of ACh. All five parameters are maximally reduced at 5-7 days after lesion and the magnitude of the decrease correlates well with the extent of lesion as shown for changes in muscarinic receptors (Fig. 1). The first three parameters have been demonstrated by a number of research groups (Wenk et al., 1980; Johnston et al., 1981; McKinney and Coyle, 1982; Pedata et al., 1982) but, more recently, we have characterised the two latter processes, mAChR and ACh release.

The magnitude of the decrease in mAChR following lesion is small (15-20%) compared with that of ChAT, for example, (50-60%) but significant. Modest changes in mAChR of this order are also shown in AD (Reisine et al., 1978; Wood et al., 1983; Mash et al., 1985). Analysis of the particular receptor subtype affected by lesion was carried out either by competition binding studies using [^{3}H]-N methylscopolamine [^{3}H]NMS over a wide range of carbachol concentrations or by using low concentrations of pirenzepine (3×10^{-10} M) to selectively label M_1 binding sites (Fig. 2). M_1 receptors are the predominant subtype found in cerebral cortex and hippocampus accounting for approximately 70% of the total mAChR number and a slightly larger proportion in man. The results obtained from both approaches showed that both M_1 and M_2 receptors were reduced by lesion whilst the K_D for neither subtype was significantly changed (de Belleroche et al., 1986). Thus, quantitatively, the M_1 receptor accounted for most of the decrease in receptor number. However, each subtype showed the same percentage decrease. Although the M_1 receptor has been shown to mediate a number of postsynaptic effects in the CNS, e.g. the facilitation of the depolarisation-induced release of dopamine in nucleus accumbens (de Belleroche and Gardiner, 1982; 1985), it does not appear to be responsible for the autoregulation of ACh release by presynaptic receptors which would be depleted by cholinergic deafferentation.

In contrast to the modest reduction in mAChR after lesion, the evoked release of ACh is substantially affected, decreasing by approximately 80% in frontal cortex (Fig. 3).

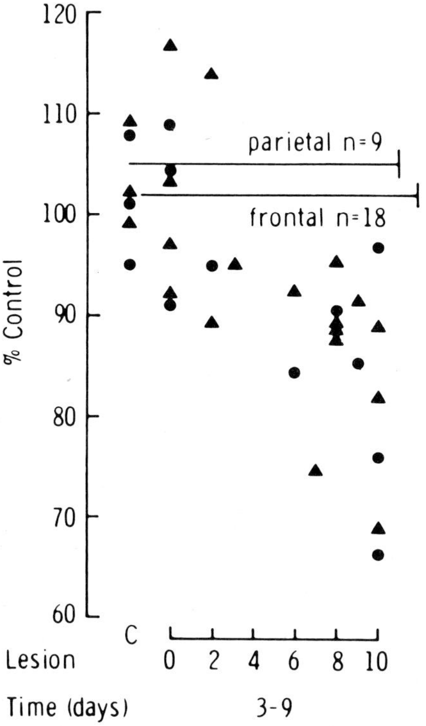

Figure 1. Effect of lesion of nucleus basalis on muscarinic receptor number in frontal and parietal cortex of rat. Unilateral kainate lesions of nucleus basalis were made and muscarinic receptor number was measured at 3-9 days after the lesion in frontal (▲) and parietal (●) cortex. Receptor number was analysed using [^{3}H]N-methylscopolamine (3 nM) and quinuclidinyl benzilate (1 μM) to define specific binding. Receptor number on the lesioned side is expressed as a percentage of that on the contralateral side and compared with the size of lesion assessed from histological examination. Values obtained for animals receiving vehicle injection only are indicated by C. Muscarinic receptor number contralateral to the lesion did not differ from that of unlesioned animals. Mean values obtained from unlesioned animals in each region are given by horizontal lines, S.E.M.s being indicated by the bars. Data from de Belleroche et al. (1985).

RECOVERY OF CHOLINERGIC PARAMETERS

Evidence from these studies indicates that considerable recovery of cholinergic parameters occurs in terminal regions after lesion (Gage et al., 1983; Wenk and Olton, 1984; Stephens et al., 1985; de Belleroche et al., 1985; Gardiner et al., 1987). The recovery of cholinergic enzymes such as ChAT and AChE which occurs from about one month after lesion appears to be due to the sprouting of spared axons which reoccupy the deficient synapses. Further, similar changes have been shown to occur in AD, whereby increased AChE activity is detected in the dentate gyrus in patients dying early in the course of the disease (Geddes et al., 1985). We have also shown that complex phenomena such as the depolarisation-induced release of acetylcholine (Fig. 4) which is reduced more than 80% by the first week after lesion is similarly reversed by 150 days in line with a parallel increase in AChE to normal levels (Gardiner et al., 1987). This time course of recovery corresponds well with that of the return of morphologically demonstrated synapses in the hippocampus after lesion of the analogous cholinergic septal input (120 days). Similar recovery is seen following lesions of inputs to dentate gyrus from the entorhinal cortex (Cotman et al., 1973) and in NB after cortical ablation (Stephens et al., 1985).

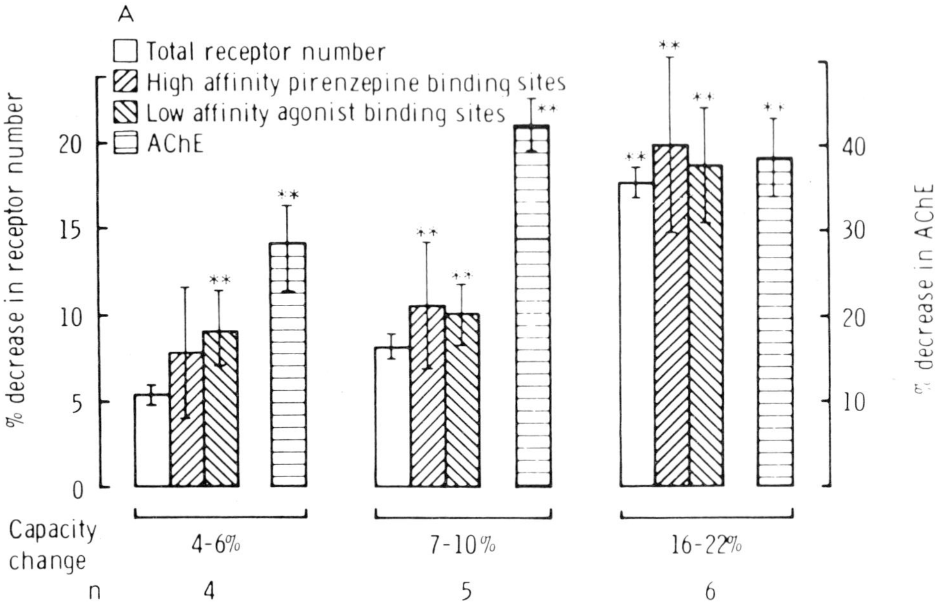

Figure 2. Effect of lesion of nucleus basalis on muscarinic receptor number, subtypes and AChE activity in frontal cortex of the rat. Unilateral lesions of nucleus basalis were made and receptor analysis and AChE activity were measured in frontal cortex at 14 days. Animals were grouped according to capacity change (total receptor number) which corresponded to histological assessment. Low affinity agonist binding sites were analysed using [^{3}H]NMS (3 nM) in the presence of carbachol (1 mM) and high affinity pirenzepine binding sites (M_1 receptors) using [^{3}H]pirenzepine (0.3 nM). Values (means ± S.E.M.s for animals) are expressed as the percentage decrease on the lesioned side compared to the contralateral side. Lesion caused a significant decrease on the ipsilateral side compared to the contralateral side (paired t-test): *$p<0.05$, **$p<0.001$. Data from de Belleroche et al. (1985).

POSTSYNAPTIC FUNCTION

The most important question that arises from these findings is whether this recovery of cholinergic parameters plays a significant role in alleviating the deficiencies of the lesion. To answer this question, we have looked at the postsynaptic response in cerebral cortex following lesion. The postsynaptic action of acetylcholine in cerebral cortex is mediated by a muscarinic receptor linked to the polyphosphoinositide (PPI) system in which two second messengers, inositol trisphosphate (IP_3) and diacylglycerol (DAG) are released by the hydrolysis of phosphatidylinositol bisphosphate (PIP_2).

This process is conveniently measured by the accumulation of IP_1 in the presence of LiCl, which is elicited by carbachol in a time and dose-dependent manner (Fig. 5). We have found that early after the lesion (1-2 weeks) there is a significant enhancement in the IP_1 produced in response to carbachol stimulation (Fig. 6). This is not due to an increase in receptor number or agonist affinity since both M_1 and M_2 receptors are

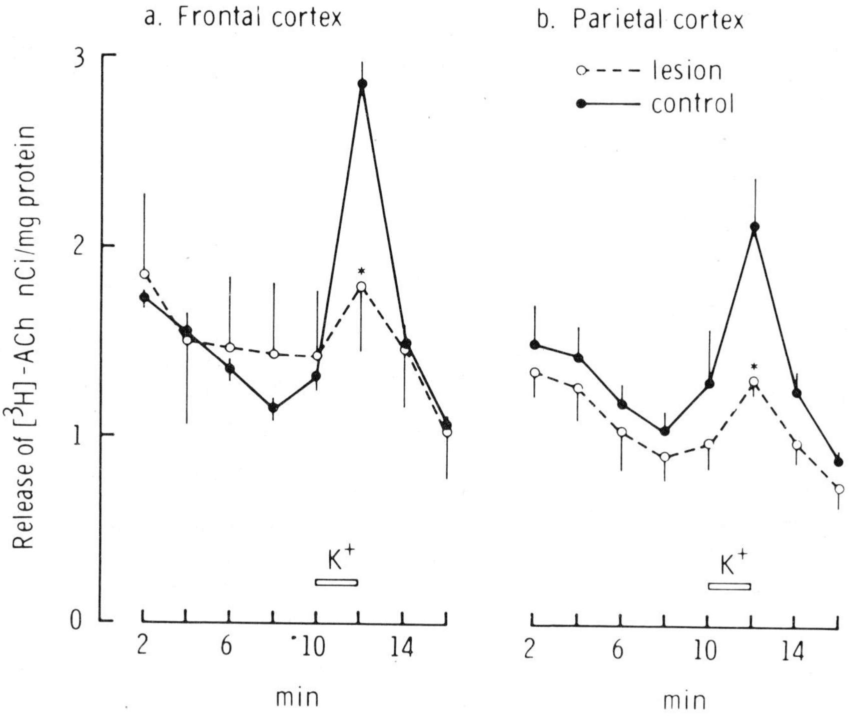

Figure 3. Release of [^{3}H]acetylcholine (nCi/mg protein) from tissue slices of rat cerebral cortex, 21 days after lesion of NB. Tissue slices of (a) frontal cortex, and (b) parietal cortex from the control hemisphere (solid lines) and the hemisphere ipsilateral to the NB lesion (dotted lines) were superfused. A pulse of 34 mM K^+ was applied during the period indicated by the bar. Values (release of [^{3}H]ACh nCi/mg protein) are means from 3 animals with the S.E.M.s indicated by bars. *Indicates that lesion caused a significant decrease in release of [^{3}H]ACh. $p<0.05$. Data from Gardiner et al. (1987).

decreased in number with no change in K_D under these conditions (de Belleroche et al., 1985a). Hence it appears that the post receptor mechanism that couples receptor activation by a cholinergic agonist to phospholipase C activity is enhanced on the lesion side rising to a maximal level twice that of the control (Bolam et al., 1986; Reed and de Belleroche, 1988). This enhancement is likely to depend on components of the coupling mechanism, e.g. G proteins, rather than the muscarinic receptor.

This conclusion is supported by the fact that other receptors in the cerebral cortex linked to the PPI system, e.g. histamine H_1 receptors, are also similarly affected by lesion. The increased generation of IP_1 in response to histamine in cerebral cortex ipsilateral to the lesion was of a similar magnitude to that obtained in response to carbachol, one week after lesion (Fig. 7). The nature and mechanism of this increased responsiveness is currently under investigation.

This marked increase in responsiveness in the postsynaptic cell potentially offers a

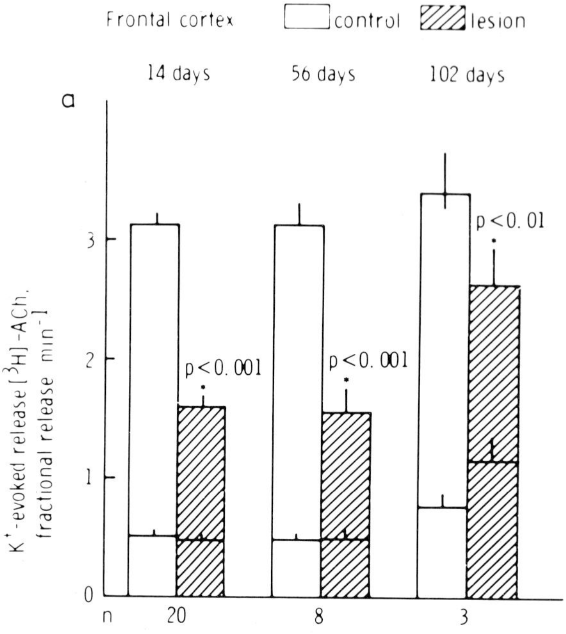

Figure 4. Effect of lesion of nucleus basalis on the K+-evoked release of [^{3}H]acetylcholine, expressed as fractional release/min at different periods after lesion. Tissue slices of frontal cortex from the control hemisphere (open histograms) and the hemisphere ipsilateral to the NB lesion (hatched histograms) were incubated at 37°C and stimulated with 34 nM K+. Values (fractional release of [^{3}H]ACh min^{-1}) are means with S.E.M.s indicated by bars and numbers of animals (n) indicated below the histograms. The basal level of release is superimposed on the K+-evoked value of release. The time after lesion is indicated in days above the histogram. *Indicates that the lesion caused a significant reduction in release with the P value shown. Data from Gardiner et al. (1987).

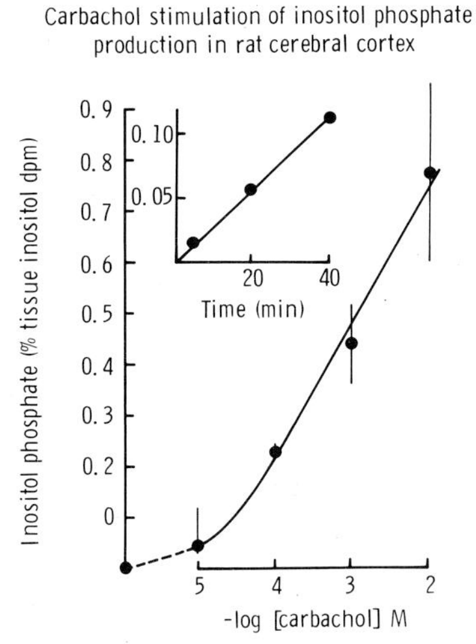

Figure 5. Carbachol stimulation of [^{3}H]-inositol phosphate generation in rat cerebral cortex. Tissue slices of rat cerebral cortex. Tissue slices of rat cerebral cortex were incubated with [^{3}H]-inositol in the presence of Li^{++} and challenged with various concentrations of carbachol for 40 min or other times as indicated in the inset. Inositol phosphates were fractionated by anion exchange chromatography and the generation of [^{3}H]-inositol phosphate is expressed as a percentage of tissue [^{3}H]-inositol. •Values are means ± S.E.M.s for 4 experiments. Data is taken from Reed and de Belleroche (1988).

valuable compensatory mechanism that will in part overcome the deficit produced by lesion. The period of this response is, however, limited and by the time the presynaptic cholinergic parameters have returned to normal, i.e. 150 days, the increased responsiveness has also decreased to normal levels. However, this period of increased responsiveness is likely to represent a significant period, possibly of several years' duration if extrapolated to man.

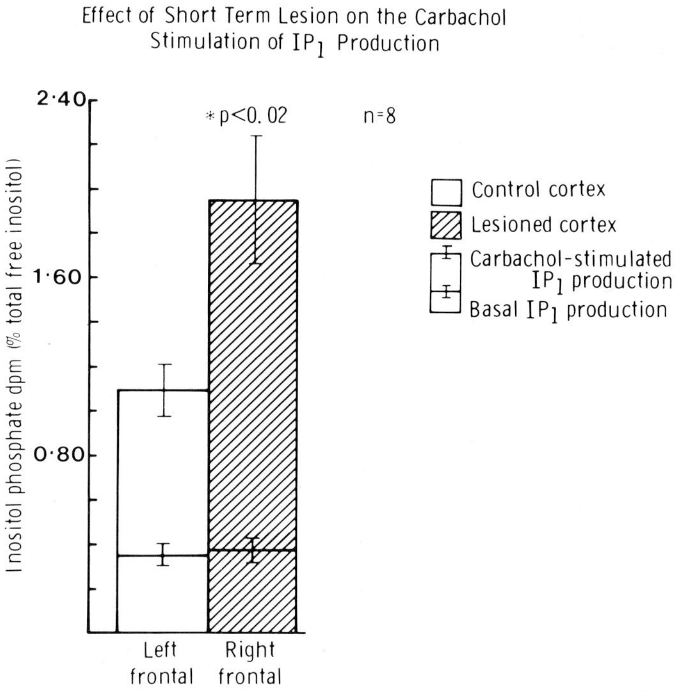

Figure 6. Effect of lesion of nucleus basalis on the carbachol stimulation of [^{3}H]-inositol phosphate generation. Tissue slices of rat frontal cortex ipsilateral to NB lesion (lesioned cortex) or contralateral to the lesion (control) were incubated and analysed as described in Figure 5. Values of [^{3}H]-inositol phosphate (% tissue [^{3}H]-inositol) generated in the absence of carbachol are superimposed on those obtained in the presence of carbachol. Values are means $\pm$ S.E.M.s for the number of experiments indicated. *Indicates that there was a significant increase in the carbachol stimulated response on the lesioned side compared to the control side. Data is taken from Reed and de Belleroche (1988).

CONCLUDING REMARKS

The changes that occur after nerve cell death are clearly enormously diverse and include the release of trophic substances such as peptide growth factors which may promote axonal sprouting and other modulators which may be responsible for the enhanced PPI responsiveness seen after experimental lesion. An understanding of these processes and the factors involved is likely to be important in treating degenerative diseases.

SUMMARY

A consistent finding in Alzheimer's disease is the cholinergic deficit in the cerebral cortex. We have investigated the consequences of this deficit on pre- and postsynaptic cholinergic properties in an animal model. Immediately following lesion of the nucleus

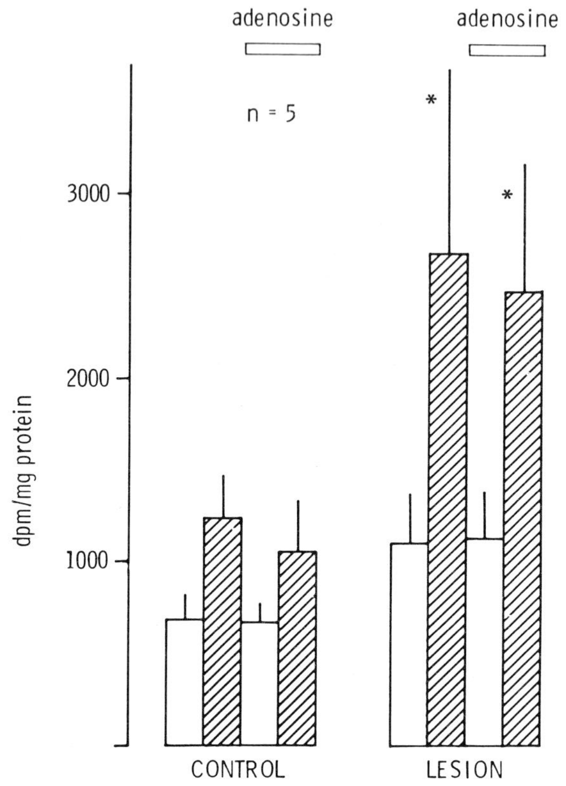

Figure 7. Effect of lesion of nucleus basalis on the histamine-induced generation of [^{3}H]-inositol phosphate. Tissue slices from rat cerebral cortex ipsilateral (lesion) and contralateral (control) to the lesion of nucleus basalis were incubated with [^{3}H]-inositol and challenged with 1 mM histamine (hatached histograms) in the presence or absence of adenosine. Values of [^{3}H]-inositol phosphate are expressed as dpm/mg protein. Values are means $\pm$ S.E.M.s for the number of experiments indicated. *Indicates that the histamine-induced generation of [^{3}H]-inositol was significantly greater on the lesioned side compared to the control side. Adenosine produced no significant effect.

basalis in the rat basal forebrain, cholinergic enzymes and muscarinic receptors are significantly reduced in frontal and parietal cortex. In addition, the depolarisation-induced release of acetylcholine is markedly reduced. This loss is accompanied by a greatly enhanced response to muscarinic receptor stimulation as measured by the carbachol activation of inositol phosphate production. This compensatory postsynaptic effect declines with time in phase with the significant reversal of the cholinergic deficit. The latter is likely to be due to the "sprouting" of spared axons which occurs during this period. These results indicate that loss of the cholinergic cells in Alzheimer's disease may be accompanied by compensatory processes occurring at both pre- and postsynaptic sites. Treatment with cholinergic agonists *early* in the disease would be particularly effective due to the initial enhanced responsiveness but this state would only be maintained for a limited period.

REFERENCES

Bolam S, Premi B, de Belleroche J (1986) Effect of kainate lesion of substantia innominata on the polyphosphoinositide response to muscarinic receptor stimulation in rat cerebral cortex. Biochem Soc Trans 14:687-688.

Cotman CW, Nieto-Sampedro M (1984) Cell biology of synaptic plasticity. Science 225:1287-1297.

Cotman CW, Matthews DA, Taylor D, Lynch G (1973) Synaptic rearrangements in the dentate gyrus: histochemical evidence of adjustments after lesions in immature and adult rats. Proc Natl Acad Sci USA 70:3473-3477.

de Belleroche J, Gardiner IM (1982) Cholinergic action in the nucleus accumbens: modulation of dopamine and acetylcholine release. Br J Pharmacol 75:359-365.

de Belleroche J, Gardiner IM (1985) Muscarinic receptors discriminated by pirenzepine are involved in the regulation of neurotransmitter release in rat nucleus accumbens. Br J Pharmacol 86:505-508.

de Belleroche J, Gardiner IM, Hamilton MH, Birdsall NJM (1985) Analysis of muscarinic receptor concentration and subtypes following lesion of rat substantia innominata. Brain Res 340:201-209.

Gage FH, Bjørklund A, Stenevi U, Dunnett B (1983) Functional correlates of compensatory collateral sprouting by aminergic and cholinergic afferents in the hippocampus formation. Brain Res 268:39-47.

Geddes JW, Monaghan DT, Cotman CW, Lott IT, Kim RC, Chui HC (1985) Plasticity of hippocampal circuitry in Alzheimer's disease. Science 230:1179-1181.

Johnston MV, McKinney M, Coyle JT (1981) Neocortical cholinergic innervation: a description of extrinsic and intrinsic components in the rat. Exp Brain Res 43:159-172.

McKinney M, Coyle JT (1982) Regulation of neocortical muscarinic receptors: effects of drug treatments and lesions. J Neurosci 2:77-105.

Maragos WF, Greenamyre T, Penney JB, Young AB (1987) Glutamate dysfunction in Alzheimer's disease: an hypothesis. Trends Neurosci 10:65-68.

Mash DC, Flynn DD, Potter LT (1985) Loss of M_2 muscarine receptors in the cerebral cortex in Alzheimer's disease and experimental cholinergic denervation. Science 228:1115-1117.

Morris RGM, Anderson E, Lynch G, Baudrey M (1986) Selective impairment of learning and blockade of long term potentiation by an N-methyl-D aspartate receptor antagonist AP5. Nature 319:774-776.

Pedata F, Lo Conte G, Sorbi S, Marconcini-Pepeu I, Pepeu G (1982) Changes in high affinity choline uptake in rat cerebral cortex following lesions of the magnocellular forebrain nuclei. Brain Res 233:359-367.

Reed L, de Belleroche J (1988) Increased polyphosphoinositide responsiveness induced by denervation. J Neurochem 50:1566-1571.

Reisine TD, Yamamura HI, Bird ED, Spokes E, Enna SJ (1978) Pre-and post-synaptic neurochemical alterations in Alzheimer's disease. Brain Res 159:477-480.

Stephens PH, Cuello AC, Sofroniew MV, Pearson RCA, Tagiari P (1985) Effect of unilateral decortication on choline acetyltransferase activity in the nucleus basalis and other areas of the rat brain. J Neurochem 45:1021-1026.

Wenk GL, Olton DS (1984) Recovery of neocortical choline acetyltransferase activity following ibotenic acid injection into the nucleus basalis of Meynert in rats. Brain Res 293:184-186.

Wenk H, Bigl V, Meyer U (1980) Cholinergic projections from magnocellular nuclei of the basal forebrain to cortical areas in rats. Brain Res Rev 2:295-316.

Wood PL, Etienne P, Lal S, Nair WPV, Finlayson MH, Gauthier S, Palo J, Maltia M, Paetau A, Bird ED (1983) A post mortem comparison of the cortical cholinergic system in Alzheimer's disease and Pick's disease. J Neurol Sci 62:211-217.

New Trends in Aging Research
G. Pepeu, B. Tomlinson, C.M. Wischik (eds)
Fidia Research Series, vol. 15
Liviana Press, Padova © 1988

PHARMACOLOGY OF AGE-RELATED MEMORY DISTURBANCES: REFINING THE CHOLINERGIC HYPOTHESIS

Richard M. Mangano and Raymond T. Bartus

American Cyanamid Company, Medical Research Division,
Lederle Laboratories, Department of Central Nervous System Research,
Pearl River, NY 10965, USA

THE CHOLINERGIC HYPOTHESIS OF GERIATRIC MEMORY LOSS

Abundant evidence exists in the scientific literature to suggest that significant functional disturbances in cholinergic activity occur in the brains of aged and especially demented subjects and that these disturbances play an important role in memory loss and cognitive problems associated with old age and dementia (see recent reviews by Bartus et al., 1987; 1986; 1985; 1982; Coyle et al., 1983; Davies, 1981). These observations form the basis of the cholinergic hypothesis of geriatric memory loss. In its simplest form, the cholinergic hypothesis states that:

— significant, functional disturbances in cholinergic activity occur in the brains of aged and particularly demented subjects;

— these disturbances play an important role in geriatric memory loss and related cognitive problems associated with dementia; and,

— proper enhancement or restoration of cholinergic function may significantly reduce the severity of cognitive loss.

It is important to realize that the cholinergic hypothesis is not concerned with the etiology of age-associated memory impairments or dementia. Neither does this hypothesis attempt to address the additional roles that cholinergic dysfunction may play

Abbreviations: AD, Alzheimer's disease; mAChR, Muscarinic acetylcholine receptor.

in other neurobehavioral disturbances of aging and dementia. Nor is any claim made by the hypothesis that the cholinergic system is exclusively involved in age-related memory loss. Indeed, it is well accepted that other neurotransmitter systems are also likely to be involved. What the hypothesis *does* imply is that the relationship between neurotransmitter dysfunction and age-related memory loss is most clearly established for the cholinergic system.

Several therapeutic possibilities for treating age-related memory disorders are suggested by the cholinergic hypothesis. These approaches include:

1. Improve the pharmacokinetics of cholinomimetics;
2. Develop newer cholinergic agents with greater specificity or selectivity for:
   — receptor subtypes, and/or
   — brain regions;
3. Develop non-traditional cholinergic agents to modulate:
   — muscarinic acetylcholine receptor affinity, and/or
   — acetylcholine release; and
4. Develop and evaluate more innovative combination therapies.

As would be expected from any working hypothesis, these therapeutic approaches are necessarily broad in scope and should not be considered mutually exclusive from each other.

Thus far, while the available clinical studies with cholinergic agents offer little immediate promise of effective therapeutic intervention, they do offer hope for future drug development. One must recognize that the currently available cholinergic agents possess clear deficiencies that may contribute to their lack of efficacy (most recently reviewed by Bartus et al., 1987). Among these deficiencies are:

— extremely short half life;
— lack of specificity to the CNS or poor penetration of the blood-brain barrier;
— high incidence of adverse side effects; and
— extremely narrow therapeutic window.

It is likely that newer compounds which correct these deficiencies may help to reduce the clinical symptoms related to age-associated memory impairment.

Basic pharmacological and biochemical research has suggested the existence of at least two and perhaps three distinct subtypes of mAChR (for reviews see Hirschowitz et al., 1984; Levine et al., 1986). Confirmation of the existence of two subtypes of mAChR has recently come from several labs utilizing recombinant DNA technology. Significantly, two distinct cDNAs have been sequenced and expressed for the porcine atrial (Peralta et al., 1987; Kubo et al., 1986a) and porcine brain mAChR (Kubo et al., 1986b).

The existence of molecular heterogeneity among mAChRs provides the potential to develop drugs targeted with greater specificity toward a particular subclass of receptor. If different subtypes are associated with different functional roles, one could reasonably expect to achieve greater selectivity of function and/or site of action from such drugs.

Thus, in order to develop more specific cholinergic agonists, newer methods of characterizing cholinergic activity will be required. A number of intracellular biochemical changes, for example, are associated with signal transduction mediated by mAChR occupancy (Downes, 1980). One of the most consistent biochemical events mediated by muscarinic agonists is stimulation of phosphatidate and phosphatidylinositol metabolism (Abdel-Latif, 1983; Downes, 1983; Fisher et al., 1984). Although the precise functional role of this response has yet to be determined, its involvement in the events culminating in post-synaptic receptor firing is gaining acceptance (Brown and Masters, 1984; Downes, 1983; Fisher and Agranoff, 1985; Fisher et al., 1984; Nishizuka, 1984). For these reasons, methods of quantifying phosphoinositide turnover following mAChR occupancy provide and independent and perhaps functionally relevant means of assessing and defining muscarinic agonists.

REFINING THE CHOLINERGIC HYPOTHESIS

Studies using these techniques indicate the existence of at least two broad classes of muscarinic agonists (Fisher et al., 1983; Fisher et al., 1984). One group of agonists (Class A) stimulate phospholipid turnover two to three times control levels versus those that are only partially active, stimulating turnover by 10% to 15% (Class B). The Class B agonists, in fact, can block the maximal effects of class A agonists when both are combined. Figure 1 illustrates that these profound differences in muscarinic agonists are not revealed by the conventional methods of receptor-ligand analysis (Fisher and Bartus, 1985; Fisher et al., 1984). Additionally, there is evidence of regional differences in coupling of mAChRs to phosphoinositide turnover within the CNS (Fisher and Bartus, 1985). Observations such as these provide the basis for developing more specific and unique muscarinic agonists.

There remains, however, an empirical question concerning the physiological response of enhanced inositol phospholipid turnover and its possible relationship to the therapeutic goal.

Preliminary experiments in our laboratory suggest that potential functional advantages may exist with muscarinic agonists which have enhanced effects on inositol phospholipid turnover (Bartus et al., 1986). Aged rats exhibit a robust deficit in the retention of a single trial passive avoidance task (Bartus et al., 1983; Gold and McGaugh, 1975; Lippa et al., 1980; Zornetzer et al., 1982) and that muscarinic agonists produce a modest, but reliable, improvement (Bartus et al., 1983).

Using aged rats in this task, we have recently compared the effects of oxotremorine with two close analogues of oxotremorine (oxotremorine-2 and oxotremorine-M). Both oxotremorine-2 and oxotremorine-M are structurally similar to oxotremorine, but differ in the number of methyl groups attached to the side chain (two and three, respectively). More importantly, the three compounds differ dramatically in their ability to stimulate turnover of phosphatidate, with oxotremorine-M being most effective, oxotremorine-2 being modestly effective, and oxotremorine only weakly effective. The results of this behavioral comparison are shown in Figure 2 and reveal clearly superior effects of the two analogues. These preliminary data, therefore, raise the possibility that muscarinic agonists that are able to induce large biochemical signals between the site of the receptor and the eventual physiological response, may be far more efficacious in improving overall cholinergic function and perhaps reducing the cognitive disturbances associated with old age and AD. Furthermore, they suggest that one practical way of accomplishing this might be by increasing the degree to which muscarinic agonists enhance phosphatidylinositol breakdown within the neuronal membrane.

We wish to emphasize that the experiments discussed above are just one example among many possibilities of how new observations of central cholinergic function can be tested within the framework of the cholinergic hypothesis. Given the diversity of cholinergic receptors and their associated signal transduction mechanisms and second messengers, many additional possibilities remain to be examined. The goal of this "refining" process is the development of different and hopefully superior cholinergic

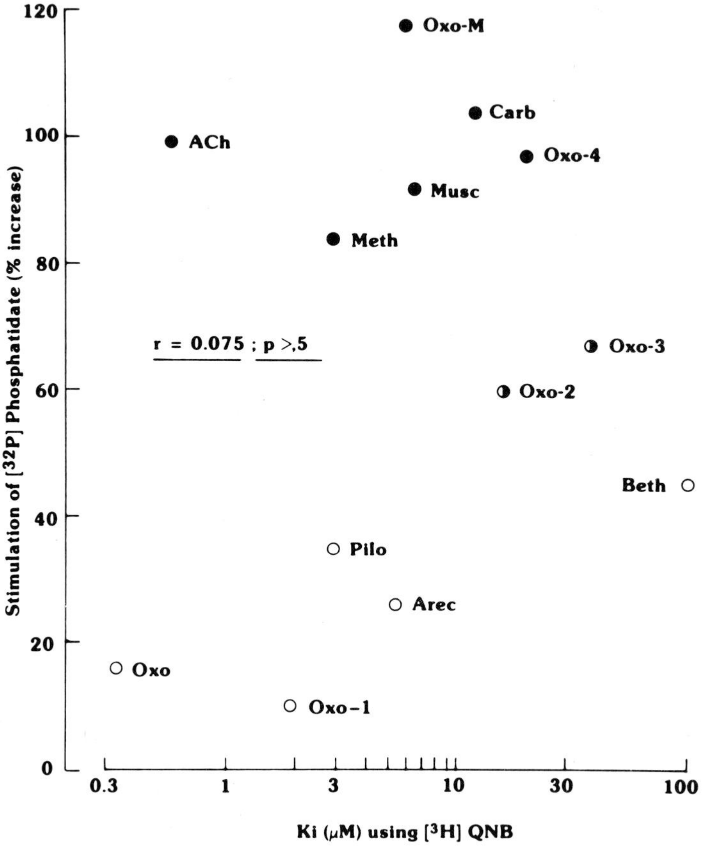

Figure 1. Effects of various muscarinic agonists on ability to stimulate phosphatidate turnover (plotted along abscissa) versus an inverse plot of ability to bind to the muscarinic receptor, measured by displacement of the muscarinic antagonist quinuclidinylbenzilate (QNB). Note that, although wide variation occurs among the agonists in their ability to stimulate phosphatidate, as well as in their affinity for the muscarinic receptor (Ki), no correlation exists between these two variables. However, a relationship does exist in the apparent ability of the agonists to induce a conformational change in the receptor, suggested by their ability to bind to high and low affinity forms of the receptor. This is depicted by the solid circles for full agonists, that bind to both interconvertible forms (and are, therefore, presumed to induce a conformational change) vs. open circles for partial agonists, that bind to a single form of the receptor (and are therefore presumed not to induce change). The results for OXO-2 and OXO-3 yielded mixed data (reprinted from Bartus et al., 1986).

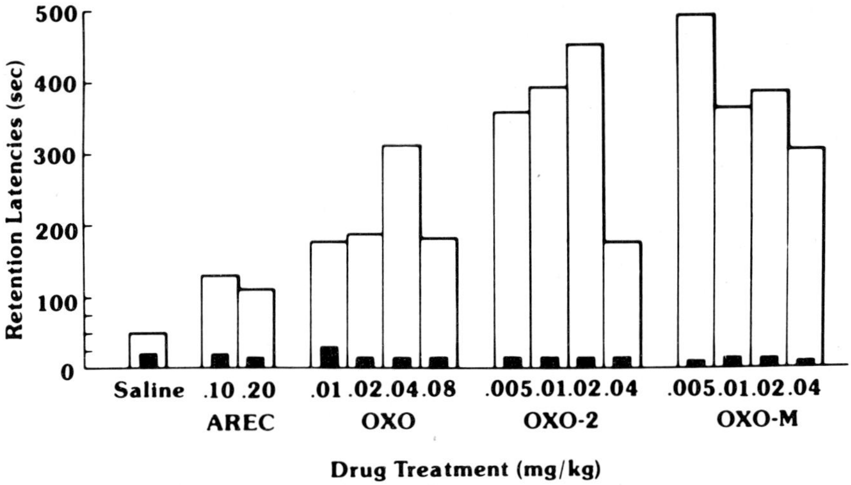

Figure 2. Effects of various doses of the traditional muscarinic agonists, arecoline and oxotremorine vs. two close analogues of oxotremorine (oxotremorine-M and oxotremorine-2) on passive avoidance retention in aged rats (open bars). Note superior efficacy and potency of the two analogues [closed bars representing pre-training, (i.e.,-day one) latencies] (reprinted from Bartus et al., 1986).

drugs. Such drugs should allow us to gain new insight into cholinergic function and hopefully provide more effective symptomatic treatment for age-associated memory impairments.

ACKNOWLEDGEMENTS

The authors wish to acknowledge the contributions of R. Dean, J.C. Figueiredo, S.K. Fisher, C. Flicker and M. Pontecorvo. We gratefully acknowledge the help of Carmela Nardella in the preparation of this manuscript.

REFERENCES

Abdel-Latif AA (1983) Metabolism of phosphoinositides. In: Lajtha A (ed): Handbook of Neurochemistry, Vol. 3. Plenum Press, New York, pp. 91-131.

Bartus RT, Dean RL, Beer B, Lippa AS (1982) The cholinergic hypothesis of geriatric memory dysfunction. Science 217: 408-417.

Bartus RT, Dean RL, Fisher SK (1986) Cholinergic treatment for age-related memory disturbances: dead or barely coming of age? In: Crook T, Bartus RT, Ferris S, Gershon S (eds): Treatment Development Strategies for Alzheimer's Disease. Mark Powley Associates, Connecticut, pp. 421-450.

Bartus RT, Dean RL, Flicker C (1987) Cholinergic psychopharmacology: an integration of human and animal research on memory. In: Meltzer HY (ed): Psychopharmacology: A Third Generation of Progress. Raven Press, New York, pp. 219-232.

Bartus RT, Dean RL, Pontecorvo MJ, Flicker C (1985) The cholinergic hypothesis: a historical overview, current perspective and future direction. In: Olton D, Gamzu E, Corben S (eds): Memory Dysfunctions: Integration of Animal and Human Research from Clinical and Preclinical Perspectives. New York Academy of Sciences, New York, pp. 332-358.

Bartus RT, Flicker C, Dean RL (1983) Logical principles in the development of animal models of age-related memory impairments. In: Crook T, Ferris S, Bartus RT (eds): Assessment in Geriatric Psychopharmacology. Mark Powley Associates, Inc. Connecticut, pp. 267-299.

Brown JH, Masters SB (1984) Does phosphoinositide hydrolysis mediate "inhibitory" as well as "excitatory" muscarinic responses? Trends in Pharmacological Sciences 5:417-419.

Coyle JT, Price DL, DeLong MR (1983) Alzheimer's disease: A disorder of cortical cholinergic innervation. Science 219:1184-1190.

Davies P (1981) Theoretical treatment possibilities for dementia of the Alzheimer's type: The cholinergic hypothesis. In: Crook T, Gershon S (eds): Strategies for the Development of an Effective Treatment for Senile Dementia. Mark Powley Associates, Connecticut, pp. 19-32.

Downes CP (1983) Inositol phospholipids and neurotransmitter-receptor signalling mechanisms. Trends in Neurosciences 6:313-316.

Fisher SK, Agranoff BW (1985) The biochemical basis and functional significance of enhanced phosphatidate and phosphoinositide turnover. In: Eichberg J (ed): Phospholipids in the Nervous System. John Wiley & Sons, New York, pp. 241-296.

Fisher SK, Figueiredo JC, Bartus RT (1984) Differential stimulation of inositol phospholipid turnover in rat brain by analogs of oxotremorine. J Neurochem 43:1171-1179.

Fisher SK, Klinger PD, Agranoff BW (1983) Muscarinic agonist binding and phospholipid turnover in brain. J Biol Chem 258:7358-7363.

Gold PE, McGaugh JL (1975) Changes in memory and learning during aging. In: Ordy JM, Brizee FR (eds): Neurobiology of Aging. Plenum Press, New York, pp. 53-57.

Hirschowitz BI, Hammer R, Giachetti I, Keerns JJ, Levine R (1984) Subtypes of Muscarinic Receptors. Trends in Pharmacological Sciences (Supplement), Elsevier, Amsterdam.

Kubo T, Maeda A, Sugimoto K, Akiba I, Mikami A, Takahashi H, Haga T, Haga K, Ichiyama A, Kangawa K, Matsuo H, Hirose T, Numa S (1986a) Primary structure of porcine cardiac muscarinic acetylcholine receptor deduced from the cDNA sequence. FEBS Letters 209:367-372.

Kubo T, Fukuda K, Mikami A, Maeda A, Takahashi H, Mishina M, Haga T, Haga K, Ichiyama A, Kangawa K, Kojima M, Matsuo H, Hirose T, Numa S (1986b) Cloning, sequencing and expression of complementary DNA encoding the muscarinic acetylcholine receptor. Nature 323:411-416.

Levine RL, Birdsall NJM, Giachetti A, Hammer R, Iversen LL, Jenden DJ, North RA (1986) Subtypes of Muscarinic Receptors II. Trends in Pharmacological Sciences (Supplement), Elsevier, Amsterdam.

Lippa AS, Pelham RW, Beer B, Critchett DJ, Dean RL, Bartus RT (1980) Brain cholinergic dysfunction and memory in aged rats. Neurobiol Aging 1:13-19.

Nishizuka Y (1984) Turnover of inositol phospholipids and signal transduction. Science 225:1365-1370.

Peralta EG, Winslow JW, Peterson GL, Smith DH, Ashkenanzi A, Ramachandran J, Schimerlik MI, Capon DJ (1987) Primary structure and biochemical properties of an M_2 muscarinic receptor. Science 236:600-605.

Zornetzer SF, Thompson R, Rogers J (1982) Rapid forgetting in aged rats. Behav Neural Biol 36:49-60.

New Trends in Aging Research
G. Pepeu, B. Tomlinson, C.M. Wischik (eds)
Fidia Research Series, vol. 15
Liviana Press, Padova © 1988

STRUCTURAL CHANGES OF BASAL FOREBRAIN CHOLINERGIC NEURONS IN THE AGED RAT. EFFECT OF PHOSPHATIDYLSERINE ADMINISTRATION

Fabrizio Milan, Diego Guidolin, Patrizia Polato, Maria Grazia Nunzi and Gino Toffano

Fidia Research Laboratories
Abano Terme, Italy

INTRODUCTION

Within the basal forebrain of the rat is a core of cholinergic neurons that has been divided into several regions which include the medial septum (MS), the diagonal band of Broca (DB) (vertical and horizontal limbs, VDB and HDB, respectively), and the nucleus basalis magnocellularis (NBM) (Sofroniew et al., 1982; Mesulam et al., 1983). The MS and VDB send their afferents mainly to the hippocampal formation (Meibach and Siegel, 1977; Segal and Landis, 1974). This cholinergic system contributes to important behavioral functions since its structural and functional integrity has been related to learning and memory capacities (Hepler et al., 1985; Kesner et al., 1986). In Alzheimer's disease, which is characterized by a primary loss of memory function, structural alterations of MS (Nakano and Hirano, 1982) and DB (Whitehouse et al., 1982) have been correlated with reduction of choline-acetyltransferase (ChAT) activity in the hippocampus (Perry et al., 1977; Reisine et al., 1978; Perry et al., 1978). Changes in cholinergic markers, occurring also in physiologic aging, support a role for cholinergic dysfunctions in age-dependent memory disturbances (Bartus et al., 1982).

Abbreviations: BC-PS, phosphatidylserine; MS, medial septum; DB, diagonal band of Broca; VDB and HDB, vertical and horizontal limbs of diagonal band; ChAT, choline-acetyltransferase; PAP, peroxidase anti-peroxidase; NGF, nerve growth factor.

Taken together, these lines of evidence suggest that any pharmacological treatment capable of enhancing cholinergic functions and/or preventing basal forebrain structural alterations, might ameliorate higher cognitive functions in old age and related disorders.

Phosphatidylserine (BC-PS), a pharmacologically active phospholipid (see Toffano and Bruni, 1980) has been reported to normalize the impaired release of acetylcholine in the cerebral cortex of old rats (Pedata et al., 1985). Furthermore, BC-PS increases learning and memory functions in old rats (Drago et al., 1981; Corwin et al., 1985) and prevents the age-related decay in active avoidance behaviour (Zanotti et al., 1986). Recently, BC-PS treatment has been shown to elicit improvement of cognitive functions in elderly human patients affected by moderate deterioration of cognitive capacities (Villardita et al., 1987; Palmieri et al., 1987).

The aim of this study was to investigate structural alterations in the cholinergic neuronal population of the basal forebrain in aged rats, and the possible counteracting effect of long-term BC-PS administration.

MATERIALS AND METHODS

Animals

Five male Sprague-Dawley rats for each of the following groups were used: young adults (3 months), old-untreated (27 months) and old (27 months) which received BC-PS treatment. Animals were kept on 12 hr light: 12 hr dark cycle, with food (Standard Diet # 4RF18, Italiana Mangimi, Milano) and water *ad libitum*. Starting at the age of 15 months, rats belonging to the treated group were given an aqueous suspension of BC-PS in place of water.

Phosphatidylserine (BC-PS) Preparation and Administration

Brain phosphatidylserine of bovine cortical origin (BC-PS) was prepared and purified as described elsewhere (Lees, 1957). Average daily water consumption and body weight were monitored weekly, over the one-year study, across the rats of the untreated group. On the basis of the weekly recorded parameters, the concentration of BC-PS in water was adjusted throughout the treatment, in order to have an average daily intake of 50 mg/kg of the phospholipid per rat.

A concentrated aqueous suspension of BC-PS was prepared once a week by Vortex mixing and the diluted solution distributed to animals every second day. Thin layer chromatography following chloroform-methanol extraction did not show any hydrolysis of the phospholipid during storage in water.

Tissue Preparation and Immunocytochemistry

Animals were anesthetized with Pentothal (Abbott, 0.04 gr/100 gr b.w., i.p.) and perfused at room temperature through the left ventricle, first with Tyrode's solution (gassed with 95% 0_2/5% CO_2 mixture) and then with a fixative containing 4% paraformaldehyde (Serva) and 0.05% glutaraldehyde (Merck) in 0.1 M phosphate buffer (pH 7.4).

Following perfusion, the brains were removed from the skull and postfixed for 3-5 hours, at 4°C, and then transferred to phosphate buffer overnight at 4°C.

The following day, brains were hand-sliced in a coronal plane, in order to obtain a block limited rostrally by the oflactory tubercle and caudally by the crossing of the anterior commissure. The tissue block was then sectioned in a coronal plane on a Vibratome (Oxford Instrument) set at 40 μm. Sections were sequentially placed in numbered 16 mm tissue culture wells containing phosphate-buffered saline (PBS). Every third section was processed for immunocytochemistry. A monoclonal antibody to choline acetyltransferase (ChAT) (Boehringer; Type I; see Eckenstein and Thoenen, 1982) and the peroxidase anti-peroxidase (PAP) method (Sternberger et al., 1970) were used to reveal ChAT immunoreactivity. Sections were free floating and the staining procedure was carried out in the following order, at room temperature, unless otherwise specified:

1. normal goat serum (NGS) (Sigma), diluted 1:5 for 1 hour;

2. primary antiserum dissolved in phosphate buffer 0.1 M, (pH 7.4), at the concentration of 2.5 μg/ml, overnight at 4°C;

3. goat anti-rat serum (Sternberger-Meyer) diluted 1:20 overnight at 4°C;

4. PAP complex (Sternberger-Meyer) diluted 1:20, for 6 hours.

To check for specificity of the immunostaining some sections were incubated in phosphate buffer instead of the primary antiserum. PBS containing 1% of NGS was used for dilution of goat anti-rat serum and for each washing after each antiserum. Only PBS was used for PAP dilution. For visualization of the peroxidase, the sections were preincubated for 30-45' in 0.05 M 3,3' diaminobenzidine tetrahydrocloride (Sigma) dissolved in 0.05 M tris-HCl buffer (pH 7.4) and subsequently reacted for 4-6 minutes in the same solution containing 0.01% hydrogen peroxide. Sections were then sequentially mounted on gelatine-coated slides, reacted for 15' with 2% osmium tetroxide in 0.1 M phosphate buffer (pH 7.4) and processed by standard procedures for light microscopic observations.

Morphometric Analysis

Morphometric analysis of ChAT-immunoreactive cells was performed on MS, VDB and HDB. Four parameters were analyzed: the number of ChAT-positive cells, the area occupied by the immunoreactive profiles (i. e., cell bodies, dendrites and fibers), the somatic cross-sectional area and the mean maximum diameter of the immunoreactive neurons. Cell count and morphometry were carried out by means of a computerized image analysis system (IBAS, Kontron, Zeiss) coupled to a Zeiss photomicroscope. Cell count and total immunoreactive area were estimated at a ×10 objective magnification, single cell morphometry at ×40. The data of the analysis on MS and DB were pooled together. Among the sections processed for immunocytochemistry, the morphometric analysis was performed on three consecutive sections (80 μm apart each other) starting approximately at level A 7890, according to Koenig and Klippel (1963) (Fig. 1). At this level, each of the selected sections contains MS, VDB and HDB nuclei in their greatest extension.

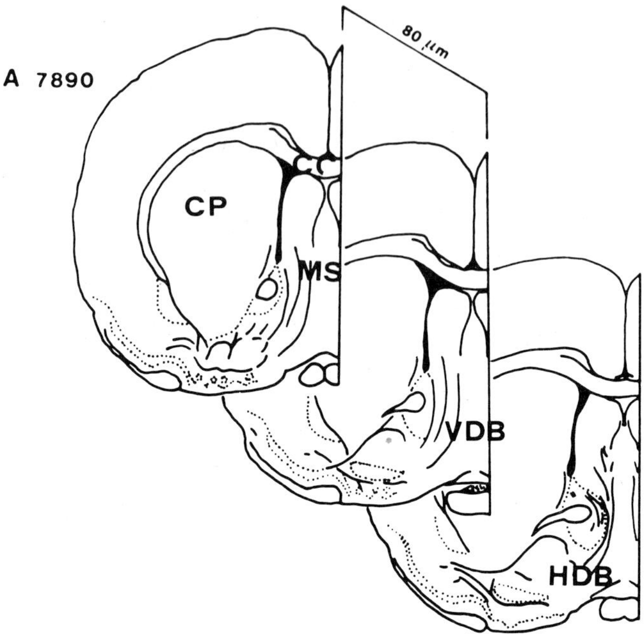

Figure 1. Coronal sections through the rat basal forebrain indicating where cell count and morphometry of ChAT-immunoreactive neurons were performed in the medial septum (MS) and both vertical and horizontal limbs of diagonal band. (VDB and HDB respectively). The approximate level of the sections (A 7890) is indicated according to stereotaxis atlas coordinates (Koenig and Klippel, 1963). CP, caudate putamen; CC, corpus callosum.

Statistical Analysis

For each animal the mean of the three sections was considered. Differences across the animal groups were tested by means of the Student's t test.

RESULTS

In all three animal groups, light microscopic analysis revealed ChAT-immunoreactive cell bodies throughout the MS and both HDB and VDB. In addition, many vertically oriented fibers were seen coursing through these nuclei. From a qualitative examination, topography and morphology of ChAT-immunoreactive neurons were similar among the animal groups and comparable to those described elsewhere (Sofroniew et al., 1982; Mesulam et al., 1983) (Fig. 2).

Morphometric analysis of the cholinergic neuronal population demonstrated that structural alterations occurred in old animals. However, the age-related alterations appeared to be counteracted by long-term BC-PS oral treatment. The results expressed

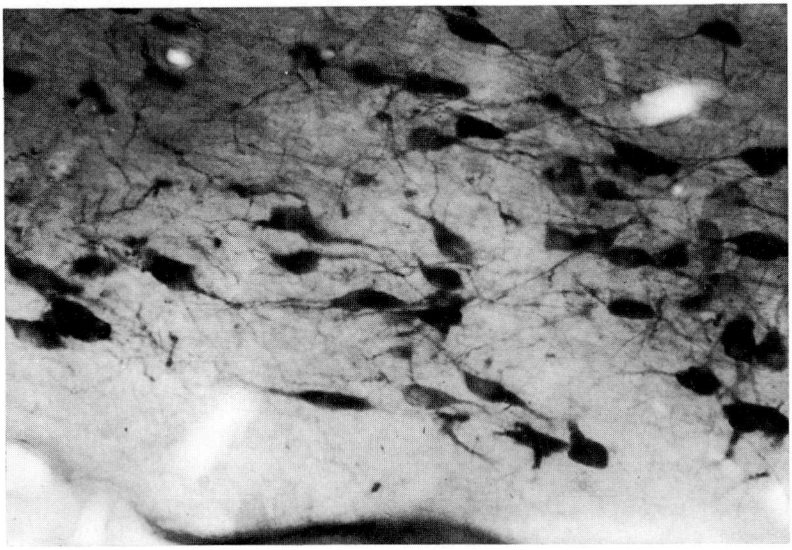

Figure 2. Light micrograph of ChAT-positive neurons of the basal forebrain (**HDB**) of a 3-month-old rat. (× 250).

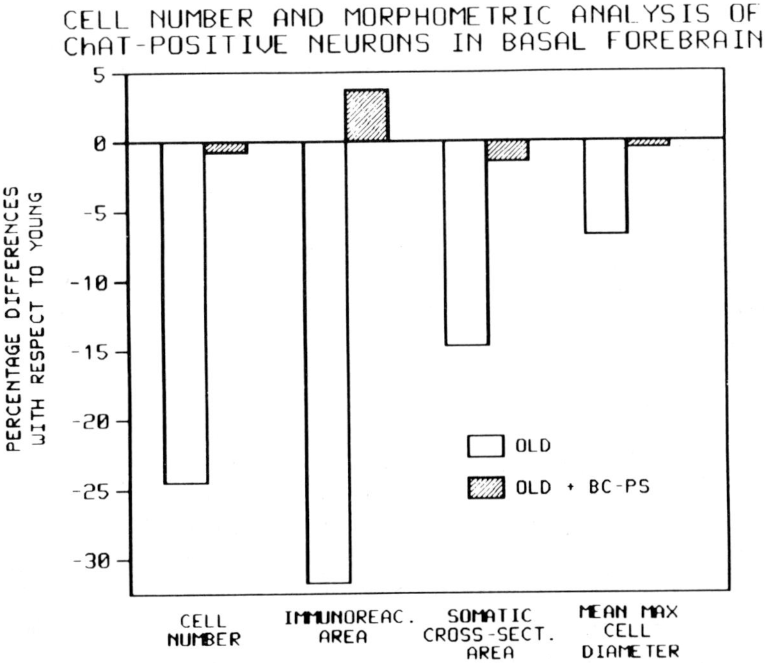

Figure 3. Morphometric analysis and count of ChAT positive neurons in the basal forebrain of old untreated and old BC-PS treated rats. Values are expressed as percentage difference with respect to the values found in young 3-month-old rats, assumed as baseline (young = 0).

as percentage differences with respect to the values of the group of young animals are summarized in Figure 3.

The cholinergic neuronal population in the basal forebrain appeared unstable throughout old age, because a marked decrease in cell number was found in the old untreated group (– 24.5% with respect to young animals, $p < .01$). On the contrary, no statistically significant differences were observed between young and old BC-PS treated rats (–.72%). In old animals the area covered by the immunoreactive profiles decreased significantly by 31.7% ($p < .05$), but no significant decrement could be observed in the old BC-PS treated group when compared with the young one (+ 3.8%). Similarly, soma size decreased in old age; old-untreated animals exhibited values in somatic cross-sectional area and mean maximum diameter, that were significantly lower than those of young rats (–14.8%, $p < .05$ and – 6.7%, $p < .01$, respectively). For the two latter parameters no statistically significant differences were present between old BC-PS-treated and young animals.

DISCUSSION

This study provides evidence that a deterioration of ChAT positive neurons of the basal forebrain occurs in old rats. In particular, from the morphometric analysis it is apparent that: a) a significant reduction in the number of ChAT-immunoreactive neurons, together with atrophic changes in the surviving cholinergic cell population, occur in old age; b) the structural alterations do not occur in animals which have received long-term BC-PS administration.

The age-related structural alterations of rat cholinergic neurons are consistent with the results obtained by others in the rodent basal forebrain, demonstrating a reduction in size (Hornberger et al., 1986) and number (Biegon et al., 1986) of AChE-containing neurons in old age. The atrophic changes may be due to a slowing of neuronal metabolism since decreased ChAT (Luine et al., 1986) and AChE activity (Biegon et al., 1986) have been reported in the basal forebrain nuclei of aged rats.

In the hippocampal formation of old rats, reduced synaptic efficacy (De Toledo-Morrel and Morrel, 1985) has been related to a reduction in synaptic density (Geinisman et al., 1977). In addition, changes in number and morphology of synapses — supposed to be cholinergic — have been reported by Bertoni-Freddari et al. (1986) in the hippocampus of aged rats. Therefore, the structural derangements of cholinergic neurons may represent also a secondary event due to age-induced changes at presynaptic terminals. In this regard, it has been suggested that in Alzheimer's disease structural alterations in the basal forebrain are a consequence of a retrograde degeneration process beginning at the nerve terminals (Arendt et al., 1985; Pearson et al., 1983).

The impaired capacity of nerve cells to support synaptic turnover with advancing age may result either from a failure of the target area (i. e. hippocampus) to sustain renewal of synapses, or from inadequacy of presynaptic components to maintain functional integrity of synaptic terminals.

In view of the role that synaptic activity can play in stabilizing synaptic contacts (Changeux and Danchin, 1976) the atrophy of cholinergic neurons may reflect an impairment in neurotransmitter functions. This conclusion is further confirmed by the finding that acetylcholine release is reduced in the hippocampus of aged rats (Consolo et al., 1986).

Recently, we have provided evidence of a reduction in the density of dendritic spines of pyramidal neurons in the hippocampus of old rats (Milan et al., 1986). Since dendritic spines have been shown to be sensitive to both structural and functional integrity of their afferent fibers (Globus and Scheibel, 1967; Parnavelas et al., 1974), loss of these post-synaptic structures may be the result of a partial deafferentation and/or functional impairment at the synaptic terminals.

The reported changes in basal forebrain cholinergic neurons may therefore be involved in deterioration of the dendritic spine population, since cholinergic fibers synapse with dendritic spine of hippocampal pyramidal cells (Frotscher and Leranth, 1985).

The effect of BC-PS on survival and trophic degree of cholinergic neurons may correlate with the capability of the phospholipid to prevent in the aged hippocampus the decrement in dendritic spine density (Milan et al., 1986). This phenomenon might reflect the maintenance through old age of those mechanisms underlying formation, stabilization and renewal of synaptic contacts. Since synaptic remodelling plays a major role in cognitive functions, the prevention by BC-PS of the decay of learning capacities in old age (Zanotti et al., 1986) may have a basis on the morpho-functional effects of BC-PS on interneuronal connectivity.

Although the mechanism(s) by which BC-PS may exert its beneficial effect on cholinergic neurons and neuronal connectivity is at present unknown, several hypotheses have to be considered.

According to Sun and Sun (1979), changes in membrane lipid composition may have a key role in old age. In rat synaptosomal membranes, changes in phospholipid content (Crews et al., 1981) and metabolism (Porcellati et al., 1982), and increases in the cholesterol/phospholipid ratio (Calderini et al., 1985) occur with age. These alterations can be explained by a decreased capacity of the aging cell membrane to incorporate fatty acids into phospholipids (Gaiti et al., 1981). Recently, lysophosphatidylserine, an active intermediate of BC-PS (Bruni and Toffano, 1982), has been shown to increase the incorporation of polyunsatured fatty acids into phosphatidylcholine and phosphatidylinositol (Sbashing-Agler and Pullarkat, 1985). Futhermore, BC-PS reduces the membrane cholesterol/phospholipid ratio and increases the specific activity of the Na^+-K^+ dependent ATPase (Calderini et al., 1985).

In adult animals, BC-PS has been shown to enhance acetylcholine output from rat cerebral cortex (Casamenti et al., 1979). In addition, long-term BC-PS administration is capable of restoring the age-related reduction of acetylcholine release from rat cortical slices (Pedata et al., 1985).

Since synaptic function has a major role in stabilization of synaptic elements (Changeux and Danchin, 1976) the effects of BC-PS on neuronal membranes and/or the increased activity of cholinergic synapses may be factors relevant in old age for renewal of synaptic connections and maintenance of trophic degree of cholinergic neurons.

It has been reported that lysophosphatidylserine enhances the nerve growth factor (NGF)-dependent release of histamine from rat mast cells (Bruni et al., 1982). It is known that NGF acts as a neuronotrophic factor for forebrain cholinergic neurons (Hefti, 1986). Age-dependent decrement in NGF levels and/or activity may therefore be involved in deterioration of cholinergic neurons in old age. BC-PS could ensure trophic support to cholinergic neurons through advancing age by enhancing their responsiveness to limiting levels of NGF.

The positive effect of BC-PS administration on age-dependent alterations of membrane properties and functions and/or the proposed interaction with NGF may be important factors for remodelling of synaptic connections. This is reflected by maintenance in old age of both pre- and post-synaptic structures and trophic degree of cholinergic neurons. These lines of evidence suggest the use of BC-PS as a potential therapeutic agent for treatment of memory and cognitive disturbances in both normal and pathological aging.

SUMMARY

Age-related structural alterations of basal forebrain cholinergic neurons were studied in three animal groups: young (3-month-old), old (27-months) and old age-matched phosphatidylserine (BC-PS) treated rats. BC-PS (50 mg/kg/die), suspended in tap water, was administered from the age of 15 months. In 27-month-old animals cell number is significantly decreased (-21.3% $p < .01$) when compared to that of the young ones. Likewise, mean cross sectional somatic area and diameter are severely affected. These parameters are reduced by 14.85% and 6.77%, respectively ($p < .05$ and $p < .01$) as compared with those of young rats. On the contrary, old BC-PS-treated rats exhibited no statistically significant differences in the above parameters when compared with young animals.

The results suggest that long-term BC-PS oral treatment is capable of preventing cholinergic cell loss and atrophy in the basal forebrain of aged rats.

Furthermore, the findings correlate with the capability of the phospholipid to prevent age-related degeneration of post-synaptic structures in the hippocampus (Milan et al., 1986), a major target area for the cholinergic innervation of basal forebrain.

The mechanism(s) by which BC-PS exerts its effects at structural level may be related to its pharmacological actions on neuronal membranes, neurotransmission and/or interaction with NGF.

REFERENCES

Arendt T, Bigl V, Tennstedt A, Arendt A (1985) Neuronal loss in different parts of the nucleus basalis is related to neuritic plaque formation in cortical target areas in Alzheimer's disease. Neuroscience 14:1-14.

Bartus RT, Dean III RL, Beer B, Lippa AS (1982) The cholinergic hypothesis of geriatric memory dysfunction. Science 217: 408-416.

Bertoni-Freddari C, Giuli C, Pieri C, Paci D (1986) Quantitative investigation of the morphological plasticity of synaptic junctions in rat dentate gyrus during aging. Brain Res 366: 187-192.

Biegon A, Greenberger V, Segal M (1986) Quantitative histochemistry of brain acetylcholinesterase and learning rate in the aged rats. Neurobiol Aging 7: 215-217.

Bruni A, Bigon E, Boarato E, Mietto L, Leon A, Toffano G (1982) Interaction between nerve growth factor and lysophosphatidylserine on rat peritoneal mast cells. Febs Lett 138: 190-192.

Bruni A, Toffano G (1982) Lysophosphatidylserine, a short lived intermediate with plasma membrane regulatory properties. Pharmacol Res Comm 14: 469-484.

Calderini G, Aporti F, Bellini F, Bonetti AC, Rubini R, Teolato S, Xu C, Zanotti A, Toffano G (1985) Phospholipids as pharmacological tools in the aging brain. In: Horrocks LA, Kaufer JN, Porcellati G (eds): Phospholipids in the nervous system, Vol. 2. Raven Press, New York, pp. 11-19.

Casamenti F, Mantovani P, Amaducci L, Pepeu G (1979) Effect of phosphatidylserine on acetylcholine output from the cerebral cortex of the rat. J Neurochem 32: 529-533.

Changeux J, Danchin P (1976) Selective stabilization of developing synapses as a mechanism for the specification of neuronal networks. Nature 264: 705-712.

Consolo S, Wang JX, Fiorentini F, Vezzani A, Ladinsky H (1986) In vivo and in vitro studies on the regulation of cholinergic neurotransmission in striatum, hippocampus and cortex of aged rats. Brain Res 374: 212-218.

Corwin J, Dean III RL, Bartus RT, Rotrosen J, Watkins DL (1985) Behavioral effects of phosphatidylserine in the aged Fischer 344 rat: amelioration of passive avoidance deficits without changes in psychomotors task performance. Neurobiol Aging 6: 11-15.

Crews FT, Calderini G, Battistella A, Toffano G (1981) Age dependent changes in the methylation of rat brain phospholipids. Brain Res 229: 256-259.

De Toledo-Morrel L, Morrel F (1985) Electrophysiological markers of aging and memory loss in rats. Ann NY Acad Sci 444: 296-311.

Drago F, Canonico PL, Scapagnini U (1981) Behavioral effects of phosphatidylserine in aged rats. Neurobiol Aging 2: 209-213.

Eckenstein F, Thoenen CH (1982) Production of specific antisera and monoclonal antibodies to choline-acetyltransferase. Characterization and use for identification of cholinergic neurons. EMBO J 1: 363-368.

Frotscher M, Leranth C (1985) Cholinergic innervation of the rat hippocampus as revealed by choline acetyltransferase immunocytochemistry: a combined light and electron microscopic study. J Comp Neurol 239: 237-246.

Geinisman Y, Bondareff W, Dodge J (1977) Partial deafferentiation of neurons in the dentate gyrus of the senescent rat. Brain Res 134: 541-545.

Globus A, Scheibel AB (1967) The effect of visual derivation on cortical neurons: a Golgi study. Exp Neurol 19: 331-345.

Hefti F (1986) Nerve growth factor promotes survival of septal cholinergic neurons after fimbrial transection. J Neurosci 6: 2155-2162.

Hepler DJ, Olton DS, Wenk GL, Coyle JT (1985) Lesions in nucleus basalis magnocellularis and medial septal area of rats produce qualitatively similar memory impairments. J Neurosci 5: 866-873.

Hornberger JC, Buell SJ, Flood DG, McNeill TH, Coleman PD (1985) Stability of number but not size of mouse forebrain cholinergic neurons to 53 months. Neurobiol Aging 6: 269-275.

Kesner RP, Crutcher KA, Measom MO (1986) Medial septal and nucleus basalis magnocellularis lesions produces order memory deficits in rats which mimic symptomatology of Alzheimer's disease. Neurobiol Aging 7: 287-295.

Koenig JFR, Klippel RA (1963) The rat brain. A stereotaxic atlas of the forebrain and lower parts of the brain stem. Williams and Williams, Baltimore.

Lees WG (1957) Preparation and analysis of phosphatides. Meth Enzymol 3: 328-345.

Luine VN, Renner KJ, Heady S, Jones KJ (1986) Age- and sex-dependent decreases in ChAT in basal forebrain nuclei. Neurobiol Aging 7: 193-198.

Meibach RC, Siegel A (1977) Efferent connections of the septal area in the rat: an analysis utilizing retrograde and anterograde transport methods. Brain Res 119: 1-20.

Mesulam M, Mufson ES, Levey AI, Weiner BH (1983) Cholinergic innervation of cortex by the basal forebrain: cytochemistry and cortical connections of cortex of the septal area, diagonal band nuclei, nucleus basalis (substantia innominata) and hypothalamus in the Rhesus monkey. J Comp Neurol 214: 170-197.

Milan F, Nunzi MG, Guidolin D, Calderini G, Toffano G (1986) Age-related loss of dendritic spines in rat Hippocampus: effect of phospatidylserine administration. In: Bes A, Cahn J, Cahn R, Hoyer S, Marc-Vergnes JP, Wisniewski MM (eds): Senile dementias: early detection. John Libbey Eurotext, London, Paris, pp. 488-413.

Nakano I, Hirano A (1982) Loss of large neurons in the medial septal nucleus in an autopsy case of Alzheimer's disease. J Neuropathol Exp Neurol 41: 341.

Palmieri G, Palmieri R, Inzoli MR, Lombardi G, Sottini C, Tavolato B, Giometto B (1987) Double blind controlled trial of phosphatidylserine in patients with senile mental deterioration. Clinical Trials Journal 24: 73-83.

Parnavelas J, Linch G, Brecha N, Cotman CW, Globus A (1974) Spine loss and regrowth in hippocampus following deafferentation. Nature 248: 71-73.

Pearson RCA, Sofroniew MV, Cuello AC, Powell TPS, Eckenstein R, Esiri M, Wilcock GK (1983) Persistence of cholinergic neurons in the basal nucleus in a brain with senile dementia of the Alzheimer's type demonstrated by immunohistochemical staining for choline acetyltransferase. Brain Res 289: 375-379.

Pedata F, Giovannelli L, Spignoli G, Giovannini MG, Pepeu G (1985) Phosphatidylserine increases acetylcholine release from cortical slices in aged rats. Neurobiol Aging 6: 337-339.

Perry EK, Perry RH, Blessed G, Tomlinson BE (1977) Necropsy evidence of central cholinergic deficits in senile dementia. Lancet 1: 189.

Perry EK, Tomlinson BE, Blessed G, Bergman K, Gibson PH, Perry PH (1978) Correlation of cholinergic abnormalities with senile plaques and mental test scores in senile dementia. Br Med J 2: 1457-1459.

Porcellati G, Gaiti A, Brunetti M (1982) Phospholipid biosynthesis in the aging brain. In: Giacomini E, Filogamo G, Giacobini G, Vernadakis A (eds): The aging brain: cellular and molecular mechanisms of aging in the nervous system, Vol. 20. New York, Raven Press, pp. 77-86.

Reisine TD, Kamamura HI, Bird ED, Spokes E, Enna SJ (1978) Pre - and postsynaptic neurochemical alterations in Alzheimer's disease. Brain Res 159: 477-481.

Sbashing-Agler M, Pullarkat RK (1985) Lysophosphatidylserine-dependent incorporation of Acyl CoA into phospholipids in rat brain microsomes. Neurochem Int 7: 295-300.

Segal M, Landis S (1974) Afferents to the hippocamus of the rat studied with the method of retrograde transport of horseradish peroxidase. Brain Res 78: 1-15.

Sofroniew MV, Eckenstein F, Thoenen H, Cuello AC (1982) Topography of choline acetyltransferase-containing neurons in the forebrain of the rat. Neurosci Lett 33: 7-12.

Sternberger LA, Hardy PH, Curculis JJ, Heyer HG (1970) The unlabelled antibody enzyme method of immunocytochemistry. Preparation and properties of soluble antigen-antibody complex (horseradish peroxidase) and its use in identification of spirodeches. J Histochem Cytochem 18: 315-333.

Sun AY, Sun GY (1979) Neurochemical aspects of the membrane hypothesis of aging. Interdiscipl Top Geront 15: 34-53.

Toffano G, Bruni A (1980) Pharmacological properties of phospholipid liposomes. Pharmacol Res Commun 12: 829-845.

Villardita C, Grioli S, Salmeri G, Nicoletti F, Pennisi G (1987) Multicentral clinical trial of brain phosphatidylserine in elderly patients with intellectual deterioration. Clinical Trials Journal 24: 84-93.

Whitehouse PJ, Price DL, Struble RG, Clark AW, Coyle JT, De Long MR (1982) Alzheimer's disease and senile dementia: loss of neurons in the basal forebrain. Science 215: 1237-1239.

Zanotti A, Aporti F, Rubini R, Toffano G (1986) Learning and memory deficits in rats during aging: effect of phosphatidylserine treatments. In: Biggio G, Spano PF, Toffano G, Gessa GL (eds): Modulation of central and peripheral transmitter function. Liviana Press, Padova, pp. 323-330.

SUBJECT INDEX

Finito di stampare
nel mese di dicembre 1988
dalla tipolitografia «La Grafica & Stampa ed. s.r.l.» di Vicenza
per conto della Liviana Editrice s.p.a. di Padova